METHODS IN PHARMACOLOGY AND TOXICOLOGY

Series Editor
Y. James Kang
Department of Pharmacology & Toxicology
University of Louisville
Louisville, Kentucky, USA

For further volumes:
http://www.springer.com/series/7653

Methods for Stability Testing of Pharmaceuticals

Edited by

Sanjay Bajaj

Select Biosciences India Private Limited, Chandigarh, India

Saranjit Singh

Department of Pharmaceutical Analysis, National Institute of Pharmaceutical Education and Research (NIPER), Mohali, Punjab, India

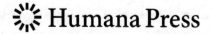 Humana Press

Editors
Sanjay Bajaj
Select Biosciences India Private Limited
Chandigarh, India

Saranjit Singh
Department of Pharmaceutical Analysis
National Institute of Pharmaceutical Education
and Research (NIPER)
Mohali, Punjab, India

ISSN 1557-2153   ISSN 1940-6053   (electronic)
Methods in Pharmacology and Toxicology
ISBN 978-1-4939-9258-4   ISBN 978-1-4939-7686-7   (eBook)
https://doi.org/10.1007/978-1-4939-7686-7

Preface

We, as pharmaceutical scientists, have always seen stability testing as a vital part of any drug development process. From the very basic level of experimentation, like stability of suspensions and emulsions in undergraduate laboratory, to stability testing of active pharmaceutical ingredients and conventional products containing them, and further to highly technical novel drug delivery systems, a thorough investigation on stability of every kind of product is desired for the benefit of the patients. Every product is supposed to be labeled with a valid expiry date and storage conditions, which are established through systematic stability studies. Due to many product failures and recalls happening for the reasons of instability, carrying out a successful stability program in the pharmaceutical industry has become very vital. Stability testing hence has to be a very well-organized activity, supported with due resources, which even stands up to critical regulatory scrutiny.

A lot of information, literature articles, and books regarding stability testing are already available, and lots of regulatory efforts have been made for harmonization of the stability testing requirements within different countries and regions. As this book is a part of the series *Methods in Pharmacology and Toxicology*, it was the intention of the editors to seek methods and protocols related to different aspects of stability programs that are followed practically in development laboratories in industry. Considering the fact that regulatory guidelines provide few experimental details, implementation of a successful stability program requires critical and logical thinking that is beyond the regular documented protocols and methods. Therefore, we have made efforts to collect the experiences from 15 organizations belonging to 9 different countries to encapsulate not all, but many, aspects of the stability testing program. We expect that this treatise will be a useful addition to the existing armamentarium of resources available to stability testing personnel, and even to students, owing to coverage of first-hand experience of international experts with many years of bench experience. Of course, making the experts agree to pen down their vital experience is always a herculean task, but we are fortunate that each contributor to this volume gave his/her best. The editors have full appreciation for each one of them. It is anticipated that the treatise will be found useful and interesting by the readers.

Of course, the editors also thankfully received great support from their families and all others connected with this compilation.

Chandigarh, India   *Sanjay Bajaj*
Punjab, India   *Saranjit Singh*

Editor's Note

This book involves contributions by authors from different organizations and multiple countries, wherein effort has been made to make best use of their practical experience in stability testing. Therefore, there always exists a possibility of some degree of variations and disagreements in similar topics covered by different individuals or difference in the views expressed and protocols/procedures followed within different organizations. The editors have attempted to harmonize many of them in discussion with the authors but do not claim any responsibility for the contents submitted by individual authors in their chapters. If any of the methods cited are different from the documented protocols, the authors can be contacted directly at the addresses given separately.

Acknowledgments

The editors express their heartfelt appreciations for all the authors and reviewers who have contributed their time, experience, and intellect to see this book in reality. We also express our gratitude to the organizations for allowing their scientists to contribute to this project. The editing work involved a lot of communication, type setting, and formatting jobs, and we appreciate the support extended to us by Ms. Bina Khanal and Ms. Richa Rani, making things simpler for us. Ms. Pooja Sharma contributed several scientific contents and we appreciate her support. We have spent a lot of our personal time in making this happen, and our parents and families have always stood beside us and had to bear with us. We deeply appreciate their support and patience. Finally, we would like to extend our sincere gratitude to all our mentors and teachers who have developed us and made us competent enough to take on this challenge and make sure this becomes a reality.

Contents

Contributors

MOHAMMED A. ALI • *Lhasa Limited, Leeds, UK*

SANJAY BAJAJ • *Select Biosciences India Private Limited, Chandigarh, India*

GULSHAN BANSAL • *Department of Pharmaceutical Sciences and Drug Research, Punjabi University, Patiala, Punjab, India*

CHRISTINE P. CHAN • *Global Manufacturing Science & Technology, Specialty Care Operations, Sanofi, Framingham, MA, USA*

SUSAN CLEARY • *Novatek International, Saint-Laurent, QC, Canada*

PARSA FAMILI • *Novatek International, Saint-Laurent, QC, Canada*

ASHISH GOGIA • *Medreich Limited, Bengaluru, Karnataka, India*

MONA GOGIA • *Cadila Pharmaceuticals Limited, Ahmedabad, India*

MARIO HELLINGS • *Janssen: Pharmaceutica NV, Beerse, Belgium*

RACHEL HEMINGWAY • *Lhasa Limited, Leeds, UK*

STEVEN HOSTYN • *Janssen: Pharmaceutical Companies of Johnson & Johnson, Beerse, Belgium*

SHALU JHAJRA • *Janssen Pharmaceutica NV, Beerse, Belgium*

PEDRO JORGE • *BMC, Winnipeg, MB, Canada*

JASMEEN KAUR • *Department of Pharmaceutical Sciences and Drug Research, Punjabi University, Patiala, Punjab, India*

SARABJEET KAUR • *Department of Pharmaceutical Sciences and Drug Research, Punjabi University, Patiala, Punjab, India*

PRIYANK KULSHRESTHA • *Novartis Healthcare Pvt. Ltd, Hyderabad, India*

PAUL MARSHALL • *DLRC Ltd., Letchworth Garden City, UK*

RAHUL SINGH NEGI • *Department of Pharmaceutical Sciences and Drug Research, Punjabi University, Patiala, Punjab, India*

MARTIN A. OTT • *Lhasa Limited, Leeds, UK*

KAMLA PATHAK • *Department of Pharmaceutics, Pharmacy College Saifai, Uttar Pradesh University of Medical Sciences, Saifai, Uttar Pradesh, India*

SATYANARAYAN PATTNAIK • *Department of Pharmaceutics, Pharmacy College Saifai, Uttar Pradesh University of Medical Sciences, Saifai, Uttar Pradesh, India*

PETER PERSICH • *Janssen Pharmaceutica NV, Beerse, Belgium*

PRADEEP PHALKE • *Janssen Pharmaceutica NV, Beerse, Belgium*

SRINIVASAN RAJAMANI • *Medreich Limited, Bengaluru, Karnataka, India*

SUMATHI V. RAO • *Medreich Limited, Bengaluru, Karnataka, India*

SANDEEP SHIROMANI • *Novartis Healthcare Pvt. Ltd., Hyderabad, India*

DILIP KUMAR SINGH • *Department of Pharmaceutical Analysis, National Institute of Pharmaceutical Education and Research (NIPER), Mohali, Punjab, India*

SARANJIT SINGH • *Department of Pharmaceutical Analysis, National Institute of Pharmaceutical Education and Research (NIPER), Mohali, Punjab, India*

B.V. SURESH KUMAR • *Novartis Healthcare Pvt. Ltd., Hyderabad, India*

NANCY SUTHAR • *Department of Pharmaceutical Sciences and Drug Research, Punjabi University, Patiala, Punjab, India*

KOEN VANHOUTTE • *Janssen Pharmaceutica NV, Beerse, Belgium*

HELEN WILLIAMS • *AstraZeneca, Macclesfield, UK*

MANUEL ZAHN • *3R Pharma Consulting GmbH, Dobel, Germany*

MARKUS ZIMMER • *Sanofi, Montpellier, France*

Chapter 1

Regulatory Guidelines on Stability Testing and Trending of Requirements

Dilip Kumar Singh, Saranjit Singh, and Sanjay Bajaj

Abstract

Stability of drug substances and their products is required to be ensured throughout their retest period/shelf-life. Various guidelines explaining the concept, procedures, and protocols have been developed and issued by international, regional, and national regulatory agencies to help the manufacturers in the generation of valid and acceptable stability data. This chapter enlists and briefly discusses the available stability guidelines, and also outlines the trends of emerging requirements.

Key words Regulatory guidelines, Stability testing, Stability guidelines, ICH guidelines, WHO guidelines, USFDA guidelines

1 Introduction

Stability is an unequivocally important attribute of drug substances and their products, because of the potential impact of unstable products on the patient health and safety. Therefore, stability testing is an important activity during drug discovery and development process. Stability testing involves significant costs, time, and scientific skills, so as to ensure that the finished pharmaceutical product (FPP) will retain desired quality during its life cycle. Successful journey of a pharmaceutical product can only be achieved if an in-depth understanding on inherent stability of the drug substance and its products is obtained pre-hand [1]. The World Health Organization (WHO) clearly highlights the rationale of stability testing by stating that "the purpose of stability testing is to provide evidence of how the quality of an active pharmaceutical ingredient (API) or FPP varies with time under the influence of a variety of environmental factors such as temperature, humidity and light. The stability program also includes the study of product-related factors that influence its quality, for example, the interaction of API with excipients, container closure systems, and packaging materials. In FPPs containing drugs in fixed-dose combination (FDC), the

Sanjay Bajaj and Saranjit Singh (eds.), *Methods for Stability Testing of Pharmaceuticals*, Methods in Pharmacology and Toxicology, https://doi.org/10.1007/978-1-4939-7686-7_1, © Springer Science+Business Media, LLC, part of Springer Nature 2018

interaction between two or more APIs also has to be considered"
[2]. In addition, regulatory approval of any drug or formulation
requires submission of entire stability data generated during stability testing in a common technical document (CTD) format for
review by the regulatory agencies [3].

Various international, regional, as well as national regulatory
groups/agencies have published guidelines for stability testing,
which outline the protocols and expected information so that the
manufacturers are able to generate the right-first-time stability data.
The evolution of regulatory guidances and study protocols has
happened as a result of tremendous efforts of regulatory, industry,
and academic experts over the years. To protect the manufacturers
from the generation of stability data that are different in small
variables, experts from within the countries or regional groups
have worked together to design the requirements most suited for
their countries and regions. On a broader perspective, International
Conference on Harmonisation (ICH) and WHO have also made
good efforts to develop harmonized guidelines, which industry all
over the world is really depending upon for planning of the stability
studies. The WHO guideline of 2009 [2], and its very recent
revised draft of July 2017 [4], is modeled on ICH guidelines,
with even the same language, but only differing with respect to a
few additional aspects, not touched by ICH, like ongoing stability
studies, and in-use and hold-time stability.

The intention of this chapter is to list and briefly discuss available drug stability testing guidelines, representing physical and
geographical diversity. The readers are requested to follow the
most accepted guidance document in consultation with the local
authorities. Moreover, as newer guidelines are being introduced,
and also revisions of old guidelines are happening regularly, the
readers must again check whether any latest versions are available,
before their adoption and implementation into the stability testing
program.

2   International Stability Testing Guidelines

Stability testing guidelines that can be truly considered "international" are those established by ICH, VICH, and WHO. ICH had
focused on harmonization of stability testing requirements in the
United States, Europe, and Japan. The three regions have been
associated with most new drug innovations and new product
launches; hence there was rationale for them to make uniform
standards for stability testing for registration of new pharmaceuticals for human use, so as to ease the sale of drug substances and
products across their borders. WHO has always been concerned
with the world countries under its umbrella, and owing to less
prevalence of new drugs in WHO member countries, therefore,

after release of ICH Q1A in 1993, WHO brought its own guideline in 1996 focusing on well-established drug substances in conventional dosage forms [5], which of course underwent revision in 2009 [2], and lately a further revised draft has been issued in July 2017 [4].

2.1 International Conference on Harmonisation (ICH) and Veterinary International Cooperation on Harmonisation (VICH) Guidelines

The first ICH meeting was hosted by the European Federation of Pharmaceutical Industries and Associations (EFPIA) in Brussels in April 1990 with the objective to initiate the harmonization of regulatory requirements for registration of pharmaceuticals for human use. After 25 years of its existence, ICH decided to make several organizational changes, including adoption of a new name "International Council for Harmonisation of Technical Requirements for Registration of Pharmaceuticals for Human Use (ICH)", and its registration as an international nonprofit association under the Swiss law [6]. With this, ICH now wishes to go ahead to achieve harmonization of regulatory standards even beyond the three regions, so that safe, effective, and high-quality medicines are developed and registered in the most resource-efficient manner all over the globe [7].

At the time of its birth in 1990, ICH opted "stability" as the first topic for harmonization, and subsequently multiple stability testing guidelines were developed with an underlying principle that the stability data generated in any one of the three regions of the United States, Japan, and the European Union (EU) on new drugs will be acceptable to the other two regions. The ICH guidelines have got widely accepted over the period, and have been utilized by WHO, regional groups, and individual country authorities as the parent guidelines for developing, modifying, and customizing their local drug stability testing requirements.

The current list of ICH guidelines (Q1A-Q1F, Q5C) is given in Table 1. Evidently, the parent guideline Q1A was revised twice. The ICH Steering Committee allowed the withdrawal of the Q1F guideline at its meeting in Yokohama in June 2006 and decided to leave the definition of storage conditions in climatic zones III and IV to the respective regions and WHO [8]. The United States Food and Drug Administration (USFDA) adopted all ICH guidelines mentioned in Table 1, except Q1F. The same was the case of European Medicines Agency (EMA), which adopted all ICH stability guidelines, except Q5C. Japan has included all of them in its regulations.

For veterinary medicines, stability testing guidelines have been published separately by the International Cooperation on Harmonisation of Technical Requirements for Registration of Veterinary Medicinal Products (VICH). The list is provided in Table 2. Except GL17 guideline entitled "Stability testing of new biotechnological/biological veterinary medicinal products", which has not been adopted by the USFDA and the EMA till now, others are already part of regulations in the three regions.

Table 1
ICH stability testing guidelines

ICH code	Document title	Publication year	Ref.
ICH Q1A(R2)	Stability Testing of New Drug Substances and Products	2003	[9]
ICH Q1B	Stability Testing: Photostability Testing of New Drug Substances and Products	1996	[10]
ICH Q1C	Stability Testing for New Dosage Forms	1996	[11]
ICH Q1D	Bracketing and Matrixing Designs for Stability Testing of New Drug Substances and Products	2002	[12]
ICH Q1E	Evaluation of Stability Data	2003	[13]
ICH Q1F*	Stability Data Package for Registration Applications in Climatic Zones III and IV	2003	[14]
ICH Q5C	Stability Testing of Biotechnological/Biological Products	1995	[15]

Note: * Withdrawn in 2006.

Table 2
VICH stability testing guidelines [16, 17]

VICH code	Document title	Publication year
VICH GL8	Stability Testing for Medicated Premixes	1999
VICH GL4	Stability Testing: Requirements for New Dosage Forms	1999
VICH GL3 (R)	Stability Testing of New Veterinary Drug Substances and Medicinal Products (Revision)	2007
VICH GL5	Stability Testing: Photostability Testing of New Drug Substances and Products	1999
VICH GL45	Bracketing and Matrixing Designs for Stability Testing of New Veterinary Drug Substances and Medicinal Products	2010
VICH GL51	Statistical Evaluation of Stability Data	2013
VICH GL17	Stability Testing of New Biotechnological/Biological Veterinary Medicinal Products	2000

2.2 World Health Organization (WHO) Stability Requirements

WHO initiated work on development of guidance document on stability testing of pharmaceuticals in 1988 [18]. After the first ICH stability guideline Q1A was published in 1993, WHO speeded up the activity and came out with the guideline entitled "Guidelines for Stability Testing of Pharmaceutical Products Containing Well Established Drug Substances in Conventional Dosage Forms" in

1996 [5]. This document provided stability data requirements for products that were already registered and available in the market, and also allowed for an appropriate transition period upon re-registration or upon re-evaluation. The study of product-related factors with influence on the quality was also covered, e.g., the interaction of API with excipients, container closure systems, and packaging materials, as well as the interaction between two or more APIs (in case of FDCs).

The withdrawal of Q1F in 2006 [8] entrusted responsibility on WHO to propose long-term stability testing conditions for all the world countries. With the help of feedback from stakeholders and independent experts, WHO drew a list, which was made part of its revision issued in 2009 [2]. In this document, WHO proposed subdivision of climatic zone IV countries into zones IVa and IVb to suit conditions in the nations where there was extreme humidity condition of 75% RH throughout the year, like ASEAN and some parts of South America.

The stability guidelines issued by WHO till date are listed in Table 3.

Table 3
Stability guidelines issued by World Health Organization (WHO)

Code	Document title	Publication year	Ref.
WHO Technical Report Series, No. 863, 1996, Annex 5	Guidelines for Stability Testing of Pharmaceutical Products Containing Well Established Drug Substances in Conventional Dosage Forms	1996	[5]
WHO Technical Report Series, No. 953, 2009, Annex 2	Stability Testing of Active Pharmaceutical Ingredients and Finished Pharmaceutical Products	2009	[2]
WHO Technical Report Series, No. 962, 2006, Annex 3	Guidelines on Stability Evaluation of Vaccines	2006	[19]
Technical Guidance Series (TGS)-2	Establishing Stability of an *In Vitro* Diagnostic for WHO Prequalification (Draft)	2015	[20]
WHO Technical Report Series No. 999, 2016, Annex 5	Guidelines on the Stability Evaluation of Vaccines for Use Under Extended Controlled Temperature Conditions	2016	[21]
Working document QAS/16.694/Rev. 1	Stability Testing of Active Pharmaceutical Ingredients and Finished Pharmaceutical Products	2017	[4]

3   Regional and National Stability Guidelines

Despite the availability of ICH/WHO international guidelines for both new and established human drugs and products, the activity by regional groups and at the national level has been ongoing in parallel. Hence, a multitude of documents is available today.

The emergence of regional and national stability test guidelines mostly happened around 2005. The ICH stability guidelines had the limitation of applicability to newer drug substances and products only, while WHO guideline of 1996 was modeled differently to ICH, and did not cover storage conditions for all regions, and even aspects covered in multiple ICH guidelines. So the regional and national agencies were forced to develop their own guidelines. The same are enlisted in Table 4. Table 5 lists guidelines issued by

Table 4
Major regional guidelines on stability testing

Region	Regulatory agency	Title	Update	Ref.
Arab States	Cooperation Council for the Arab States of the Gulf	The GCC Guidelines for Stability Testing of Active Pharmaceutical Ingredients (APIs) and Finished Pharmaceutical Products (FPPs)	Version 3.1, Updated 24 February 2013	[22]
ASEAN	Association of Southeast Asian Nations	ASEAN Guideline on Stability Study of Drug Product (Version 6.0)	Updated revision: 15 May 2013	[23]
EAC	East African Community Partner States' National Medicines Regulatory Authorities (NMRAs)	PART II: EAC Guidelines on Stability Testing Requirements for Active Pharmaceutical Ingredients (APIs) and Finished Pharmaceutical Products (FPPs)	September 2014	[24]
SADC	Registration of Medicines	SADC Guideline for Stability Testing	2004	[25]
WHO Eastern Mediterranean Region	World Health Organization	Stability Testing of Active Substances and Pharmaceutical Products	DRAFT 2.0 19 April 2006	[26]
LATAM	Pan American Health Organization via PANDRH	Requirements for Medicines Registration in the Americas	PANDRH Series— Technical Document No. 10, June 2013	[27]

Table 5
The European Medicines Agency's stability guidelines on drug substances and drug products for human medicines and on the non-immunologicals for veterinary medicines

Code (reference number)	Document title	Publication year	Ref.
CPMP/QWP/159/96 corr.	Maximum Shelf Life for Sterile Products for Human Use After First Opening or Following Reconstitution	1998	[29]
CPMP/QWP/2934/99	In-Use Stability Testing of Human Medicinal Products	2001	[30]
CPMP/QWP/609/96/ Rev.2	Declaration of Storage Conditions for Medicinal Product Particulars and Active Substances (Annex)	2003	[31]
CPMP/QWP/122/02, Rev. 1 corr.	Stability Testing of Existing Active Ingredients and Related Finished Products	2003	[32]
EMA/HMPC/3626/2009	Reflection Paper on Stability Testing of Herbal Medicinal Products and Traditional Herbal Medicinal Products	2010	[33]
EMA/CHMP/CVMP/ QWP/441071/2011-Rev.2	Stability Testing for Applications for Variations to Marketing Authorization	2014	[34]
EMEA/CVMP/422/99/ Rev.3	Declaration of Storage Conditions: 1. In the Product Information of Pharmaceutical Veterinary Medicinal Products, 2. for Active Substances (Annex)	2007	[35]
EMEA/CVMP/424/01	In-Use Stability Testing of Veterinary Medicinal Products (Excluding Immunological Veterinary Medicinal Products)	2002	[36]
EMEA/CVMP/198/99	Maximum Shelf Life for Sterile Medicinal Products after First Opening or Following Reconstitution	2001	[37]
EMEA/CVMP/846/99-Rev.1	Stability Testing of Existing Active Substances and Related Finished Products	2008	[38]
EMEA/CVMP/IWP/ 250147/2008	Data Requirements to Support In-Use Stability Claims for Veterinary Vaccines	2010	[39]

EMA that are different from ICH and VICH. The individual country guidelines are separately enumerated in Table 6. All of them are discussed below individually.

3.1 Regional Guidelines

3.1.1 European Union

The EMA works across the EU and globally to protect public and animal health by assessing medicines to rigorous scientific standards [28]. The authority has equally well focused on stability testing and did adopt almost all core ICH guidelines, being party to the agency. It also has come out with multiple documents on topics not covered by ICH or even VICH. The list is provided in Table 5.

Table 6
National guidelines on stability testing

Region	Regulatory agency	Title	Update	Ref.
Australia	Therapeutic Goods Administration	Stability Testing for Prescription Medicines	Version 1.1, March 2017	[40]
Brazil	ANVISA	Guide for Stability Studies	Resolution: RE N° 1, of July 29th, 2005	[41]
Canada	TPD, Health Canada	Guidance for Industry: Stability Testing of Existing Drug Substances and Products	23 April 2003	[42]
China	Chinese Pharmacopoeia	Guidelines for the Stability Testing of Drug Substances and Preparations	Appendix XXC	[43]
Ghana	Food and Drugs Board	Stability Testing of New Drug Substances and Products	–	[44]
India	IDMA-APA	Stability Testing of Existing Drug Substances and Products	Draft 02, 8 April 2002	[45]
	CDSCO	Guidelines for Stability Testing of Pharmaceutical Products	–	[46]
	CDSCO	Schedule Y, Appendix IX, Stability Testing of New Drugs	2005	[47]
Mexico	Health Department, Mexico	Stability of Drugs And Medicine	Official Mexican Standard NOM-073-SSA1-2005, 4 January 2006	[48]
Panama	Ministry of Health	Untitled	9 November 2005	[49]
South Africa	Medicines Control Council	Stability	Version 7.1, August 2012	[50]

Evidently, other than WHO, EMA is the second agency to bring out a guideline on stability testing of existing drugs and products, and on topics like in-use stability, post-approval changes, and stability testing post-reconstitution of drugs for injection.

3.1.2 Gulf Cooperation Council

In May 2005, Gulf Cooperation Council (GCC) established a general guideline for stability studies for products manufactured in the GCC states (Bahrain, Kuwait, Oman, Qatar, Saudi Arabia, and the United Arab Emirates). The guideline has been updated periodically and its final version 3.1 was issued in February 2013 by Executive Board of the Health Ministers' Council of GCC States. Major contents of this guidance have been adapted from 2009

WHO guideline on stability testing of active pharmaceutical ingredients and finished pharmaceutical products. The countries in the GCC states are categorized under either climatic zone III (hot/dry climate) or IVa (hot/humid climate), based on analysis of the effects of climatic conditions [22].

3.1.3 Association of Southeast Asian Nations (ASEAN)

ASEAN comprises ten member states including Singapore, the Philippines, Thailand, Indonesia, and Malaysia as major ones, besides five others. The sea area of ASEAN is about three times larger than its land counterpart, due to which ASEAN countries fall in climatic zone IV (hot and humid climate). Therefore, the group rightly focused on long-term stability test storage conditions in their region, and also on harmonization of general stability testing requirements. The second meeting of ASEAN was held on 5 and 6 March 2000 in Bangkok, Thailand, to discuss important issues in the context of harmonization of requirements, and this meeting was followed by another technical meeting of Pharmaceutical Product Working Group (PPWG) on product information and stability at Siem Reap, Cambodia, on 4–6 September, 2002. It primarily focused on the first draft of working guidelines namely "Draft Guidelines on Stability Studies-Indonesia". Also, PPWG developed the ASEAN Common Technical Requirements (ACTR) and associated guidelines. The ACTR is a set of written material intended to guide applicants to prepare an application that is consistent with the expectations of all ASEAN Drug Regulatory Authorities. A meeting was again held at Jakarta from 12 to 14 January 2004, where harmonization status of stability requirements was discussed [51]. It was strongly put forward that ICH and WHO stability testing guidelines did not adequately address the climatic conditions prevalent in the majority of ASEAN countries. Therefore, in this meeting, a long-term testing condition of 30 °C $\pm$ 2 °C/ 75% RH $\pm$ 5% RH was proposed, which was different from the one established earlier by ICH and WHO for Zone IV countries, viz., 30°C/65% RH. The ASEAN Guideline on Stability Study of Drug Product was formalized on 22 February 2005 at 9th ACCSQ-PPWG meeting held at the Philippines from 21 to 24 February 2005. This guideline was suggested to be followed for all product classifications, including new chemical entities, biotechnology-derived drugs, generics, and variations, but excluding biologicals and drug products containing vitamin and mineral preparations. The good point of ASEAN guidelines is specific recommendations on several different dosage forms, including transdermal patches, metered-dose inhalations, nasal aerosols, and suppositories; inclusion of examples of a protocol for stability study; a report format; reduced design and extrapolation of data; and examples of types; thickness, and permeability coefficient. An updated revision of the same guideline was finalized in 20th

ACCSQ-PPWG meeting held in Bali, Indonesia, from 13 to 17 May 2013. The new guideline clearly mentions that long-term stability testing for ASEAN region is to be done in accordance with the Zone IVb condition of 30 °C/75% RH [23].

3.1.4 East African Community

The East African Community (EAC) is an intergovernmental organization mandated by the governments of Burundi, Kenya, Rwanda, Uganda, and Tanzania. EAC Medicines Registration Harmonization project was an outcome of African Medicines Regulatory Harmonization Initiative (AMRHI), which got started on 30 March 2012 at Arusha, Tanzania. In 2014, EAC issued "Guideline on Stability Testing of Active Pharmaceutical Ingredients (API) and Finished Medicinal Products", which is a part of the Common Technical Document for National Medicines Regulatory Authorities (NMRAs) of EAC partner states. This guideline was adapted from WHO Technical Report Series, No. 953, Annex II. The required long-term storage conditions for APIs by EAC countries are either 30 °C ± 2 °C/65% RH ± 5% RH or 30 °C ± 2 °C/75% RH ± 5% RH. The purpose cited for the development of the guideline has been to enable uniform evaluation and registration of APIs and finished medicinal products in the EAC partner states [24].

3.1.5 Southern African Development Community

Southern African Development Community (SADC) includes 15 states (i.e., Angola, Botswana, Democratic Republic of Congo, Lesotho, Madagascar, Malawi, Mauritius, Mozambique, Namibia, Seychelles, South Africa, Swaziland, United Republic of Tanzania, Zambia, and Zimbabwe). The community issued "SADC Guideline for Stability Testing" in 2004, which defined the stability data package for new API and medicinal products (Part A), and also existing APIs and products (Part B). However, it is claimed that the guideline does not cover the stability requirements for abbreviated or abridged applications, variations, clinical trial applications, etc. The storage conditions for long-term stability studies mentioned are 25 °C ± 2 °C/60% RH ± 5% RH and 30 °C ± 2 °C/65% RH ± 5% RH. These conditions are very similar to climatic zone II and IVa of WHO stability testing guidelines [25].

3.1.6 Eastern Mediterranean Region (EMR)

The countries situated in Eastern Mediterranean Region (EMR) fall geographically to the east of the Mediterranean Sea. The region comprises 22 countries, most of which are Arab countries together with Afghanistan, Iran, and Pakistan. WHO Regional Office for the Eastern Mediterranean, vide its efforts to contribute to regional harmonization, organized a consultation on Regional Guidelines on Stability Studies of Medicines on 25–28 February 2006 at Jeddah in Saudi Arabia. The consultation reviewed and discussed relevant national, regional, and international guidelines. The consultation also discussed climatic conditions in the region, with particular emphasis on determining the mean kinetic temperature (MKT) and the appropriate climate zone for each country. The draft regional guideline entitled "Stability Testing of Active Substances and Pharmaceutical Products" was the enormous effort of the consultation [26]. These guidelines were based in part on existing guidelines of ICH, EMA, and GCC. The final draft 2.0 was recommended for adoption in countries of the Eastern Mediterranean Region. This guidance provided long-term testing conditions in each country of the region, after evaluation of their climatic conditions. The guideline also recommended acceptance of stability data for studies conducted at higher temperatures and humidities, e.g., at 30 °C/75% RH. This guideline later became the starting point for the development of new WHO guideline, which was finalized in 2009 [2].

3.1.7 Latin American (LATAM) Countries

All LATAM countries are situated in Central America, South America, or the Caribbean, with the exception of Mexico, located in North America. The regulatory process in the region has been highly country specific. Many countries, especially in Central America, require the data from stability studies to be formatted under country-specific guidelines. Unlike the EU or the ASEAN countries, LATAM drug registration processes are not harmonized, though extensive efforts have been ongoing, mainly through the initiative of the Pan American Health Organization (PAHO) via the Pan American Network for Drug Regulatory Harmonization (PANDRH). The lack of country-specific stability data requirements is a real challenge for the drug registration across LATAM nations. A brief of stability requirements of selected LATAM countries is mentioned in Table 7. The PANDRH Series Technical

Table 7
Key stability study requirements and considerations for selected LATAM countries [52]

Countries	Stability study requirements/considerations
Argentina	Climatic zone: Local market, zone II. Zone IV is also accepted
Brazil	Climatic zone: Primarily zone IV (30 °C ± 2 °C/75% RH ± 5% RH). Stress studies for biologic/biotech (possible exposure of the product outside recommended conservation care should be evaluated, such as high temperatures and/or freezing)
Chile	Climatic zone: Primarily I and II. It accepts stability data generated for zones III and IV for exportation, if other requirements are fulfilled
Colombia	Climatic zone: Zone IVa (zone IVb is also acceptable)
Mexico	Climatic zone: Primary zone II (zones III and IV may be accepted). Norm NOM-073-SSA1-2005 defines long-term storage condition for the country as 30 °C ± 2 °C/ 65% RH ± 5% RH
Peru	Climatic zone: for the most part zone IVa
Venezuela	Climatic zone: for the most part zone IVb

Document No. 10 entitled "Requirements for Medicines Registration in the Americas" discusses about key stability study requirement to some extent [52].

3.2 National Stability Guidelines

3.2.1 Australia

Therapeutic Goods Administration (TGA) is part of the Australian Government Department of Health and is responsible for regulating medicines and medical devices. The TGA guideline "Stability Testing for Prescription Medicines" addresses concern that the major population centers in Australia experience a combination of high humidity and high temperature during the summer. Accordingly, TGA defines stability requirements as given for Zone IV regions. In addition to that, TGA has adopted maximum number of the stability guidelines issued by EMA, even retaining the same reference number.

3.2.2 Brazil

The Brazilian Health Surveillance Agency (ANVISA) issued guidance for stability studies under circular "RESOLUTION—RE N° 1, OF JULY 29th 2005". The shelf-life of a product to be marketed in Brazil is determined by a long-term stability study at 30 °C ± 2 °C/75% RH ± 5% RH for solid and semisolid pharmaceuticals.

3.2.3 Canada

The ICH harmonized tripartite guidance "Stability Testing of New Drug Substances and Products" was originally adopted by Health Canada in 1994. Additionally, the Canadian agency published "Guidance for Industry-Stability Testing of Existing Drug Substances and Products" in April 2004. It recommended that submissions shall contain data from 6-month studies at 25 °C ± 2 °C/60% RH ± 5% RH and/or 30 °C ± 2 °C/65% RH ± 5% RH, as applicable. This guidance provides additional clarification on examples of various scenarios for stability designs (e.g., multiple strengths of identical or closely related formulations).

3.2.4 China

Chinese Pharmacopoeia, appendix XX C, provides "Guidelines for the Stability Testing of Drug Substances and Preparations". The defined long-term condition is 25 °C ± 2 °C/60% RH ± 10% RH. The condition for long-term stability testing is adopted on the basis of the international climatic zone; China is mostly in the region of subtemperate zone, which is consistent with ICH.

3.2.5 Ghana

The Food and Drugs Board, Ghana, has guidance on "Stability Testing of New Drug Substances and Products", which describes an approach to the broader use of WHO and ICH guidelines on stability testing. The guideline addresses the information to be submitted in registration application for new molecular entities and associated drug products, and generic products for registration in territories in climatic zones III and IV. The new feature in this guidance has been insistence on fixed relative humidity (RH) level of 70%, rather than the stipulated range of 60–70% RH indicated in the table by the WHO/ICH guidelines. This is because the RH level in Ghana is claimed to hardly fall below the 70% level. In the same guidance, the Board has proposed fees for stability as well as stress testing.

3.2.6 India

Indian stability guideline is encompassed in Appendix IX of schedule Y issued on 20.1.2005. The section is entitled "Stability Testing of New Drugs". It describes long-term stability conditions, *viz.* 30 °C ± 2 °C/65% RH ± 5% RH(Table 6). Otherwise, the long-term testing condition stated for India in the WHO list is 30 °C/ 70% RH [2]. A guidance manual for compliance of Indian Pharmacopoeia by drugs regulatory bodies, drugs testing laboratories & pharmaceutical industry [46] was released by the Indian Pharmacopoeia Commission on 12 December 2012. As a part of contents, the manual outlines a guidance on stability testing of pharmaceutical products,which is modelled on 1996 stability testing guideline of WHO. However, the regulatory status of the manual itself is not clear.

3.2.7 Mexico

The official Mexican Standard NOM-073-SSA1-2005 is entitled "Stability of Drugs and Medicine", whereby requirements of the stability studies that should be performed to the drugs and medications commercialized in Mexico have been established. Long-term stability testing conditions mentioned in the guidance are 25 °C ± 2 °C/60% RH ± 5% RH or 30 °C ± 2 °C/65% RH ± 5% RH that belong to both Zones II and IV.

3.2.8 Panama

Panama belongs to climatic zone IV, which is the most critical in matters of temperature and humidity and represents a risk factor for drug stability. Executive Decree No. 178, dated 12 July 2001, regulates Law N°. 1, dated 10 January 2001, and considers stability norms in Title II, Chapter I, Section III. It declares that Panama has adopted the WHO and the ICH modifications for stability studies for pharmaceutical products for climatic zones IV. Article 9 of the same document states that "The long-term or real-time studies must be carried out under controlled storage conditions, at a temperature of 30 °C ± 2 °C and a relative humidity of 70% RH ± 5% RH or 65% RH ± 5% RH, or those storage conditions harmonized for Climatic Zone IV that Panama may adopt posterior to the stipulations of this Decree".

3.2.9 South Africa

The stability guideline of South Africa has been adopted with only minor modifications of the ICH and WHO guidelines. It contains aspects relating to testing conditions, numbers of batches to be tested, and requirements regarding follow-up stability data. The South African Weather Service (SAWS) classifies climate of South Africa as ranging from "Desert (arid)" in the west to "All-

Table 8
Stability guidelines issued by USFDA

FDA organizations	Document title	Publication year	Ref.
ORA	CPG Sec. 480.100 Requirements for Expiration Dating and Stability Testing	1995	[57]
ORA	CPG Sec. 480.300 Lack of Expiration Date of Stability Data	1995	[58]
CDER	Expiration Dating and Stability Testing of Solid Oral Dosage Form Drugs Containing Iron	1997	[59]
ORA	CPG Sec. 280.100—Stability Requirements—Licensed In Vitro Diagnostic Products	2000	[60]
CBER, CDER, CDRH, CVM	Container and Closure System Integrity Testing in Lieu of Sterility Testing as a Component of the Stability Protocol for Sterile Products	2008	[61]
CBER	Guidance for Industry: Testing Limits in Stability Protocols for Standardized Grass Pollen Extracts	2008	[62]
CVM	Guidance for Industry: Drug Stability Guidelines	2008	[55]
CDER	Guidance for Industry: ANDAs—Stability Testing of Drug Substances and Products	2013	[56]
CDER	Guidance for Industry: ANDAs—Stability Testing of Drug Substances and Products, Questions and Answers	2014	[63]

Note: ORA: Office of Regulatory Affairs; CDER: Center for Drug Evaluation and Research; CVM: Center for Veterinary Medicine; CBER: Center for Biologics Evaluation and Research; CDRH: Center for Devices and Radiological Health

year rain with hot summers" in the eastern coastal region. WHO classifies South Africa in zone IVa [2]. However, the country accepts data generated even under zone IVb condition.

3.2.10   United States of America

Prior to ICH guidelines, the USFDA had in place "Guideline for Submitting Documentation for Stability of Human Drug and Biologics" issued in 1987, which was followed extensively. From 1993 onwards, FDA adopted and implemented ICH Q1 guidelines, and hence the use of original 1987 guideline was abandoned. Subsequently, the agency planned for issuing a combined document incorporating all ICH guidelines and recommendations for all content issues that were not settled at the ICH forum. Accordingly, it issued a draft FDA stability guideline in 1998 [53], but due to pressure from ICH member states, the guideline could not be finalized for many years and was finally withdrawn on June 1, 2006. This document included all content topics like stability testing requirements during all phases of drug discovery and development, site-specific stability testing, stability testing re-workup requirements on post-approval changes, etc. Table 8 lists all non-ICH guidelines issued by USFDA related to stability testing from time to time. Other than these, the Office of Generic Drugs (ODG) of USFDA introduced the concept of Quality by Design (QbD) in 2006, wherein it expressed the belief that the stability of drug products could be best ensured through QbD [54]. The agency's Center for Veterinary Medicine (CVM) also issued "Guidance for Industry: Drug Stability Guidelines" on 9 December 2008 to establish drug stability in support of original, abbreviated, or supplements to new animal drug applications (NADAs/ANADAs) [55]. The Center for Drug Evaluation and Research (CDER) further released "Guidance for Industry ANDAs: Stability Testing of Drug Substances and Products" for generic drugs in June 2013 [56].

4 Another Set of Guidelines Related to Ensuring Stability of Pharmaceutical Products

With multiple recalls of drug products and warning letters being issued owing to reasons of product instability and deficiencies in stability testing programs, respectively, it is prudent for industry to pay attention even to other international and national guidelines, whose concepts have a direct bearing on their stability testing practices. The relevant guidelines and specific aspects are discussed below:

4.1 ICH Guidelines Q2, Q3, and Q6–Q11

Various other ICH guidelines, even not on the topics of stability testing, can be used in an effective way for completion of stability testing program on drug substances or products. A specific and stability-indicating procedure is supposed to be used for the determination of the drug content and quantitation of impurities/degradation products in the stability samples. The method has to be duly validated, for which one can apply validation protocol outlined in Q2(R1) [64]. Similarly, any degradation product observed in stability studies at recommended storage conditions, at a level greater than the identification threshold, should be identified in accordance with Q3A(R2) and Q3B(R2) [65, 66]. Reporting of impurity content of each batches on stability testing is required to be done. Q3B(R2) suggests that stability-indicating chromatograms for long-term and accelerated stability studies should be peaks labelled, including chromatograms from validation studies [66]. ICH Q6A guideline on specifications suggests establishing the single set of global specification in terms of acceptance criteria for the degradation product(s), formed during stability studies in a new drug substance or product. It also suggests that results from accelerated and long-term stability studies are helpful to justify the acceptance criteria [67]. Q7 guidance "Good Manufacturing

Practice Guide for Active Pharmaceutical Ingredients" suggests that complete records of stability testing and out-of-specification (OOS) results should be maintained [68]. It also highlights about following of best practices during stability monitoring of APIs, like documentation, retest dating, and stability indication method validation.

The concept of QbD was first introduced by FDA in 2006, and thereafter it was followed in Q8(R2). The guidance defines "stability" as the "quality target product profile" and hence lays down the need to identify critical quality attributes, which could affect the product stability [69]. Guideline Q9, which mainly focuses on quality risk management, also emphasizes on mitigation of risks during pharmaceutical development and hence on stability testing to ensure stability of product till the shelf-life period [70]. The guideline Q10 "Pharmaceutical Quality System" on product life cycle builds up the link between pharmaceutical development and manufacturing activities, wherein also the stability of the product can be affected [71]. The role of stability studies in identifying the critical quality attributes is also highlighted in the recently introduced Q11 guideline "Development and Manufacture of Drug Substances (Chemical Entities and Biotechnological/Biological Entities)" [72].

4.2 Data Integrity Guidelines

In recent years, other than noncompliance to current good manufacturing practices (cGMP), data integrity violations are a good reason for frequent regulatory actions, including issue of warning letters, import alerts, and consent decrees. Many examples exist where warning letters have been issued owing to stability testing-linked data integrity issues, or problems in the conduct of stability testing. Select examples are cited in Table 9. The Medicines and Healthcare Products Regulatory Agency (MHRA) of the UK first discussed "Data Integrity" in their document "MHRA GMP Data Integrity Definitions and Guidance for Industry" in March 2015 [73]. The Agency published a new version of the document entitled "GxP Data Integrity Definitions and Guidance for Industry: Draft version for consultation" in July 2016 [74]. The USFDA issued a draft on "Data Integrity and Compliance with cGMP" in April 2016. This guidance states that "Data integrity refers to the completeness, consistency, and accuracy of data. Complete, consistent, and accurate data should be attributable, legible, contemporaneously recorded, original or a true copy, and accurate (ALCOA)" [75]. On 10 August 2016, the Pharmaceutical Inspection Convention (PIC/S) issued a first draft "Good Practices for Data Management and Integrity in Regulated GMP/GDP Environments" and simultaneously the EMA extended their "Questions and Answers: Good Manufacturing Practices" web page by 23 answers on data integrity-related questions [76, 77]. The WHO Technical Report Series No. 996, 2016,

Table 9
Specific recent examples where warning letters have been issued owing to stability testing-linked data integrity issues

Warning Letter No. Date	Comment	Ref.
320-16-12 May 16, 2016	Failure to follow a documented, ongoing stability testing program to monitor the stability characteristics of API and to use the results to confirm appropriate storage conditions and retest or expiry dates. You did not follow your stability program, SOP No. Q-0007. According to your SOP, you must fully test at least (b)(4) batch of (b)(4) API (b)(4) for stability at defined stability intervals. Your firm could not provide any stability data to support the (b)(4) expiration date assigned to your (b)(4) API	[79]
320-16-13 May 19, 2016	One of your analysts acknowledged falsifying test data for (b)(4) stability batch (b)(4) in August 2012. The analyst substituted a reference standard chromatogram in place of the 12-month stability interval chromatogram. You also submitted this data to FDA in support of drug master file (DMF) (b)(4) In your response, you stated that laboratory management did not discover the discrepancy until the 24-month stability interval. You also stated that the batch quality is unaffected because subsequent test results met specifications at the 24- and 36-month stability intervals	[80]
320-16-19 June 21, 2016	"For example, our investigator reviewed a data file audit trail that showed that during impurities analysis of an 18-month stability sample of (b)(4) crude batch (b)(4), your analyst aborted the injection before the test was complete, set the HPLC PC clock back, and then repeated the injection. Your analyst only reported the results of the second injection in the quality control data package. This test, for which your computerized system did not retain original data about the quality of your (b)(4) crude, had been performed as part of a stability study your firm executed in response to FDA's previous inspection in July, 2013. Our investigator observed the same technique for data manipulation and deletion in multiple other impurities analyses for (b)(4) When our investigator asked your staff about these instances of falsification and manipulation, your quality control manager stated that your firm 'forgot' to perform stability testing and therefore created falsified results for each missed time point by manipulating the controlling PC clock"	[81]
320-16-26 August 11, 2016	For example, during the inspection, we reviewed electronic data from your high-performance liquid chromatography (HPLC) system. An unknown impurity peak was present when the original 3-month stability sample of (b)(4) batch (b)(4) was run on October 9, 2014. This unknown peak was OOS and would have caused the sample to fail for unknown impurities, but it was not included in the official record for this stability test. Instead, an analyst ran a new sample to obtain a passing result on October 10, 2014, and only the passing result from the second sample was reported in the official record	[82]
320-16-27 August 12, 2016	Our inspection documented that you modified the manufacturing process multiple times for (b)(4) API. Your quality unit did not approve these changes, nor did you document them through a change control review process. Furthermore, you did not place samples from any of the batches produced through modified processes in your stability monitoring program to assess the effects of these changes on the quality of your API throughout the expiry period	[83]

(continued)

Table 9
(continued)

Warning Letter No. Date	Comment	Ref.
	In your response you referenced stability data from batches not manufactured using the modified processes discussed above. Your response is inadequate because you do not have stability data to demonstrate that your API meets specifications throughout its expiry period	
16-PHI-10 August 15, 2016	You did not adequately investigate the stability failure of lot (b)(4) of felodipine 2.5 mg tablets for an unknown impurity. The product specification for unknown impurities is (b)(4) percent, but your 3-month stability test result for this lot was (b)(4) percent impurities. You opened an investigation into the stability failure on February 12, 2015. Your own records indicate that as of April 29, 2015, you were aware that benzophenone had leached into the tablets from the ink and varnish on the primary container label, but you did not recall this lot until July 16, 2015, during the FDA inspection	[84]
320-16-30 August 25, 2016	Your firm failed to ensure that its drug product bore an expiration date that was supported by appropriate stability testing (21 CFR 211.137(a)). Your firm had no stability data to support your expiration date	[85]
320-17-16 January 6, 2017	Your firm failed to establish and follow an adequate written testing program designed to assess the stability characteristics of drug products and to use results of such stability testing to determine appropriate storage conditions and expiration dates (21 CFR 211.166(a)) You did not retain any samples to test and evaluate product stability and had no data to support the (b)(4) shelf-life claim of your products	[86]

included requirements on data integrity in Annex 5 entitled "Guidance on Good Data and Record Management Practices", which outlines expectations and examples of special risk management considerations for the implementation of ALCOA principles in paper-based and electronic systems. Therefore, it is onus on industry to follow ALCOA principles to ensure avoidance of problems due to reasons of data integrity [78].

4.3 Quality Metrics Requirements

For the last few years, FDA has increased its emphasis on auditing of global pharmaceutical industry, and it has been facing difficulty in evaluation of the data presented by the latter. Hence it proposed the industry to provide quality metrics data, to help improve the efficiency and effectiveness of inspection. Accordingly, FDA released draft guidance (revision 1) on "Submission of Quality Metrics Data" in November 2016 [87]. The agency requested the companies to follow quality metrics as part of its analysis for stability testing with respect to the following:

(a) The number of out-of-specification (OOS) results for the product, including stability testing.

(b) The number of lot release and stability tests conducted for the product.

(c) The number of OOS results for lot release and stability tests for the product, which are invalidated due to lab error.

4.4 ANVISA Forced Decomposition Guideline

In December 2015, ANVISA of Brazil approved "Resolution RDC 53/15", which outlined specific requirements for product registration and post-approval change submission with regard to reporting, identification, and qualification of degradation products in the drug products. These new rules have a significant impact on the forced degradation practices of the pharmaceutical industry, as they emphasize that the extent of drug degradation in the product should be greater than 10%, and if it is less than 10%, the company must submit justified technical justification. It also highlights that any change and inclusion of synthetic route of the active pharmaceutical ingredient, or quantitative and qualitative changes of excipient in the final drug product, should lead to a new forced degradation study. The guidance suggests conduct of forced degradation study on placebo, API (representative of manufacturing process), formulation (single active) representative of manufacturing process, and fixed-dose combination formulation (active alone and together). Hence, applicants for marketing authorization in Brazil need to critically understand and implement ANVISA registration filing requirements for forced degradation studies, as they are different from other regulatory agencies [88].

4.5 Stability Requirements Subsequent to Post-approval Changes

After the regulatory permission, multiple forced causes can lead to post-approval changes of various types. These changes/variations can variably impact the stability of the product. The significant changes tend to trigger regeneration of substantial amount of stability data, while minor changes call for only a written stability commitment. USFDA initially had a detailed portion on the subject in its draft 1998 guideline [53], but owing to its non-finalization, it introduced guidance for industry "Changes to an Approved NDA or ANDA" in April 2004, which offered a significant amount of information to guide the sponsor in filing and data requirements related to stability study [89]. Health Canada also introduced guidance document on "Post-Notice of Compliance (NOC) Changes: Quality Document" in 2009, which was periodically amended and recently revised in July 2016 [90]. This guidance highlighted change to the post-approval stability protocol or stability commitment in details. In between, the WHO Prequalification Team: medicines (PQTm) issued guidance entitled "Guidelines on Variations to a Prequalified Product" (Annex 3) in 2013 [91]. Sections 3.2.S.7 and 3.2.P.8 of this guidance discuss in details the stability requirements on post-approval changes in case of the drug substance as well as the product.

5   Stability Guidelines for Other/Specific Product Categories

While the above discussion revolves around stability testing requirements for new and existing drug substances and products, there are many other documents that lay down specific stability testing protocols for other types of products, like OTCs, cosmetics, transdermal patches, in vitro diagnostic reagents, excipients, and homeopathic drugs. The list is provided in Table 10. These are discussed below individually.

Table 10
Stability guidelines/documents on miscellaneous topics

Guidelines	Regulatory agency	Publication year	Ref.
Australian Regulatory Guidelines for Sunscreens	TGA	2012	[92]
Cosmetic Products Stability Guide	ANVISA	2005	[93]
Guidelines on Stability Testing of Cosmetic Products	The Cosmetic, Toiletry, and Fragrance Association (CTFA) and the European Cosmetic, Toiletry and Perfumery Association (COLIPA)	2004	[94]
Guideline on Quality of Transdermal Patches	EMA/CHMP/QWP/911254/2011	2014	[95]
Evaluation of Stability of In Vitro Diagnostic Reagents	Clinical and Laboratory Standards Institute	2009	[96]
The IPEC Excipient Stability Program Guide	International Pharmaceutical Excipients Council (IPEC)	2010	[97]
Guideline for the Stability Testing of Nonprescription (OTC) Drug Products not Regulated by an NDA/ANDA	Consumer Healthcare Products Association	2012	[98]
Homeopathic Drug Stability Guidelines	Homoeopathic Pharmacopoeia Convention of the United States	2014	[99]
Stability Testing for Medicinal Products Prepared in Accordance with Homoeopathic Manufacturing Procedures	–	–	[100]
Medical Device Registration Guideline	Registration and Drug Control Department Ministry of Health—UAE	2011	[101]
Guidance for Conducting Stability Testing to Support an Expiration Date Labelling Claim for Medical Gloves (Draft)	USFDA	–	[102]
Stability Testing of Dietary Supplements	NSF International	2011	[103]

5.1 Nonprescription Over-the-Counter (OTC) Drug Products

The lone guideline on OTC drug products is the one established by the Consumer Healthcare Products Association (CHPA) of the United States. It is titled as "Guideline for the Stability Testing of Nonprescription (OTC) Drug Products Not Regulated by a NDA/ANDA". The primary objective of this guideline has been to define the minimum stability data package to support the commercial distribution of OTC monograph drug products in the United States per climatic zone II. As per this guidance, photostability testing may be omitted with scientific justification; otherwise, ICH Q1B should be followed for the same. The criteria of selection of batches, batch size, and testing time points for long-term as well as accelerated stability testing are laid down differently from ICH Q1A(R2). The guidance suggests assignment of 24-month expiry period upon successful completion of 3-month accelerated testing, which is quite different from ICH expiry dating policy.

5.2 Cosmetic Products

The Cosmetic, Toiletry and Fragrance Association (CTFA) of the United States and the European Cosmetic, Toiletry and Perfumery Association (COLIPA) jointly developed a guideline for cosmetic products in March 2004, which was titled "Guidelines on Stability Testing of Cosmetic Products". The guidance covers important topics like cosmetic stability study design and prediction of functionality under stress conditions. The guideline suggests that "accelerated stability test studies be done at 37 °C, 40 °C or 45 °C during 1, 2, 3 ... months, but the temperature used and the duration will depend on the product type". Another cosmetics-focused stability guideline is from ANVISA under the name "Cosmetic Products Stability Guide", which was released in 2005. In this guideline, the main objective has been to ensure quality of cosmetics, and includes good emphasis on stability studies. An important suggestion is this: "For the stability tests, the most common storage conditions for samples to be considered are temperature of environment, high and low temperature, exposure to light and freezing and defrosting cycles". The TGA of Australia also introduced "Australian Regulatory Guidelines for Sunscreens" in November 2012. It covers stability test requirements, stability protocol, and shelf-life prediction from short-term testing at elevated temperatures. This is a revised form of the parent document "Guidelines for Stability Testing of Sunscreens April 1994", which was developed by the Australian industry peak bodies and accepted by TGA. The Personal Care Products Council (PCPC), formerly known as CTFA, recently issued "Guideline for Industry: The Stability Testing of Cosmetic Products", which has been more focused on photostability testing and even has been aligned to ICH Q1B. PCPC recommends that stability testing should cover a minimum of 12-month duration on at least one batch, while the manufacturer decides the appropriate humidity conditions to use, based generally on formulation, package type, intended use, and the market.

5.3 Transdermal Patches

EMA issued "Guideline on quality of transdermal patches" on 23 October 2014, which addresses new marketing authorization applications (including generic or abridged applications) and subsequent variation submissions for transdermal patches for systemic delivery. The guideline does not cover stability requirements for transdermal patches, but it suggests to follow the stability testing guideline ICH Q1A(R2) [9]; Stability Testing: Requirements for New Dosage Forms (ICH Q1C) [11]; Stability Testing of Existing Active Ingredients and Related Finished Products, CPMP/QWP/122/02 Rev. 1 corr., etc.

5.4 In Vitro Diagnostic Reagents

Clinical and Laboratory Standards Institute (CLSI) of the United States has on its list an approved guideline on "Evaluation of Stability of In Vitro Diagnostic Reagents (EP25-A)". This document provides guidance for establishing shelf-life and in-use stability claims for in vitro diagnostic reagents, such as reagent kits, calibrators, control products, and sample diluents. The design, implementation, data analysis, and documentation needed for studies also find mention in the guideline.

5.5 Excipients

International Pharmaceutical Excipients Council (IPEC), which is an association comprising four regional pharmaceutical excipient industry associations covering the United States, Europe, China, and Japan, issued a guidance "The IPEC Excipient Stability Program Guide" in 2010. This guideline is applicable to all the excipients, including those that are new or novel chemicals. It acknowledges that the stipulations in ICH Q1A(R2) are not appropriate for excipients, because the ICH document is intended for drug substances and drug products. In this guideline, three options are mentioned for the stability studies on excipients:

1. Utilize historical data including that found in the literature and generate a report summarizing the data and drawing conclusions about excipient stability.

2. Conduct a study using the excipient packed in the commercial packaging placed in one or more warehouses, which are used to hold commercial stocks, and where the temperature of the warehouse is known and monitored.

3. Conduct a study using the conditions and recommendations in ICH Q1A(R2).

4. Option 3 is normally necessary for novel and new excipients where stability data in accordance with options 1 or 2 are unavailable.

5.6 Homeopathic Drugs

Stability testing for medicinal products prepared in accordance with homeopathic manufacturing procedures is recommended to be done according to "Guideline on Stability Testing: Stability Testing of Existing Active Substances and Related Finished Products" (CPMP/QWP/122/02, Rev. 1 corr.). This document suggests that no stability tests on active substances are required if their starting materials are monographed in the German Homeopathic Pharmacopoeia (GHP). The recommended long-term storage conditions are 25 °C ± 2 °C/60% RH ± 5% RH or 30 °C ± 2 °C/65% RH ± 5% RH for finished products.

The Homeopathic Pharmacopeia of the United States (HPUS) also introduced "Homeopathic Drug Stability Guideline" in April 2014. This guidance claims that "homeopathic marketed dosage forms must meet the requirements for drug product stability in 21 CFR 211.166 with a written assessment of stability based on testing or examination of product".

5.7 Medical Devices and Gloves

The Registration and Drug Control Department, Ministry of Health of the United Arab Emirates (UAE) issued a "Medical Device Registration Guideline" in 2011. The medical device product registration/listing requirements cover stability study with shelf-life specifications according to ICH guidelines for Zone IV, covering full shelf-life, accelerated study for 6 months, in-use stability studies, etc. A draft document "Guidance for Conducting Stability Testing to Support an Expiration Date Labeling Claim for Medical Gloves" was released by Center for Devices and Radiological Health (CDRH), USFDA, which covers stability testing protocols and requirements for gloves made from synthetic materials.

5.8 Dietary Supplements/ Nutraceuticals

The stability testing requirements for dietary supplements in the United States have been hanging for long, as there has not been sufficient agreement whether the products shall be labelled by the term "Expiry date" or "Best used by". One finds mention of this fact in the Department of Health and Human Services, FDA, final rule titled "Current Good Manufacturing Practice in Manufacturing, Packaging, Labeling, or Holding Operations for Dietary Supplements" of 2007 [104]. The content issue has been that biological activity of certain dietary ingredients used in supplements was unknown, therefore, it was practically difficult for the manufacturers to propose a definite date on the label. So, the final rule did not require establishment of an expiration date, and hence no guidance was included on the type of data that were acceptable to support an expiration date.

However, NSF International of the United States, whose earlier name was the National Sanitation Foundation (NSF), created a stability testing working group, which finalized the document, entitled "Stability Testing Guideline for Dietary Supplements" in January 2011. This guidance applies and extends the principle and concept of ICH Q1E "Evaluation for Stability Study" to dietary supplements. For long-term stability testing, 20–25 °C $\pm$ 2 °C/ 60% RH $\pm$ 5% RH has been recommended. The guidance also covers a topic like open package testing and excursion testing. The United States Pharmacopeia (USP) general chapter <2750> on "Manufacturing Practices for Dietary Supplements" also includes a few elements of stability testing for dietary supplements [105]. Otherwise, USP has a "USP Verified" marking program, under which the agency also carries out market surveillance to ensure that the dietary supplement products with "USP Verified" logo continue to retain quality and stability over their shelf-life [106].

6   Summary of Trends

The stability testing requirements have been evolving for about last 25 years, and have been revised frequently to broaden their scope and make them absolute with time. Recently, the focus of stability studies has shifted from how to conduct stability studies to how best to implement successful stability study programs. Some of the current trends are highlighted below:

1. Implementation of risk-based strategies in the stability program after the ICH Q8-11 guidelines had come into effect.

2. Introduction of science-based quality-by-design concept to stability-indicating method development for assay and impurity controls in stability test samples.

3. Due to the introduction of FDA guidance on "Data Metrics", huge emphasis has come on identification and resolution of OOS and OOT in stability testing.

4. The alignment with "Data Integrity" principles during stability testing is now compulsory.

5. Maintaining of high levels of compliance of the stability systems and operations to regulatory requirements is the order of the day. It calls for constant training of staff and implementation of Quality Management Systems (QMS) in stability departments. The issuance of an ever-increasing number of warning letters, product recalls, notices for suspension of production, and even orders for plant closures, in many cases due to stability failures, can only be halted if the manufacturers are alert and allocate enough resources for making their stability testing programs all-encompassing.

7   Conclusions

Stability testing, which is an indispensable activity to ensure quality of products and hence patient safety, has increasingly been of regulatory interest, as evident from above-discussed large number of international, regional, and country guidelines issued from time to time. Though sincere efforts have been made to bring out a universal guideline, the same has been elusive still. In general, ICH guidelines are the mainstay in stability testing practices throughout the globe. The newer ICH guidelines from Q8 to Q10 also have a good stake towards ensuring quality of drugs and products. Equally important are quality metrics and data integrity considerations, for which guidelines have been issued lately. Sticking to recommendations is a necessity, in view of the multiple warning letters being issued to industry worldwide and associated product recall notices. It is good to see emergence of guidelines on other product categories, not covered by ICH, VICH, FDA, EMA, or WHO, and it might be desirable that official guidelines are also developed in due course on the mentioned product types. The covered recent trends highlight the requirement of paying real focus on application of right principles to stability testing, and also on stringent control of stability testing operations. Many aspects have been covered in details as independent chapters in this book.

References

1. Bajaj S, Singla D, Sakhuja N (2012) Stability testing of pharmaceutical products. J Appl Pharm Sci 2:129–138

2. Expert Comittee on Specification for Pharmaceutical Preparations, WHO Technical Report Series 953, Annex 2, Stability Testing of Active Pharmaceutical Ingredients and Finished Pharmaceutical Products (2009) WHO, Geneva, Switzerland. http://www.ich.org/fileadmin/Public_Web_Site/ICH_Products/Guidelines/Quality/Q1F/Stability_Guideline_WHO.pdf. Accessed 10 June 2017

3. Singh S, Bakshi M (2000) Stress test to determine inherent stability of drugs. Pharm Technol 4:1–14

4. Expert Comittee on Specification for Pharmaceutical Preparations, Working document QAS/16.694/Rev. 1, Stability Testing of Active Pharmaceutical Ingredients and Finished Pharmaceutical Products (2017) WHO, Geneva, Switzerland. http://www.who.int/medicines/areas/quality_safety/quality_assurance/StabilityAPIsandFPPS-QAS16-694Rev1-26072017.pdf. Accessed 15 Janurary 2018

5. Expert Committee on Specification for Pharmaceutical Preparations, WHO Technical Report Series, No. 863, Thirty Fourth Report, Annex 5-Guidelines for Stability Testing of Pharmaceutical Products Containing Well Established Drug Substances in Conventional Dosages Forms (1996) WHO, Geneva, Switzerland. http://apps.who.int/medicinedocs/pdf/s5516e/s5516e.pdf. Accessed 8 June 2017

6. http://www.ich.org/about/history.html. Accessed 21 Sept 2017

7. http://www.ich.org/about/mission.html. Accessed 20 Sept 2017

8. http://www.ich.org/fileadmin/Public_Web_Site/ICH_Products/Guidelines/Quality/Q1F/Q1F_Explanatory_Note.pdf. Accessed 18 Sept 2017

9. Stability Testing of New Drug Substances and Products Q1A(R2) (2003) In: International conference on harmonization, Geneva, Switzerland. http://www.ich.org/fileadmin/Public_Web_Site/ICH_Products/Guidelines/Quality/Q1A_R2/Step4/Q1A_R2__Guideline.pdf. Accessed 2 June 2017

10. Stability Testing: Photostability Testing of New Drug Substances and Products Q1B (1996) In: International conference on harmonization, Geneva, Switzerland. http://www.ich.org/fileadmin/Public_Web_Site/ICH_Products/Guidelines/Quality/Q1B/Step4/Q1B_Guideline.pdf. Accessed 3 June 2017

11. Stability Testing for New Dosage Forms Q1C (1996) In: International conference of harmonization, Geneva, Switzerland. http://www.ich.org/fileadmin/Public_Web_Site/ICH_Products/Guidelines/Quality/Q1C/Step4/Q1C_Guideline.pdf. Accessed 4 June 2017

12. Bracketing and Matrixing Designs for Stability Testing of New Drug Substances and Products Q1D (2002) In: International conference on harmonization, Geneva, Switzerland. http://www.ich.org/fileadmin/Public_Web_Site/ICH_Products/Guidelines/Quality/Q1D/Step4/Q1D_Guideline.pdf. Accessed 5 June 2017

13. Evaluation of Stability Data Q1E (2003) In: International conference on harmonization, Geneva, Switzerland. http://www.ich.org/fileadmin/Public_Web_Site/ICH_Products/Guidelines/Quality/Q1E/Step4/Q1E_Guideline.pdf. Accessed 6 June 2017

14. Stability Data Package for Registration Applications in Climatic Zones III and IV Q1F (2003) In: International conference on harmonization, Geneva, Switzerland.

15. Stability Testing of Biotechnological/Biological Products Q5C (1995) In: International conference on harmonization, Geneva, Switzerland. https://www.ich.org/fileadmin/Public_Web_Site/ICH_Products/Guidelines/Quality/Q5C/Step4/Q5C_Guideline.pdf. Accessed 1 June 2017

16. http://www.vichsec.org/guidelines/pharmaceuticals/pharma-quality/pharma-stability.html. Accessed 14 Aug 2017

17. http://www.vichsec.org/guidelines/biologicals/bio-quality/stability.html. Accessed 13 Aug 2017

18. http://www.who.int/medicines/areas/quality_safety/quality_assurance/RAJ2006WHOStability.pdf. Accessed 22 Sept 2017

19. Expert Comittee on Specification for Pharmaceutical Preparations, WHO Technical Report Series 962, Annex 3, Guidelines on Stability Evaluation of Vaccines (2006) WHO, Geneva, Switzerland. http://www.who.int/biologicals/vaccines/Annex_3_WHO_TRS_962-3.pdf. Accessed 9 June 2017

20. Technical Guidance Series (TGS-2), Establishing stability of an in vitro diagnostic for WHO Prequalification (2015) WHO, Geneva, Switzerland. http://www.who.int/diagnostics_laboratory/guidance/160613_tgs2_stability.pdf?ua=1. Accessed 13 June 2017

21. Expert Committee on Biological Standardization, WHO Technical Report Series 999, Annex 5, Guidelines on the Stability Evaluation of Vaccines for Use under Extended Controlled Temperature Conditions (2016) WHO, Geneva, Switzerland. http://apps.who.int/medicinedocs/documents/s22428en/s22428en.pdf. Accessed 11 June 2017

22. The GCC Guidelines for Stability Testing of Active Pharmaceutical Ingredients (APIs) and Finished Pharmaceutical Products (FPPs) (2013) GCC, Saudi Arabia. http://www.sfda.gov.sa/en/drug/resources/Guides/The%20GCC%20Guidelines%20for%20Stability%20Testing%20%20version%203.1%2024-2-2013.pdf. Accessed 1 July 2017

23. ASEAN Guideline on Stability Study of Drug Product (2013) ASEAN, Philippines. http://www.hsa.gov.sg/content/dam/HSA/HPRG/Western_Medicine/Overview_Framework_Policies/Guidelines_on_Drug_Registration/ASEAN%20STABILITY%20GUIDELINE%20(version%206.0).pdf. Accessed 2 July 2017

24. PART II: EAC Guidelines on Stability Testing Requirements for Active Pharmaceutical Ingredients (APIs) and Finished Pharmaceutical Products (FPPs) (2014) East African Community Secretariat, Arusha, Tanzania. http://apps.who.int/medicinedocs/documents/s22312en/s22312en.pdf. Accessed 10 Apr 2017

25. http://www.ich.org/fileadmin/Public_Web_Site/ABOUT_ICH/Organisation/SADC/Guideline_for_Stability_Studies.pdf. Accessed 25 Aug 2017

26. http://www.who.int/medicines/services/expertcommittees/pharmprep/QAS06_179_StabilityGuidelineSept06.pdf. Accessed 10 Aug 2017

27. http://apps.who.int/medicinedocs/documents/s20205en/s20205en.pdf. Accessed 30 Sept 2017

28. http://www.ema.europa.eu/ema/index.jsp?curl=pages/about_us/general/general_content_000628.jsp&mid=WC0b01ac058087addd. Accessed 22 Sept 2017

29. Maximum Shelf-Life for Sterile Products for Human Use After First Opening or Following Reconstitution (1998) CPMP/QWP/159/96 corr, London, UK. http://www.ema.europa.eu/docs/en_GB/document_library/

Scientific_guideline/2009/09/WC500003
476.pdf. Accessed 10 May 2017

30. In-Use Stability Testing of Human Medicinal
Products (2001) CPMP/QWP/2934/99,
London, UK. http://www.ema.europa.eu/
docs/en_GB/document_library/Scientific_
guideline/2009/09/WC500003475.pdf.
Accessed 12 May 2017

31. Declaration of Storage Conditions for Medicinal Products Particulars and Active Substances (Annex) (2003) CPMP/QWP/609/
96/Rev 2, London, UK. http://www.ema.
europa.eu/docs/en_GB/document_library/
Scientific_guideline/2009/09/
WC500003468.pdf. Accessed 11 May 2017

32. Stability Testing of Existing Active Ingredients and Related Finished Products (2003)
CPMP/QWP/122/02, rev 1 corr, London,
UK. http://www.ema.europa.eu/docs/en_
GB/document_library/Scientific_guideline/
2009/09/WC500003466.pdf.   Accessed
9 May 2017

33. Reflection paper on stability testing of herbal
medicinal products and traditional herbal
medicinal products (2010) EMA/HMPC/
3626/2009, London, UK. http://www.ema.
europa.eu/docs/en_GB/document_library/
Scientific_guideline/2010/11/
WC500098816.pdf. Accessed 1 May 2017

34. Stability Testing for Applications for Variations to Marketing Authorisation (2014)
EMA/CHMP/CVMP/QWP/441071/
2011—Rev. 2, London, UK. http://www.
ema.europa.eu/docs/en_GB/document_
library/Scientific_guideline/2014/04/
WC500164972.pdf. Accessed 13 May 2017

35. Declaration of storage conditions: 1. in the
product information of pharmaceutical veterinary medicinal products, 2. for active substances (Annex) (2007) EMEA/CVMP/
422/99/Rev.3, London, UK. http://www.
ema.europa.eu/docs/en_GB/document_
library/Scientific_guideline/2009/10/
WC500004345.pdf. Accessed 4 May 2017

36. In-Use Stability Testing of Veterinary Medicinal Products (Excluding Immunological Veterinary Medicinal Products) (2002) EMEA/
CVMP/424/01, London, UK. http://www.
ema.europa.eu/docs/en_GB/document_
library/Scientific_guideline/2009/10/
WC500004399.pdf. Accessed 6 May 2017

37. Maximum Shelf-Life for Sterile Medicinal
Products After First Opening or Following
Reconstitution (2001) EMEA/CVMP/
198/99, London, UK. http://www.ema.
europa.eu/docs/en_GB/document_library/
Scientific_guideline/2009/10/
WC500004400.pdf. Accessed 8 May 2017

38. Guideline on Stability Testing: Stability Testing of Existing Active Substances and Related
Finished Products (2008) EMEA/CVMP/
QWP/846/99-Rev.1, London, UK. http://
www.ema.europa.eu/docs/en_GB/docu
ment_library/Scientific_guideline/2009/
10/WC500004356.pdf. Accessed 3 May
2017

39. Data Requirements to Support In-Use Stability Claims for Veterinary Vaccines (2010)
EMA/CVMP/IWP/250147/2008,
London, UK. http://www.ema.europa.eu/
docs/en_GB/document_library/Scientific_
guideline/2010/03/WC500077932.pdf.
Accessed 2 May 2017

40. https://www.tga.gov.au/sites/default/files/
stability-testing-prescription-medicines.pdf.
Accessed 3 July 2017

41. Guide for Stability Studies (2005) ANVISA,
Brazil.   http://pharmalytik.com/images/
stories/PDF/brazil%20-%20english%20-%
201%20aug%202005.pdf. Accessed 3 July
2017

42. Guidance for Industry: Stability Testing of
Existing Drug Substances and Products
(2003) TPD, Canada. https://www.canada.
ca/content/dam/hc-sc/migration/hc-sc/
dhp-mps/alt_formats/hpfb-dgpsa/pdf/pro
dpharma/stabt_stabe-eng.pdf.   Accessed
4 July 2017

43. Chinese Pharmacopoeia Commission (2011)
Appendix XXC. Chinese Pharmacopoeia,
Beijing

44. Stability Testing of New Drug Substances and
Products Food and Drugs Board, Ghana.
http://www.rrfa.co.za/wp-content/
uploads/2014/01/Ghana-Stability-Testing-
of-New-Drug.pdf. Accessed 10 Apr 2017

45. Stability Testing of Existing Drug Substances
and Products (Draft Guideline) (2002)
IDMA-APA, India. http://pharmabiz.com/
PrintArticle.aspx?aid=60682&sid=0.
Accessed 6 Apr 2017

46. Guidelines for Stability Testing of Pharmaceutical Products, In: Guidance Manual for Compliance of Indian Pharmacopoeia by Drugs
Regulatory Bodies, Drugs Testing Laboratories & Pharmaceutical Industry, The
Indian Pharmacopoeia Commission, Ghazia-
bad,   India.   http://www.ipc.gov.in/
writereaddata/newsimages/94.pdf. Accessed
15 Jan 2018

47. http://cdsco.nic.in/html/D&C_Rules_
Schedule_Y.pdf. Accessed 15 Aug 2017

48. Official Mexican Standard NOM-073-SSA1-
2005, Stability of Drugs and Medicine (2006)
Health   Department,   Mexico.   http://

pharmalytik.com/images/stories/PDF/
mexico%20nom-073-ssa1-2005%20-%
20english%20corr.pdf. Accessed 6 July 2017

49. http://pharmalytik.com/images/stories/
PDF/panama%20-%20stability%20guidelines
%20-%209%20nov%202005.pdf. Accessed
12 Aug 2017

50. Stability (2012) MCC, South Africa. http://
www.mccza.com/documents/b22b99e32.
05_Stability_Jul12_v7_1.pdf. Accessed 5 Apr
2017

51. https://open.unido.org/api/documents/
4700222/download/Medicines%20Registra
tion%20Harmonisation%20In%20the%
20Southern%20African%20Development%
20Community%20-%20Study%20com
missioned%20by%20the%20Southern%20Afri
can%20Generic%20Medicines%20Associa
tion. Accessed 1 June 2017

52. Prat AG (2013) A practical overview of
requirements for drug registration in Latin
America. Regul Rapporteur 10(9):5–10

53. http://academy.gmp-compliance.org/
guidemgr/files/1-7-3.PDF. Accessed 23 Aug
2017

54. https://www.fda.gov/downloads/Drugs/
Guidances/UCM070337.pdf. Accessed
28 Aug 2017

55. Guidance for Industry: Drug Stability Guidelines (2008) USFDA, Rockville, USA.
https://www.fda.gov/downloads/Animal
Veterinary/GuidanceComplianceEnforce
ment/GuidanceforIndustry/ucm051556.
pdf. Accessed 19 June 2017

56. Guidance for Industry ANDAs: Stability Testing of Drug Substances and Products (2013)
USFDA, Rockville, USA. https://www.fda.
gov/downloads/drugs/guidancecompliance
regulatoryinformation/guidances/
ucm320590.pdf. Accessed 17 June 2017

57. CPG Sec. 480.100 Requirements for Expiration Dating and Stability Testing (1995)
USFDA, Rockville, USA. https://www.fda.
gov/iceci/compliancemanuals/
compliancepolicyguidancemanual/
ucm074408.htm. Accessed 27 June 2017

58. CPG Sec. 480.300 Lack of Expiration Date of
Stability Data (1995) USFDA, Rockville,
USA. https://www.fda.gov/ICECI/Com
plianceManuals/CompliancePolicyGuidance
Manual/ucm074410.htm. Accessed 26 June
2017

59. Expiration Dating and Stability Testing of
Solid Oral Dosage Form Drugs Containing
Iron (1997) USFDA, Rockville, USA.
https://www.fda.gov/downloads/drugs/
guidancecomplianceregulatoryinformation/

guidances/ucm070276.pdf. Accessed
24 June 2017

60. CPG Sec. 280.100—Stability Requirements—Licensed In Vitro Diagnostic Products (2000) USFDA, Rockville, USA.
https://www.fda.gov/ICECI/Compliance
Manuals/CompliancePolicyGuidance Man
ual/ucm073881.htm. Accessed 23 June
2017

61. Guidance for Industry: Container and
Closure System Integrity Testing *in Lieu* of
Sterility Testing as a Component of the Sta-
bility Protocol for Sterile Products (2008)
USFDA, Rockville, USA. https://www.fda.
gov/downloads/RegulatoryInformation/
Guidances/UCM146076.pdf. Accessed
22 June 2017

62. Guidance for Industry: Testing Limits in Stability Protocols for Standardized Grass Pollen
Extracts (2008) USFDA, Rockville, USA.
https://www.fda.gov/downloads/Biologics
BloodVaccines/GuidanceComplianceRegu
latoryInformation/Guidances/Allergenics/
ucm078633.pdf. Accessed 20 June 2017

63. Guidance for Industry ANDAs: Stability
Testing of Drug Substances and Products,
Questions and Answers (2014) USFDA,
Rockville, USA. https://www.fda.gov/
downloads/drugs/guidancecompliance
regulatoryinformation/guidances/ucm366
082.pdf. Accessed 16 June 2017

64. Validation of Analytical Procedures: Text and
Methodology Q2(R1) (2005) In: Interna-
tional conference on harmonization, Geneva,
.Switzerland. http://www.ich.org/
fileadmin/Public_Web_Site/ICH_
Products/Guidelines/Quality/Q2_R1/
Step4/Q2_R1__Guideline.pdf. Accessed
2 Jun 2017

65. Impurities in New Drug Substances Q3A
(R2) (2006) In: International conference on
harmonization, Geneva, Switzerland. http://
www.ich.org/fileadmin/Public_Web_Site/
ICH_Products/Guidelines/Quality/Q3A_
R2/Step4/Q3A_R2__Guideline.pdf.
Accessed 2 June 2017

66. Impurities in New Drug Products Q3B
(R2) (2006) In: International conference on
harmonization, Geneva, Switzerland. http://
www.ich.org/fileadmin/Public_Web_Site/
ICH_Products/Guidelines/Quality/Q3B_
R2/Step4/Q3B_R2__Guideline.pdf.
Accessed 2 June 2017

67. Specifications: Test Procedures and Acceptance Criteria for New Drug Substances and
New Drug Products: Chemical Substances
Q6A (1999) In: International conference on
harmonization, Geneva, Switzerland. http://

www.ich.org/fileadmin/Public_Web_Site/ ICH_Products/Guidelines/Quality/Q6A/ Step4/Q6Astep4.pdf. Accessed 2 June 2017

68. Good Manufacturing Practice Guide for Active Pharmaceutical Ingredients Q7 (2000) In: International conference on harmonization, Geneva, Switzerland. http:// www.ich.org/fileadmin/Public_Web_Site/ ICH_Products/Guidelines/Quality/Q7/ Step4/Q7_Guideline.pdf. Accessed 2 June 2017

69. Pharmaceutical Development Q8(R2) (2009) In: International conference on harmonization, Geneva, Switzerland. http://www.ich. org/fileadmin/Public_Web_Site/ICH_ Products/Guidelines/Quality/Q8_R1/ Step4/Q8_R2_Guideline.pdf.   Accessed 2 June 2017

70. Quality Risk Management Q9 (2005) In: International conference on harmonization, Geneva, Switzerland. http://www.ich.org/ fileadmin/Public_Web_Site/ICH_Products/ Guidelines/Quality/Q9/Step4/Q9_Guide line.pdf. Accessed 2 June 2017

71. Pharmaceutical Quality System Q10 (2008) In: International conference on harmonization, Geneva, Switzerland. http://www.ich. org/fileadmin/Public_Web_Site/ICH_ Products/Guidelines/Quality/Q10/Step4/ Q10_Guideline.pdf. Accessed 2 June 2017

72. Development and Manufacture of Drug Substances (Chemical Entities and Biotechnological/Biological Entities) Q11 (2012) In: International conference on harmonization, Geneva, Switzerland. http://www.ich.org/ fileadmin/Public_Web_Site/ICH_Products/ Guidelines/Quality/Q11/Q11_Step_4.pdf. Accessed 2 June 2017

73. MHRA GMP Data Integrity Definitions and Guidance for Industry (2015) MHRA, UK. http://academy.gmp-compliance.org/ guidemgr/files/Data_integrity_definitions_ and_guidance_v2.pdf. Accessed 26 Sept 2017

74. MHRA GxP Data Integrity Definitions and Guidance for Industry (2016) MHRA, UK. http://academy.gmp-compliance.org/ guidemgr/files/MHRA_GxP_data_integ rity_consultation.pdf. Accessed 26 Sept 2017

75. Guidance for Industry: Data Integrity and Compliance With CGMP (2016) USFDA, Rockville, USA. https://www.fda.gov/ downloads/drugs/guidances/ucm495891. pdf. Accessed 26 Sept 2017

76. https://www.picscheme.org/layout/docu ment.php?id=714. Accessed 26 Sept 2017

77. http://www.ema.europa.eu/ema/index.jsp? curl=pages/regulation/q_and_a/q_and_a_

detail_000027.jsp#section18.   Accessed 29 Sept 2017

78. http://www.who.int/medicines/ publications/pharmprep/WHO_TRS_996_ annex05.pdf. Accessed 2 June 2017

79. https://www.fda.gov/ICECI/Enforcement Actions/WarningLetters/2016/ucm502347. htm. Accessed 29 Sept 2017

80. https://www.fda.gov/ICECI/Enforcement Actions/WarningLetters/2016/ucm503699. htm. Accessed 3 June 2017

81. https://www.fda.gov/ICECI/Enforcement Actions/WarningLetters/2016/ucm508291. htm. Accessed 4 June 2017

82. https://www.fda.gov/ICECI/Enforcement Actions/WarningLetters/2016/ucm518546. htm. Accessed 5 June 2017

83. https://www.fda.gov/ICECI/Enforcement Actions/WarningLetters/2016/ucm516883. htm. Accessed 6 June 2017

84. https://www.fda.gov/ICECI/Enforcement Actions/WarningLetters/2016/ucm516918. htm. Accessed 7 June 2017

85. https://www.fda.gov/ICECI/Enforcement Actions/WarningLetters/2016/ucm518694. htm. Accessed 8 June 2017

86. https://www.fda.gov/ICECI/Enforcement Actions/WarningLetters/2017/ucm538059. htm. Accessed 9 June 2017

87. Guidance for Industry: Submission of Quality Metrics Data (2016) USFDA, Rockville, USA.   https://www.fda.gov/downloads/ drugs/guidances/ucm455957.pdf. Accessed 26 Sept 2017

88. http://portal.anvisa.gov.br/documents/ 33836/418522/Perguntas+e+Respostas+- +RDC+53+2015+e+Guia+04+2015/ 6b3dec42-546c-4953-943f-4047b8b50f87. Accessed 27 Sept 2017

89. https://www.fda.gov/downloads/drugs/ guidancecomplianceregulatoryinformation/ guidances/ucm077097.pdf.   Accessed 12 June 2017

90. https://www.canada.ca/content/dam/hc-sc/ migration/hc-sc/dhp-mps/alt_formats/pdf/ prodpharma/applic-demande/guide-ld/post noc_change_apresac/noc_pn_quality_ac_sa_ qualite-final-eng.pdf. Accessed 13 June 2017

91. http://www.who.int/medicines/areas/qual ity_safety/quality_assurance/Annex3TRS- 981.pdf. Accessed 14 June 2017

92. https://www.tga.gov.au/sites/default/files/ sunscreens-args.pdf. Accessed 1 Aug 2017

93. http://portal.anvisa.gov.br/documents/ 106351/107910/Cosmetic+Products

+Stability+Guide/5f90ee5b-c77b-4c1e-91f9-5fa680b05022. Accessed 2 Aug 2017

94. https://www.cosmeticseurope.eu/files/5914/6407/8121/Guidelines_on_Stability_Testing_of_Cosmetics_CE-CTFA_-_2004.pdf. Accessed 3 Aug 2017

95. http://www.ema.europa.eu/docs/en_GB/document_library/Scientific_guideline/2014/12/WC500179071.pdf. Accessed 4 Aug 2017

96. https://clsi.org/standards/products/method-evaluation/documents/ep25/. Accessed 5 Aug 2017

97. http://ipec-europe.org/UPLOADS/100311_IPECStabilityGuide-Final.pdf. Accessed 6 Aug 2017

98. https://www.chpa.org/VCG_Stability Testing.aspx. Accessed 7 Aug 2017

99. http://www.hpus.com/homeopathic-drug-stability-guidelines-4-14.pdf. Accessed 8 Aug 2017

100. http://www.bfarm.de/SharedDocs/Downloads/EN/Drugs/licensing/zulassungsarten/pts/Leitf_Stabi_060623_en.pdf?__blob=publicationFile&v=2. Accessed 26 Aug 2017

101. http://www.cpd-pharma.ae/downloads/4-Medical%20Device/MD%20guide%20line.pdf. Accessed 9 Aug 2017

102. https://www.fda.gov/OHRMS/DOCKETS/98fr/994487gd.pdf. Accessed 2 July 2017

103. http://www.nsf.org/newsroom_pdf/Stability_Testing_Dietary_Supplements.pdf. Accessed 14 Aug 2017

104. https://www.fda.gov/ohrms/dockets/98fr/cf0441.pdf. Accessed 15 June 2017

105. http://www.drugfuture.com/pharmacopoeia/usp32/pub/data/v32270/usp32nf27s0_c2750.html. Accessed 16 June 2017

106. http://www.usp.org/verification-services/dietary-supplements-verification-program. Accessed 17 June 2017

Chapter 2

The Stability Dossier: Common Deficiencies and Ways to Improve

Paul Marshall

Abstract

Stability testing on pharmaceutical products is carried out to demonstrate that product quality remains fit for purpose until the end of its shelf-life when stored as recommended, and during use by healthcare professionals or patients. International and regional guidelines on stability testing have been published for over 20 years, yet despite this, regulatory authorities still find a large number of deficiencies with stability dossiers. A survey of marketing authorization (MA) applications submitted in the UK between April 2012 and March 2013 found that 96% of dossiers had deficiency points with the stability dossier for the active substance and/or the finished product, representing an average of 3–4 deficiency points per application. The survey also revealed common deficiencies in both the active substance and finished product stability dossiers. A similar survey of MA applications carried out 10 years earlier found the same deficiencies with the stability dossiers, suggesting little improvement in their quality. The common deficiencies listed in this chapter represent an excellent starting point for discussion on improving the quality of the stability dossier. In addition, more in-depth practical guidance is provided herein on ways to improve the stability summary and conclusions, post-approval commitments, and presentation of the stability data, including consideration of the different approaches for marketing authorization variations and clinical trial applications.

Key words Stability testing, Regulatory guidance, Deficiencies, Stability dossier, Stability summary and conclusions, Shelf-life, Storage, Post-approval stability commitments, Presentation of data, Marketing authorization, Variation, Clinical trial

1 Introduction

Pharmaceutical companies carry out stability testing to ensure that the pharmaceutical product (whether drug substance, finished product, or a drug–device combination), remains acceptable, safe, and efficacious, during its labelled shelf-life when stored under the recommended storage conditions, and when used by a healthcare professional or patient. As such, stability is considered a fundamental critical quality attribute (CQA) of the quality target product profile for a pharmaceutical product, whether a traditional or an enhanced quality-by-design development approach is adopted.

Sanjay Bajaj and Saranjit Singh (eds.), *Methods for Stability Testing of Pharmaceuticals*, Methods in Pharmacology and Toxicology, https://doi.org/10.1007/978-1-4939-7686-7_2, © Springer Science+Business Media, LLC, part of Springer Nature 2018

The stability dossier for a drug substance and the drug product is an important part of any submission to a regulatory authority. Its principle aim is to describe the studies undertaken to evaluate the stability of the product and their outcome, and provide a conclusion on the overall stability of the product. Regulatory authorities use the stability dossier to agree the expiry period for the product, as well as how the product should be stored.

The purpose of this chapter, therefore, is to review the common mistakes that companies have typically made when compiling the stability dossier for a marketing authorization (MA) application, using them as a starting point to look at practical guidance and advice on improving the quality of the stability dossier. The chapter also briefly touches upon stability testing during the drug product life cycle, as well as for clinical trials, as the approaches for the stability dossier are slightly different.

For simplicity and ease of reading, the chapter focuses on the drug product; however, the principles discussed here apply equally to the stability dossier of drug substances, biological products, or drug-device combinations. The principles also apply equally for stability data presented in other parts of the dossier, for example, in the pharmaceutical development or manufacturing validation (for bulk product-holding times) sections.

2   Regulatory Guidance on Stability Testing

The International Conference on Harmonisation (ICH) published parent guidance on stability testing in 1993 [1], followed by several associated guidelines and supplementary annexes (see Table 1). ICH guidelines have been adopted and form part of the regulatory requirements in many regions around the world, such as Europe, the USA, Japan, Canada, Brazil, Switzerland, Australia, New Zealand, and South Korea, as well as the World Health Organization (WHO) and the European Directorate for the Quality of Medicine and Healthcare (EDQM). The full membership list of ICH can be found on the ICH website [2]. Some regulatory authorities have also published additional region-specific guidances on stability testing, for example, the European Committee of Human Medicinal Products (CHMP) [3] and CHMP Quality Working Party Questions & Answers on stability [4] (see Chap. 1, for details).

The guidelines describe current thinking by regulatory authorities on acceptable ways to carry out stability testing, and provide detailed scientific and regulatory advice concerning the type and number of stability batches, testing frequency, duration and storage conditions, container closure system, orientation of storage, analytical methods, and stability specifications. Consequently, it is strongly advised that companies endeavor to understand and comply with these guidelines, wherever possible; though deviations from guidelines are permitted, but any variation should be fully

Table 1
ICH guidelines for stability testing

Code	Document title
Q1A(R2)	Stability testing of new drugs and products Provides recommendations on stability testing protocols including temperature, humidity, and trial duration for climatic zones I and II, and takes into account the requirements for stability testing in climatic zones III and IV in order to minimize the different storage conditions for submission of a global dossier
Q1B	Stability testing: Photostability testing of new drug substances and products Provides guidance on the basic testing protocol required to evaluate the light sensitivity and stability of new drugs and products
Q1C	Stability testing for new dosage forms Extends Q1A(R2) for new formulations of already approved medicines and defines the circumstances under which reduced stability data can be accepted
Q1D	Bracketing and matrixing designs for stability testing of new drug substances and products Describes general principles for reduced stability testing and provides examples of bracketing and matrixing designs
Q1E	Evaluation of stability data Extends Q1A(R2) by explaining possible situations where extrapolation of retest periods/ shelf-lives beyond the long-term data may be appropriate, and provides examples of statistical approaches to stability data analysis
Q1F	Stability data package for registration applications in climatic zones III and IV ICH steering committee withdrew the guideline in June 2006 and decided to leave definitions of storage conditions in climatic zones III and IV to the respective regions and WHO (WHO Technical Report Series, No. 953, 2009)
Q5C	Stability testing for biotechnological/biological products Augments Q1A(R2) and deals with the particular aspects of stability test procedures needed to take account of the special characteristics of products in which the active components are typically proteins and/or polypeptides

explained and scientifically justified in the dossier; otherwise regulatory authorities will request an explanation. It is advised that planned deviations with respect to stability testing are discussed with the authorities prior to starting a study, as errors and misunderstandings are costly in terms of time and money to rectify. Major issues with stability will delay approval of a MA application by around 9–15 months. ICH guidance Q1A(R2) [1] advises that a systematic approach should be used in the presentation and evaluation of stability data, and that the stability data should include, as appropriate, results from the physical, chemical, biological, and microbiological tests, plus any particular attributes of the dosage form that are relevant to stability (e.g., functionality testing for a device part of a drug-device combination product). The adequacy of mass balance between assay and total impurities should also be reviewed, considering the different stability and degradation performance, and different sensitivities in analytical methods. Each CQA likely to influence the quality, safety, and efficacy of the drug product should be evaluated separately, and then an overall assessment should be made of the findings for the purpose of proposing the shelf-life, which should not exceed that predicted for any single quality attribute.

The ICH guideline Q1A(R2) [1] also introduced the concept of using the results from samples stored at accelerated and intermediate storage conditions to extrapolate 12 month long-term stability data to support provisional shelf-life of 24 months. More detailed guidance on extrapolation, including considering the existence of supporting data, the underlying mechanisms of degradation, any mathematical relationships or models, and the statistical approaches used in the analysis of the data, is described in ICH Q1E [5]. This guideline also provides a useful decision tree in Appendix A to describe the extent by which the real-time data can be extrapolated under different scenarios. It is worth noting that the extent to which the long-term stability data can be extrapolated may differ from region to region, and from product to product. It should be noted that ICH guidance Q5C [6] does not permit extrapolation for biological/biotechnological products, and thus the shelf-life is limited to the time period covered by long-term stability data.

It is required that the data should be presented in an appropriate format (e.g., tabulated, graphical, narrative) and the values of quantitative attributes at all time points should be reported as measured (e.g., assay as percent of label claim). If statistical analysis is performed, the procedure used and the assumptions underlying the model should be stated and justified, together with a tabulated summary of the outcome of statistical analysis and/or graphical presentation of the long-term data. The basic concepts of stability data presentation and evaluation are the same for single- versus multifactor studies and for full- versus reduced-design studies.

In addition to the shelf-life, the stability data should be used to propose the recommended storage conditions, such as "store below 25 °C", "store below 30 °C", "do not freeze", or "protect from light and/or moisture". Companies should ensure that the format and wording of storage advice on the labelling and patient information leaflet are in line with the regional guidance.

3   Common Deficiencies with Stability Dossiers

In the UK, the regulatory authority for approving human medicinal products is the Medicine and Healthcare products Regulatory Agency (MHRA). In certain situations, the MHRA can seek advice from independent experts, such as the Commission on Human Medicines (CHM) and any of its expert advisory groups (EAG). The chemistry, pharmacy, and standards EAG (CPSEAG) is responsible for providing advice on the quality of a pharmaceutical products, including its stability.

A survey of marketing authorization (MA) applications referred to CPSEAG during April 2012 to March 2013 was carried out for the number and type of deficiencies in sections 3.2.S.7 and 3.2.P.8 of the common technical document (CTD) [7]. These sections represent the stability dossier for the drug substance and drug product, respectively. These MA applications were chosen purely from a practical perspective since the relevant assessment reports were readily available for analysis, having been collated by the CHM secretariat. It should be noted that the main reason for CPSEAG referral did not specifically relate to issues with the stability data, and thus these applications can be considered a representative subset of all MA applications received in this time period and across other regulatory authorities (since the applications had been submitted using the European centralized, decentralized, and mutual recognition, as well as UK national procedures).

The survey revealed the following results:

1. 77 submissions were referred to CPSEAG, comprising 75 MA applications and 2 MA variations.

2. 74 submissions (96%) had deficiencies with the stability dossier of the drug substance and/or the drug product.

3. 81 deficiency points were raised on the stability dossier of the drug substance.

4. 183 deficiency points were raised on the stability dossier of the drug product.

5. 264 deficiency points were raised on both stability sections in total.

6. Each application had an average of between 3 – 4 deficiency points on the stability sections of the dossier.

The types of deficiencies and their frequency are described in Tables 2 and 3. It can be clearly seen that there are a number of common deficiencies between the stability dossiers for both the drug substance and drug product, namely:

1. Insufficient stability data are provided to support proposed shelf-life.

2. Issues with stability specification (missing CQAs or unacceptably wide acceptance limits).

3. Analytical procedures (and validation data) used for stability testing are not clearly described or referenced.

4. Absence of photostability data.

5. Absence of a critical discussion of the stability data.

6. Absence of a post-approval commitment for commercial scale stability testing.

Table 2
Common deficiencies in the drug substance stability dossier in MA applications submitted to MHRA between April 2012 and March 2013

Ranking	Deficiency	MA applications (%)
1	Insufficient stability data provided to support proposed retest period (e.g., additional batches, time points)	24
2	Proposed retest period and/or storage conditions requires further amending or clarifying	17
3	Quality critical parameters missing from stability specification (e.g., polymorphic form, particle size, microbial quality)	14
4	Storage conditions, stability batch history, and container closure system not clearly described	12
5	Analytical procedures and related validation data not clearly described or shown to be stability-indicating	12
6	Photostability data or justification for its omission not provided	7
7	Critical discussion of the stability data not provided, including statistical analysis when relevant, trend analysis, extrapolation of real-time stability data, and mass balance	5
8	Stress testing of drug substance not carried out or otherwise justified (i.e., degradation pathway not discussed)	4
9	Post-approval commitment to stability test first three commercial scale batches not provided	4
10	Stability specification acceptance limits are not acceptable (i.e., limits are too generous)	1

In March 2002 and March 2004, a similar survey had been carried out on submissions referred to the CPS subcommittee of Committee on Safety of Medicines (as CPSEAG was formerly known) for advice (*see* Table 4) [8]. The survey revealed that similar, if not identical, types of deficiencies were found in the stability dossiers submitted 10 years earlier, which suggests that, during this time, pharmaceutical companies continued to make the same basic errors with their stability dossier, despite the fact that ICH stability guidelines had been published, and that companies receive regular feedback from regulatory authorities by way of deficiency letters and assessment reports.

It is worth mentioning that reviewing the stability dossier deficiencies described in Tables 2, 3, and 4 represents a solid starting point for any company wanting to improve the overall quality of their stability programs and dossier submissions, with a view to reducing the chance of receiving deficiency questions on stability from regulatory authorities.

Table 3

Common deficiencies in the drug product stability dossier in MA applications submitted to MHRA between April 2012 and March 2013

Ranking	Deficiency	MA applications (%)
1	Insufficient stability data provided to support proposed retest period (e.g., additional batches, time points)	19
2	No in-use stability data provided, and consequently in-use shelf-life and storage conditions not specified	13
3	Stability specification acceptance limits are not acceptable (i.e., limits are too generous)	11
4	Proposed shelf-life and/or storage conditions require further amending or clarifying	11
5	Critical discussion of the stability data not provided, including statistical analysis when relevant, trend analysis, extrapolation of real-time stability data, and mass balance	10
6	Photostability data or justification for its omission not provided	9
7	Quality critical parameters missing from stability specification (e.g., polymorphic form, particle size, microbial quality, physical tests, and functionality of drug-device combinations)	8
8	Post-approval commitment to stability test first three commercial scale batches not provided	6
9	Stability data on bulk products, including transportation, not provided	4
10	Confirmation that start of shelf-life is determined in line with CPMP/QWP/ 072/96 Start of shelf-life of the finished dosage form (annex to the note for guidance on the manufacture of the finished dosage form)	4
11	Analytical procedures and related validation data not clearly described or shown to be stability-indicating	2
12	Stability samples not stored in the recommended orientation	2
13	Stability data is inconsistent or illegible	1
14	Storage conditions, stability batch history, and container closure system not clearly described	1

4   Improving the Stability Dossier

Stability dossiers need to be provided for both the drug substance and drug products, in sections 3.2.S.7 and 3.2.P.8, respectively. The stability dossier is typically composed of the following sections: (a) the stability summary and conclusions; (b) the post-approval stability protocol and stability commitment; and (c) the stability

Table 4
Common deficiencies in the stability dossier of MA applications submitted to MHRA between March 2002 and March 2004

Deficiency	MA applications (%)
Specification limits not in line with the stability data – Acceptance limits for assay, related substances, fine particle mass, moisture require tightening in line with stability data	21
Insufficient stability data/incomplete results – Insufficient real-time stability data submitted – "Complies" reported where quantitative data could be provided – Stability data not obtained under ICH conditions – Small-size stability batches, different compositions, different container closure systems	12
Appropriate stability tests not conducted – Critical tests missing, e.g., dissolution, viscosity, fine particle mass, leachable – Issues with qualification of impurities – Orientation of storage not considered – Photostability data not provided	11.5
Insufficient discussion of stability results Stability data not fully discussed, e.g., out-of-specification results, obvious trends, mass balance issue	6
Queries on the start of shelf-life – Unclear that shelf-life started when drug substance is first mixed with excipients	2.8
Other deficiencies – Storage precautions not in line with stability conclusions – Not enough in-use stability testing – Inadequate information on analytical methodology – Commitments required on post-approval stability programs – Information on drug substance batches used in the drug product not provided – Problems with practicalities of storage related to product stability	Number of cases not recorded

data. All sections should be included in the MA application without exception. In the stability dossier, as with other sections of the CTD, duplication should be kept to a minimum; companies are encouraged to use cross-references and hyperlinks to other sections of the CTD to avoid presenting the same information in different sections. This reduces the chances of introducing minor variations in the information, which authorities will find and question. Minimizing duplication also improves the overall readability of the dossier, for which the assessor will be thankful.

4.1 The Stability Summary and Conclusions

The stability summary and conclusions is a critical section of the stability dossier. It describes the batches that have been stability tested (e.g., composition, container closure system, sites and method of manufacturing, date of manufacture and packing), storage conditions, testing time points (including use of matrixing and bracketing), duration of the stability study, stability specification, analytical procedures, a critical evaluation of the stability data including trends in the data, out-of-specification results, use of extrapolation and statistical analysis, and finally proposed shelf-life and storage conditions.

4.2   Declaration of Shelf-Life and Storage Conditions

It is important that the proposed shelf-life and storage conditions are clearly and unambiguously described at the beginning of the section as an executive summary. The same shall also be stated in the product information, as authorities will cross-check this and query any discrepancy. The proposed storage conditions should comply with any regional or national guidance, not forgetting pharmacopoeial requirements, where relevant. For example, the proposed storage advice in Europe should comply with CHMP guidance [9] rather than other guidelines. It is very important that only one set of proposed storage conditions, relevant to the region in which the dossier is being submitted, are declared; specifying multiple storage conditions, perhaps for different regions where the product may be sold, will not be accepted by authorities as it creates confusion over what has been authorized.

It goes without saying that the stability data must support the proposed shelf-life and storage conditions, and extrapolation of long-term data must be in line with ICH Q1E or other relevant regional or national guidance. If this is not the case, regulatory authorities will either ask for additional stability data to support the shelf-life and storage conditions, which may delay the application, or request the shelf-life be shortened in line with the stability data, or the storage conditions changed, which may have commercial ramifications for the product. Requests for additional stability data or changing the shelf-life and storage conditions were raised in 30% of drug products (*see* Table 3), and 41% of drug substance dossiers (*see* Table 2), which represents, by far, the most frequent deficiency with stability dossiers.

Finally, companies should also remember to include a statement on how the expiry date is calculated, as this is relatively minor and often overlooked, but is a standard question for some regulatory authorities. For European applications, this is achieved by simply stating compliance with CPMP/QWP/072/96 [10].

4.3   Stability Batch History

Comprehensive information on the batches that have undergone stability testing need to be provided in the form of a tabulated batch history. An exemplar batch history is provided in Table 5. This should include the batch numbers (including batch numbers of any common blends), dates of manufacture and packaging, batch size (weight and dosage units), sites of manufacture, drug substance batches used in the drug product, container closure system, pack sizes, etc. Failure to describe the batches that were stability

Table 5
An example of a tabulated history of the drug product stability batches

Stability batches—Captopril 40 mg capsules			
Batch number	0001A	0002B	0003C
Drug substance batch used in product	IAP3	IAP3	IAP4
Container closure system	HDPE bottle/PP cap 30 cc/30 capsules 100 cc/100 capsules	HDPE bottle/PP cap 30 cc/30 capsules 100 cc/100 capsules	HDPE bottle/PP cap 30 cc/30 capsules 100 cc/100 capsules
Date of manufacture	28/01/2017	28/01/2017	28/02/2017
Date of packaging	14/02/2017	14/02/2017	15/03/2017
Batch size	100,000 capsules	100,000 capsules	100,000 capsules
Site of manufacture	Contract-Pharma, Kettering, UK	Contract-Pharma, Kettering, UK	Contract-Pharma, Kettering, UK

tested appears to be more of a problem in the drug substance dossier, with 12% of dossiers having this deficiency compared to just 1% of drug product dossiers. Regulatory authorities need to assure themselves that the stability data supporting the proposed shelf-life and storage conditions have been generated on drug product that is representative of the proposed product to be marketed.

Another common error that companies make is stability testing a single pack size (e.g., a 30-capsule bottle or a 60 g tube of cream), and then including a range of pack sizes in the product information (e.g., 7-, 28-, 30-, and 60-capsule bottles or 30 g, 60 g, and 120 g tubes of cream). Regulatory authorities will refuse to approve pack sizes that are not supported by stability data, unless a bracketing approach has been used or the container closure system is unit dose. Also, authorities will be unlikely to accept stability data generated using different packaging materials to those being proposed for market, although some may accept less protective packaging as a worse-case scenario supporting a more protective packaging material, but this approach has increased risk.

Cases are known where blisters of drug product, overwrapped in aluminum foil pouches, were placed on stability test by companies to protect against moisture, improve stability, and achieve a longer shelf-life. These aluminum pouches were not declared in their stability dossier, or product information, and were not used in commercial batches. This oversight put patient safety at risk, and should not be condoned under any circumstance. Regulatory authorities treat these kinds of discrepancies very seriously and will take enforcement action, which may include criminal prosecution.

Table 6
An example of a stability protocol

Storage condition	Test time points (months)								
	0	3	6	12	18	24	36	48	72
25 °C/60% RH and/or 30 °C/ 75% RH (long-term)	C/M	C	C	C/M	C	C/M	C/M	C/M	C/M
30 °C/65% RH (intermediate)	(C/M)	(C)	(C)	(C/M)	–	–	–	–	–
40 °C/75% RH (accelerated)	C/M	C	C/M	–	–	–	–	–	–

Note: C - physical and chemical tests; M - microbiological tests. Tests in parenthesis to be carried out if testing at more extreme conditions fails specification.

4.4 Stability Protocol

The storage conditions, testing frequency and duration, and the CQAs tested at each time point should be described in a tabulated stability protocol. An exemplar stability protocol is provided in Table 6. Storage conditions and testing frequency should ideally be in line with international or national guidance, such as ICH Q1A (R2) [1] or the WHO guidance [11]. Regulatory authorities are aware that companies use global stability programs to reduce costs, but tend not to object if more rigorous stability testing is being employed than required in their respective region. However, where the stability protocol does not meet requirements, companies must scientifically justify the deviation or accept that authorities will question it.

The stability protocol is an excellent vehicle to illustrate where a reduced stability study design has been used, through matrixing and/or bracketing. The protocol should also specify the stability specification and analytical methods used to test the stability batches. The stability specification should include a list of CQAs that are likely to change on storage and/or are important for product safety, efficacy, and quality, together with the associated acceptance criteria. In 8% of drug product and 14% of drug substance dossiers, authorities found that the stability specification did not contain appropriate CQAs. A list of CQAs that should typically be considered for inclusion in the stability specification is described in Table 7.

Acceptance criteria should comply with any regional or national guidance, not forgetting any general or product-specific pharmacopoeial requirements, as well as results from development stability studies, as this is also a frequent deficiency raised by regulatory authorities (in 11% of drug product dossiers). Rectifying this deficiency is not simply a case of tightening the specification limits; the stability data will need to be reviewed again, using the tightened limits, along with the stability summary and the proposed shelf-life and/or storage conditions, which may also need amendment.

Table 7
Typical CQAs that may change on storage and should be included in a stability quality specification

Pharmaceutical product	Critical quality attributes (CQA)
Drug substance	Appearance, assay, related substances, physicochemical properties, particle size distribution, polymorphic form, chirality, water content, and microbial quality
All drug products	Appearance, assay, and related substances
Tablets and capsules	Dissolution, disintegration, hardness/friability (capsule brittleness), water content, and microbial quality
Oral liquids (solutions, emulsions, and suspensions)	pH, microbial quality, antioxidant content, antimicrobial preservative content, extractables and leachables, alcohol content, dissolution, precipitation/particle size distribution, polymorphic form, phase separation, redispersibility, reconstitution time, rheological properties, and water content
Parenteral products	pH, sterility, endotoxins/pyrogens, particulate matter, water content (for nonaqueous products), antimicrobial preservative content, antioxidant content, extractables and leachables, functionality of delivery system (e.g., prefilled syringes), osmolality, particle size distribution, redispersibility, reconstitution time, and rheological properties
Inhalation and nasal products	Moisture content, mean delivered dose, delivered dose uniformity, fine particle mass, particle/droplet size distribution, leak rate, agglomeration, microbial quality, sterility, extractables and leachables, antimicrobial preservative, delivery rate, water content, spray pattern, foreign particulate matter, and examination of the valve components/container corrosion/gasket deterioration
Topical	pH, suspendability (for lotions), consistency, rheological properties, particle size distribution (for suspensions, when relevant), microbial quality, weight loss, and sterility (for eye products)
Suppositories and pessaries	Softening range, disintegration, and dissolution
Transdermal patches	Dissolution, peel/adhesive properties of the patch, and crystal formation
Drug-device combinations	Functioning of the device, including corrosion of any electrical circuitry or component of the device

Analytical methods for assay and related substances should be shown to be stability-indicating, as this is another common deficiency raised by regulatory authorities. The stability-indicating nature of the analytical method is typically demonstrated by stress testing of the product, under different extreme storage conditions (thermal, oxidative, reductive, humidity, acid/base hydrolysis, and light), and is typically carried out as part of analytical method validation. Companies should remember to include a cross-reference to the analytical methods and method validation section in the stability dossier.

It is important that the stability protocol, including specifications and analytical methods, are established before the stability study starts, and should not be amended once the study commences, unless there is scientific justification; otherwise it places doubt on the conduct of the stability study and validity of data. Finally, the protocol should match the resulting stability data; otherwise authorities are likely to raise a question requesting an explanation.

4.5 Critical Evaluation of the Stability Data

A full and critical evaluation of the stability data should be provided, as this is missing from 10% of the drug product and 5% of drug substance dossiers, and was subsequently requested. A well-written and thorough critique of the stability data demonstrates that the company fully understands how their product is affected by storage over time and under different storage conditions, and the impact this has on product quality. It give authorities confidence in the application. It is not acceptable to state simply that "the stability data are within shelf-life specifications". Authorities want to know how each CQA changed on storage; whether the data remained unchanged, increased, or decreased with time, temperature, and/or humidity; and how any trend in the data related to the acceptance limits (for example, are the data likely to be out-of-specification in the future). Out-of-specification (OOS) results need to be clearly identified and fully explained - it is better for the company to do this, than let the assessor find an OOS result and ask a question.

However, the discussion of the stability data does not necessarily need to be lengthy and can be reasonably concise, but it does need to focus on those CQAs that change during storage e.g., it would be acceptable to state that "appearance, pH, dissolution and microbial quality changed little over the time and storage conditions. Assay values decreased on storage, in a temperature dependent manner, and did not comply with specification after 3 months storage at accelerated conditions". The above discussion would benefit from the inclusion of references to batch numbers and data values to annotate specific points, where relevant. The variability of the data also needs to be addressed, as this is relevant when the long-term stability data are extrapolated. The evaluation should finally include an overall summary of the stability of the product, concluding with the proposed shelf-life and storage condition.

4.6 Mass Balance

Mass balance is a controversial subject that is frequently discussed amongst those responsible for stability testing pharmaceutical products. Mass balance essentially looks at whether the degradation of the drug substance is matched by the increase in the level of total impurities. Regulatory authorities equate a discrepancy in mass balance with undetected impurities, which is a potential serious risk to human health on safety grounds and may lead to the eventual refusal of the MA application. However, authorities do tolerate a certain amount of mass imbalance as they accept that the analytical methods used to determine drug substance content and impurities will have different sensitivities, different degradation performance, etc. Levels around 1–2% will typically not be questioned, but higher values will start to attract attention and questions, and thus needs to be explained by the company.

4.7   In-Use Testing

If the drug product is packed in a multiple-use container (e.g., tablets in a bottle or cream in a tube), authorities will routinely expect in-use stability data to be provided, and is raised as a deficiency point in 13% of dossiers. In-use stability testing addresses the risk of multiple opening and closing of the container affecting physicochemical degradation of the product and/or microbiological proliferation and contamination. If the product decomposes or microbial quality deteriorates once the container closure system is breached for the first time, companies may need to propose a "once-opened" shelf-life. However, if the patient is likely to use the product before the in-use shelf-life expires, this may be acceptable justification for not stating an in-use storage period. Also, it has been known that some authorities do not ask for in-use shelf-lives where this exceeds 3 months, although this is a somewhat arbitrary value, and it is better to link any omission with how the product is used.

4.8   Post-approval Stability Commitments

Where long-term stability data do not cover the proposed shelf-life or are based on noncommercial/pilot scale batches, companies should remember to provide a post-approval commitment to stability test the first three commercial scale batches, together with the proposed stability protocol (which should ideally be identical to that used for the pivotal stability batches). The omission of a stability commitment is found in around 5% of applications. The post-approval stability commitment should not be confused with the annual stability testing required by good manufacturing practice (GMP); these are distinctly separate requirements, both of which need to be complied with.

4.9   Presentation of Stability Data

The stability data section of the CTD should only contain the stability study results, wherever possible (the only exception being the provision of analytical methods, and validation, that have been used for stability testing). Companies should not be tempted to duplicate information, such as batch histories and stability protocols, that have already been presented earlier in the stability dossier, as this reduces the readability of the dossier. When compiling the stability data, the assessor should be borne in mind, and the data should be presented in a way that permits an easy review. Variability in the data, trends in relation to different storage conditions and time, any difference in stability between different batches, pack presentations, strengths, orientation, etc., and any OOS results, should be easily identified. Time and care should be taken when presenting the stability data; it is not a case of simply data dumping the stability results from a laboratory information management system into the dossier. The stability data should be organized and formatted so that it is presented in the best light possible.

Stability data should be presented as numerical values, wherever possible, with the exception of appearance and any other subjective description tests, as it allows trend analysis and extrapolation of the long-term stability data. Failure to do so will either result in a request for the numerical values to be provided, or authorities will simply restrict the shelf-life to that covered by long-term data. Companies should check that the stability data are legible. This used to be a frequent issue when dossiers were mainly paper based, and were photocopied (often, many times). However, this issue has not disappeared with electronic dossiers, as the PDF rendering and CTD compilation software can often malfunction, resulting in garbled or missing text in the dossier. Therefore, it is worthwhile reading through the dossier to ensure that it is complete and legible prior to submission.

There are various ways to format and organize tabulated stability data, and no one way is better than another. Typically, stability data can be tabulated so that there is either (a) one batch/one storage condition (*see* Table 8); (b) multiple batches/one storage condition (*see* Table 9); or (c) one batch/multiple storage

Table 8
Presentation of stability data: one batch, one storage condition

Stability protocol—ACEP 40 stab EU v.1.0							
Batch 0001/17; Storage condition—25 °C/60% RH;							
Pack—HDPE bottle + PP cap (30 s); orientation—vertical							
Quality attributes **Batch 0001/17**	**Acceptance criteria**	**Time (months)**					
		0	**3**	**6**	**9**	**12**	**18**
Appearance	Round, biconvex white tablet	C	C	C	C	C	C
Assay	95–105% of target	101.0	100.9	100.5	100.5	100.1	99.7
Impurities	Single—NMT 0.10%	0.02	0.02	0.04	0.05	0.05	0.07
	Total—NMT 0.7%	0.03	0.04	0.05	0.07	0.09	0.11
Disintegration	Q = 75, 45 min	23	24	23	22	26	24
Microbial quality	TAMC—10^3/TYMC—10^2	0/0	0/0	0/0	0/0	0/0	0/0

Note: *C* - complies

Table 9
Presentation of stability data: multiple batches, one storage condition

Stability protocol—ACEP 40 stab EU v.1.0							
Storage condition—25 °C/60% RH;							
Pack—HDPE bottle + PP cap (30s); orientation—vertical							
		Time (months)					
Quality attributes and acceptance criteria	**Batch**	**0**	**3**	**6**	**9**	**12**	**18**
Appearance (round, biconvex white tablet)	0001/17	C	C	C	C	C	C
	0002/17	C	C	C	C	C	C
	0003/17	C	C	C	C	C	C
Assay (95–105% of target)	0001/17	101.0	100.9	100.5	100.5	100.1	99.7
	0002/17	100.7	100.8	100.3	100.1	99.8	99.2
	0003/17	99.6	99.3	98.9	98.8	98.6	98.3
Impurities	0001/17	0.02	0.02	0.04	0.05	0.05	0.07
(Single - NMT 0.10%		0.03	0.04	0.05	0.07	0.09	0.11
Total - NMT 0.5%)	0002/17	0.01	0.01	0.05	0.05	0.08	0.10
		0.05	0.07	0.10	0.09	0.11	0.15
	0003/17	0.02	0.03	0.04	0.05	0.06	**0.11**
		0.02	0.04	0.06	0.09	0.09	0.14
Dissolution ($Q = 75$, 45 min)	0001/17	23	24	23	22	26	24
	0002/17	30	35	24	28	22	21
	0003/17	15	23	27	19	28	27
Microbial quality (TAMC - 10^3/TYMC - 10^2)	0001/17	0/0	0/0	0/0	0/0	0/0	0/0
	0002/17	0/0	0/0	0/0	0/0	0/0	0/0
	0003/17	0/0	0/0	0/0	0/0	0/0	0/0

Note: C - complies, emboldened text - out-of-specification

conditions (*see* Table 10). The latter two formats may be more useful in certain situations where comparison of the data across different batches and storage conditions, respectively, would be beneficial.

The stability table should ideally fit onto a single page, as this avoids the assessor having to flip backwards and forwards to view and compare the data, which can be extremely frustrating if there is a large amount of data to review. If the table cannot fit onto a single page, then the quality attributes should be grouped together on one page in a logical fashion, again to facilitate easy review. Consideration should be given to the type of font and text size used in the tables, as some are easier to read than others. Likewise, format of the table (e.g., borders and their weighting, background shading) can also affect the readability of a table. The format and layout of the stability tables should be identical from batch to batch, pack type to pack type, etc., as this again helps the assessor review and compare the data. It is strongly recommended to differentiate OOS

Table 10
Presentation of stability data: one batch, multiple storage conditions

Stability protocol - ACEP 40 stab EU v.1.0							
Batch 0001/17;							
Pack - HDPE bottle + PP cap (30s); orientation - vertical							
		Time (months)					
Quality attributes	Batch	0	3	6	9	12	18
Appearance (round, biconvex white tablet)	25 °C/60% RH	C	C	C	C	C	C
	30 °C/65% RH	C	C	C	C	C	C
	40 °C/75% RH	C	C	C	C	C	C
Assay (95–105% of target)	25 °C/60% RH	101.0	100.9	100.5	100.5	100.1	99.7
	30 °C/65% RH	101.0	100.1	99.7	99.2	98.6	97.1
	40 °C/75% RH	101.00	97.2	**94.4**	–	–	–
Impurities (Single - NMT 0.10% Total - NMT 0.5%)	25 °C/60% RH	0.02	0.02	0.04	0.05	0.05	0.07
		0.03	0.04	0.05	0.07	0.09	0.11
	30 °C/65% RH	0.02	0.04	0.05	0.07	0.08	0.10
		0.03	0.07	0.15	0.20	0.31	0.4
	40 °C/75% RH	0.02	**0.15**	**0.25**	–	–	–
		0.03	0.31	**0.56**	–	–	–
Dissolution ($Q = 75$, 45 min)	25 °C/60% RH	23	24	23	22	26	24
	30 °C/65% RH	23	34	35	39	50	55
	40 °C/75% RH	23	34	40	–	–	–
Microbial quality (TAMC - 10^3/ TYMC - 10^2)	25 °C/60% RH	0/0	0/0	0/0	0/0	0/0	0/0
	30 °C/65% RH	0/0	0/0	0/0	0/0	0/0	0/0
	40 °C/75% RH	0/0	0/0	0/0	–	–	–

Note: C - complies, emboldened text - out-of-specification

results, by highlighting, emboldening, or use of parenthesis (plus including an explanatory footnote). Assessors will review the stability data for compliance with the acceptance limits, and it is better to declare and explain OOS results up front rather than let the assessor find them and ask a question.

Graphical representation of the data should be used to demonstrate increasing and decreasing trends in the data or when statistical analysis is used, particularly when extrapolation of the long-term data are being used to justify the shelf-life. The graphs should be clearly annotated with the acceptance limits. If stability data undergoes little change over time, this can be clearly seen from the tabulated data without the need to duplicate the data in a graph.

Companies should be aware that information on product stability can be requested during a GMP inspection or as part of a defective medicine investigation, and thus this information should match that provided in the MA application (inspectorate and licensing divisions work closely together).

5   How Do Authorities Evaluate Stability Data to Agree the Proposed Shelf-Life and Storage Conditions?

Regulatory authorities do not use special formulae or rules when evaluating stability data to agree a shelf-life and storage conditions for a drug product; they use scientific principles and published international, regional, and national guidance to evaluate the data on its own merits, and the same scientific principles and guidance that is also available to industry. The data will be analyzed for OOS results, trends, variability, and dependency on temperature and humidity as this will determine the extent to which the long-term data can be extrapolated. Consistency of the data across the different batches, pack sizes, packaging materials, orientation, etc. will also be considered when agreeing shelf-life.

Extrapolation of the real-time stability data will follow the flow chart in ICH Q1E [5] in the vast majority of cases. In some cases, companies rely on the simple rule of the amount of long-term data twice, up to a maximum of 12 months, when setting the shelf-life, but this should be used with caution as this represents the maximum extent of extrapolation. There are certain situations where the flow diagram indicates a shorter period of extrapolation. Where the data are variable and trends near to acceptance limits, authorities will be less likely to extrapolate data as far as when the data are less variable and well within limits. Companies should remember that authorities are likely to take a conservative approach when setting the shelf-life, but it is usually relatively easy to extend shelf-lives by variation once the initial MA has been authorized and the product is on the market.

Results from stress testing are typically not taken into account, with the exception of photostability, which should be carried out in accordance with ICH requirements. However, absence of photostability data are typically missing from 9% of MA submissions, which concerns authorities as photodegradants tend to have particular safety issues. The stability data at the different storage conditions are used to agree the proposed storage conditions. Instability at accelerated and intermediate storage conditions will prompt authorities to require special temperature storage conditions. Depending on the product, the susceptibility of the product to moisture and freezing will also be considered by assessors, and thus also needs addressing by companies.

It is worth mentioning that the proposed storage conditions will be reviewed from a practical perspective, taking into account how the drug product will be used day to day. If the proposed storage advice is impractical, authorities will request amendment accordingly. Generic products also deserve special mention with respect to the storage conditions. Whilst these products are typically evaluated on their own merits, the proposed storage advice will be compared with the reference or innovator product to see if there are any differences that may lead to detrimental medication errors in practice, which would likely to be raised as a major objection to grant of license.

6   Life Cycle Management and Stability

It is inevitable that a drug product will undergo changes during its life cycle, whether this is a change in the source of drug substance or excipients, its manufacture, specification and test methods, the container closure system, or a change in the shelf-life or storage conditions.

The general principles for presenting the stability data described above hold true for these situations. However, the stability of the proposed product should be compared to that of the original product to demonstrate that the change has no impact on product quality (and thus safety and efficacy). For the comparison exercise, the batches of the original product should be recently manufactured, that is, no more than 2 or 3 years old (the more recent, the better) - if older batches are used, authorities will request more recent batches. Graphical representations are very useful in this situation as the stability profile of the current and proposed batches can be quickly compared. Where the stability of the proposed product is comparable to the current, it will typically allow companies to continue using the existing shelf-life and storage conditions. Where this is not the case, then the impact of such a change should be considered by the company, in case this leads to detrimental medication errors, and may require additional measures to highlight the change.

7   Stability Studies in Clinical Trials

Investigational medicinal products (IMPs) used in clinical studies also deserve a brief mention. IMPs can be prototype formulations, used in phase I studies, and may have little stability data or they can be developed products that are typically used in multicenter phase III trials and have a larger stability database, or can even be authorized medicinal products. Clinical studies may also involve (modified) comparator products and placebos, for which stability data will also need to be provided. Again, the principles for presenting stability data described above are equally applicable for products used in clinical trials. It is important that the IMP dossier should contain the most up-to-date stability information and the amount of stability data should be commensurate with the clinical and formulation development stage, as this will be expected by authorities. The often used maxim "more is better" is highly relevant here.

Regulatory authorities are primarily concerned that IMPs used in clinical trials are safe to be given to trial participants. There is generally more flexibility in setting wider acceptance limits, provided that these do not put patients at risk. Authorities will usually accept extrapolation of long-term data by four times up to a maximum of 12 months without question, for both chemical and biological IMPs. Furthermore, authorities permit more freedom in extrapolating the long-term data. Stability studies will also need to be started prior to the clinical trial, and run parallel to the trial for its entire duration. To avoid having to submit substantial amendments to the dossier, a proposal for extending the shelf-life also needs to be included, together with the stability protocol covering the extrapolated shelf-life and the criteria for analysis of trends and extrapolation of data. It is sensible to limit the shelf-life of any (modified) comparator or placebo to the shelf-life of the IMP, unless it is an authorized medicinal product.

8 Conclusion

International and regional guidelines on stability testing have been available for over 20 years; however, regulatory authorities continue to find a high number of deficiencies with the stability dossier for the drug substance and drug product. These deficiencies, together with any feedback received from the authorities in deficiency letters, or assessment reports, should be used by companies as a starting point to improve their practices concerning stability dossiers, so that the same mistakes are not repeated. Whilst the advice on presenting a good stability dossier contained in this chapter is focussed on a chemical drug product, its principles are equally applicable to biological products, as well as stability dossiers for drug substances, variation applications, or investigational medicinal products. The stability dossier needs careful preparation, ensuring that all required sections are provided, are compliant with relevant regulatory and pharmacopoeial requirements, and are logically laid out, clear, and well written; duplication should be avoided wherever possible, and the dossier should be easily read. The final point to remember is be open and honest about the stability of the product. It is better to be up front about any stability issue, rather than let the assessor discover it. This will give the assessor confidence that the company has a sound and thorough understanding of their product, which is likely to carry into other areas of the dossier.

References

1. International Conference on Harmonisation (2003) Q1A(R2) Stability testing of new drug substances and products
2. International Conference on Harmonisation (2017) http://www.ich.org/home.html. Accessed 16 Feb 2017
3. European Medicines Agency (2017) Scientific guidelines/Quality/Stability. http://www.ema.europa.eu/ema/index.jsp?curl=pages/regulation/general/general_content_000361.jsp&mid=WC0b01ac0580028eb1. Accessed 16 Feb 2017
4. European Medicines Agency (2017) Scientific guidelines/Q&A on quality/Part 2. http://www.ema.europa.eu/ema/index.jsp?curl=pages/regulation/q_and_a/q_and_a_detail_000072.jsp&mid=WC0b01ac058002c2b0. Accessed 16 Feb 2017
5. International Conference on Harmonisation (2003) Q1E Evaluation of stability data
6. International Conference on Harmonisation (1995) Q5C Stability testing of biotechnological/biological products
7. Marshall P (2014) Oral presentation 'Overview of stability testing across the product lifecycle for European markets' at Informa Stability Testing Conference, London, March 2014
8. Al-hadithi D (2009) Oral presentation 'An overview of European regulatory requirements' at Royal Pharmaceutical Society course on the Stability Testing of Pharmaceuticals, Cambridge
9. Commission on Human Medicinal Products (2007) CPMP/QWP/609/96/Rev 2 Guideline on declaration of storage conditions: A: in the product information of medicinal products; B: for active substances. Annex to note for guidance on stability testing of new drug substances and products. Annex to note for guidance on stability testing of existing active substances and related finished products
10. CPMP/QWP/072/96 (2001) Start of shelf-life of the finished dosage form (Annex to the note for guidance on the manufacture of the finished dosage form)
11. World Health Organisation (2009) Technical Report Series, No 953 Annex 2. Stability testing of active pharmaceutical ingredients and finished pharmaceutical products

Chapter 3

In Silico Drug Degradation Prediction

Mohammed A. Ali, Rachel Hemingway, and Martin A. Ott

Abstract

Zeneth is an in silico tool that can provide insight into the chemical degradation of organic compounds under various environmental conditions. The program is therefore primarily employed within the pharmaceutical industry to understand and account for any potential degradation problems during drug substance development. The program uses a knowledge base of chemical transformations together with a reasoning engine to determine the likelihood of a particular degradation product. The knowledge base is continuously expanding and contains a diverse range of chemistries for many common functional groups.

Key words Zeneth, ICH, FDA, Drug substance, Forced drug degradation, Stress testing, Knowledge base, Transformation, Reasoning, Expert system, In silico prediction

1 Introduction

Stability testing or forced degradation studies are required during the development of a drug substance. The guidance on forced degradation comes mainly from the International Conference on Harmonisation (ICH) [1–4] as well as the regulatory bodies FDA [5] and ANVISA [6] and extends to the degradation products of the drug substance and even the drug product. Stability assessment is crucial as drug substance impurities can appear due to chemical breakdown. This has further implications, for example, with the ICH M7 guidelines [7] which are associated with the risk posed by mutagenic degradation products.

In-depth compound stability assessments, which are long-term (12 months) or accelerated (6 months), impact on the already heavy time constraints of drug substance development and can increase the time to get the product to market. Therefore methods for the early identification of potential impurity issues are important to the pharmaceutical scientist. This chapter details a computer-aided approach to stability or forced degradation prediction by taking into consideration the chemical structure of the drug substance.

Sanjay Bajaj and Saranjit Singh (eds.), *Methods for Stability Testing of Pharmaceuticals*, Methods in Pharmacology and Toxicology, https://doi.org/10.1007/978-1-4939-7686-7_3, © Springer Science+Business Media, LLC, part of Springer Nature 2018

1.1 Computer-Aided Reaction Tool

The vastness and complexity of organic chemistry is burdensome for any chemist and requires an encyclopedic knowledge, which only develops with years of research and experience. Computer tools present a means for scientists of various disciplines and levels of expertise to access vast amounts of chemical knowledge at the click of a mouse. Over the last 40 years mathematical chemistry and computer science have combined [8–10] and this has resulted in an increase in the predictive capabilities of in silico methodologies. There are two in silico approaches available: logic oriented and information oriented.

1.1.1 Logic Oriented

Logic-oriented systems use mathematical models to search for all possible solutions to the query. Physicochemical parameters such as bond dissociation energy, lipophilicity (LogP), and electronegativity are modelled to allow an exploration of "chemistry" as a general theory [11]. Analyses are then performed by describing reactions as rearrangements of chemical structures. Programs like IGOR [12] and its complementary tool RAIN [10, 13] were developed for this purpose by Ugi and co-workers. However, these programs never made it to the public arena and to date there is no commercial logic-oriented system available. The reader is directed to reviews for a comprehensive discussion on such systems [14–17]. Logic-oriented systems require complex properties to be estimated with high precision, which makes them hard to adjust and update, should fine-tuning be required. The level of expertise and knowledge required to be entered by the user to be able to produce meaningful results is also a limiting factor.

1.1.2 Information Oriented

Information-oriented systems, often called expert systems, have the ability to emulate the decision making process of a human brain by accessing a "library" or knowledge base of known information. Expert systems have been under development for over 45 years and much of the early development ideas are attributed to the synthesis design tool LHASA [18, 19], which was designed to aid strategic synthetic planning. Systems like CAMEO [20], EROS [21, 22], and ROBIA [23] were developed from these ideas and although these systems were not designed to predict forced degradation specifically, more to generate sequences of forward reactions to support synthetic design, they were able to predict degradation pathways with moderate success. In 2006, Pfizer developed DELPHI [24], a prediction tool dedicated to forced degradation, but it was built using proprietary data and was not easily updated resulting in its non-commercialization and ultimate discontinuation. Information-oriented systems are easily updated and refined as new data and/or knowledge becomes available but require continuous revision and are always limited by the content of their knowledge library.

<table>
<tr><td>1.1.3 The Computer
Program Zeneth</td><td>Zeneth is an information-oriented, expert knowledge-based in silico system for the prediction of forced degradation pathways [25]. It is, to our knowledge, the only commercially available, actively maintained program of its kind. The program has been designed to predict the degradation pathways of a query molecule based on its structure and user-selected processing constraints. Zeneth is an encapsulation of drug degradation knowledge from pharmaceutical reports and chemistry literature as well as from consultation with experts (S.W. Baertschi) and direct interaction with industry (GlaxoSmithKline, Eli Lilly, Pfizer, Merck, Amgen, Johnson and Johnson, and others). It is comprised of a knowledge base of transformations (what reaction can occur), which when combined with a reasoning engine (assessing how likely this reaction is to occur), generates a degradation profile under various environmental conditions, namely thermolytic, hydrolytic, oxidative, and photolytic, which align with ICH Q1A(R2) and Q1B guidelines [1, 2]. This profile can then assist in the identification of potential degradation products. Zeneth is designed to have a broad coverage outlining all the knowledge it has about a given query to aid the user [26]. However, just because a degradation product is predicted by Zeneth doesn't mean that it will be seen experimentally, simply that it has the potential to be observed. The program is not quantitative and does not give an indication of shelf-life and results on accelerated degradation nor does it give quantities, reaction rates, or other kinetic calculations.</td></tr>
</table>

2 Zeneth and Its Features

<table>
<tr><td>2.1 Methodology</td><td>The user is required to input some initial information and set certain parameters (see Fig. 1), namely a query structure, which must be in its neutral form regardless of the pH. Zeneth has design features that address the pH dependency of reactions and these are discussed in more detail later in this section. Zeneth cannot perform predictions on polymers or proteins and performs best in the area of small molecules.

Zeneth takes into account the four main pharmaceutically relevant degradation conditions: thermolytic, hydrolytic, oxidative, and photolytic. It allows temperature and pH to be selected using a numerical scale along with the presence or absence of water, oxygen, metal, radical initiator, peroxide, and light (<i>see</i> Fig. 2). It is important to note that the program requires a set of conditions to be chosen, e.g., set A in Fig. 2. This set will then be used in single-condition processing. AutoZeneth, a feature within the program, is able to run multiple sets of conditions against a query compound (<i>see</i> Sect. 2.4).

Zeneth then requires the maximum number of steps to be set. This parameter allows successive generations of degradation</td></tr>
</table>

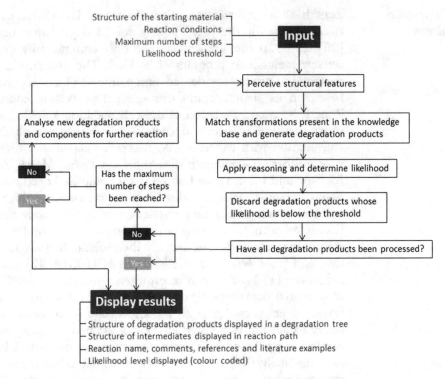

Fig. 1 Methodology outlining how the computer program Zeneth is designed to predict the degradation profile of a given starting material

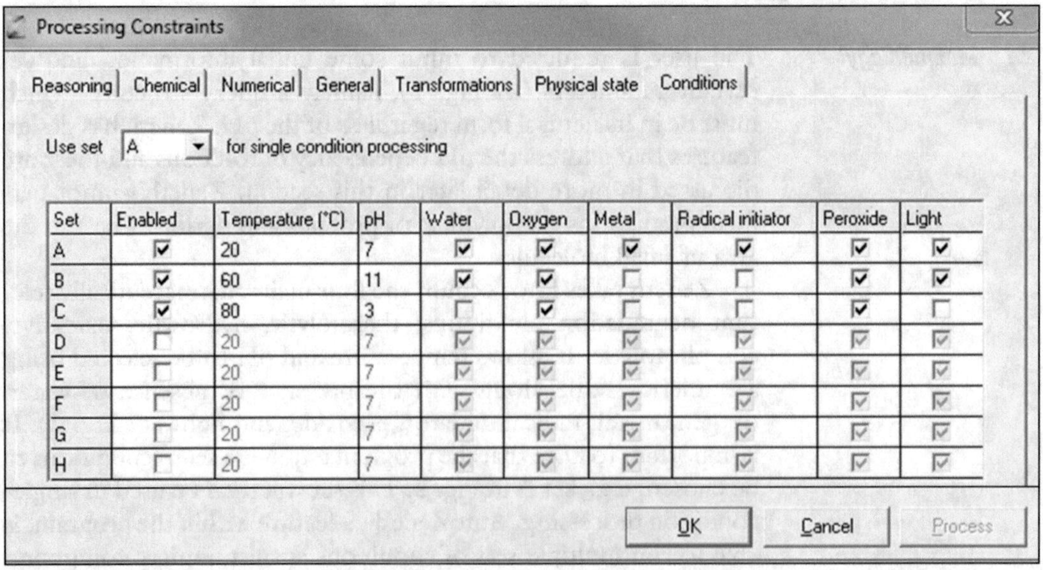

Set	Enabled	Temperature (°C)	pH	Water	Oxygen	Metal	Radical initiator	Peroxide	Light
A	☑	20	7	☑	☑	☑	☑	☑	☑
B	☑	60	11	☑	☑	☐	☐	☑	☑
C	☑	80	3	☐	☑	☐	☐	☑	☐
D	☐	20	7	☑	☑	☑	☑	☑	☑
E	☐	20	7	☑	☑	☑	☑	☑	☑
F	☐	20	7	☑	☑	☑	☑	☑	☑
G	☐	20	7	☑	☑	☑	☑	☑	☑
H	☐	20	7	☑	☑	☑	☑	☑	☑

Fig. 2 Selecting sets of reaction conditions. Set A is "default", sets B and C have been customized

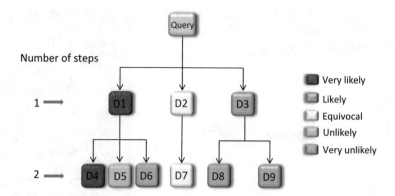

Fig. 3 An example degradation tree outlining the generations of degradation products that would be displayed at each step and their associated likelihood

products to be predicted, e.g., if the maximum number of steps is set to one, only the first generation of degradation products which directly arise from the query will be shown, but if the default of two is used, two generations of degradation products will be shown (*see* Fig. 3).

The program is designed to predict how likely a degradation product is. This likelihood threshold can be set to "very unlikely", "unlikely", "equivocal", "likely", and "very likely" and a predicted degradation product will be "binned" into one of these categories (based on chemical knowledge and literature evidence). Degradation products will only be displayed if predicted at or above the chosen threshold; the default is "likely". Once this initial information has been entered a prediction can be performed by searching the knowledge base within Zeneth.

2.1.1 The Transformation Library

Perceiving the structural features of a query compound is a function computer tools are particularly good at. Molecular perception is important for determining the structure of degradation products and the bonds that have been made or broken. Rearrangements, symmetry, and stereochemistry are often difficult for the human brain to perceive (quickly) but a program can interpret these features with ease. Once a query has been submitted, Zeneth will begin searching through its library of transformations. When a pattern in a specific transformation is "matched" and the reaction conditions are met, the corresponding rules are triggered and a degradation product is generated.

Transformation Patterns

A transformation pattern is implemented after examining all available data on a particular reaction to effectively determine a "degradophore". This is the smallest part of the molecule responsible for the degradation reaction [25] and takes into consideration an analysis of the mechanism. The pattern details atom and bond attributes (on the reactant), e.g., the number of heteroatoms that

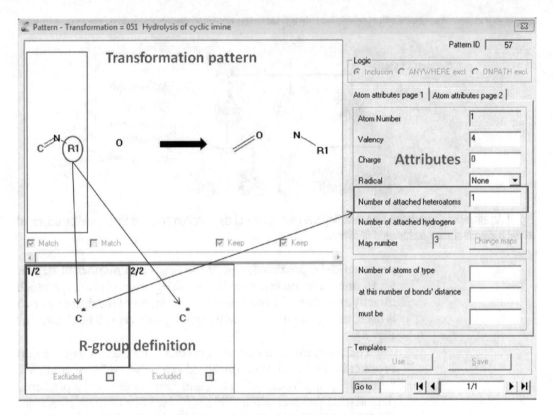

Fig. 4 Transformation pattern for transformation 051: hydrolysis of cyclic imines

can be attached to a particular atom or whether a bond can be single, double, triple, or aromatic. R groups are used to describe chemical coverage (*see* Fig. 4). The mechanistic path is proposed including intermediates (if applicable). Therefore patterns define both the transformation and the scope of the chemical reaction that can take place.

For a transformation to generate a degradation product, the query compound must "match" the pattern(s). The pattern then describes how the structure should be changed to generate the degradation product. A transformation usually contains more than one pattern to account for variations and can also contain exclusion patterns which, if matched, exclude specific areas of scope. This may be because there is evidence that the compounds covered by this scope undergo a different mechanism and cannot be included in this transformation or that they are already included in the scope of another (more likely) transformation. For example, decarboxylation of indole-2-carboxylic acid or related compounds excludes 2-hydroxyindole-2-carboxylic acid and related compounds from the scope because they decarboxylate via a different mechanism and are covered by a more likely transformation: the decarboxylation of orthocarboxyphenol or heteroaromatic analogue.

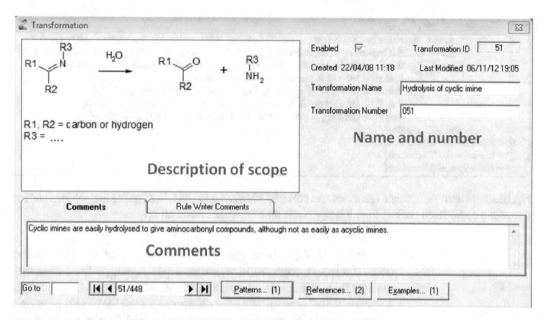

Fig. 5 User view of the transformation in the knowledge base editor

The transformation is supplemented with comments that discuss details about the mechanism as well as references and examples (*see* Fig. 5). The likelihood of a transformation and its dependency on reaction conditions are described by reasoning rules.

2.1.2 Reasoning Rules

There are two types of reasoning rules within the Zeneth framework: absolute reasoning and relative reasoning. Absolute reasoning evaluates the level of likelihood that degradation will occur and relative reasoning compares the likelihood of competing transformations.

Absolute Reasoning

There are six likelihood levels that can be applied to a transformation to predict how likely a given degradation product is: "very unlikely", "unlikely", "equivocal", "likely", and "very likely". There are also a small number of tautomerization and decarboxylation transformations deemed so likely as to be unavoidable and they have been assigned a likelihood level of "certain". Reaction conditions required for a particular chemical reaction to occur, e.g., pH (acid or base catalyzed) or presence of water, will be established from literature evidence and these dependencies will then be turned into "rules" and linked to the transformation. For example, transformation 051 in the knowledge base describes the hydrolysis of cyclic imines and the likelihood of this degradation reaction happening is dependent on the pH and the presence of water. This has been reflected in the knowledge base using rules (*see* Fig. 6). Rules are entered using a strict format: if (Grounds) are (Threshold) then (Proposition) is (Force) and readers are directed to the paper by Parenty and co-workers [25] for a detailed explanation of these terms.

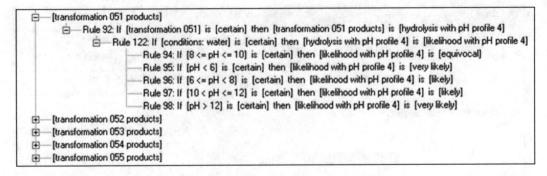

Fig. 6 Excerpt from the absolute reasoning rule editor for transformation 051, highlighting that the likelihood of a resulting degradation product from this hydrolysis reaction is dependent on pH

Rules 94–98 reflect the acid/base nature of transformation 051. If a query compound was run at pH 3, which fired transformation 051, the resulting degradation product would be predicted as "very likely"; the same query compound at pH 9 would generate an "equivocal" degradation product and at pH 11 the degradation product would be "likely".

Therefore, Zeneth has the capacity to analyze the query molecule and generate a degradation product with an associated likelihood when a transformation pattern has matched and a corresponding reasoning rule has been satisfied (*see* Fig. 7).

Relative Reasoning

Relative reasoning accounts for the relative reactivity of functional groups and again is based on literature evidence and chemical sense. All transformations in the knowledge base are linked to at least one other transformation. Relative reasoning is used to describe the most likely pathway. If Zeneth predicts that two or more transformations are likely to occur at the same time on the same compound, the relative reasoning engine assesses which transformation will take precedence relative to other transformations.

For example, if the query shown in Fig. 8 was processed in Zeneth, there are three hydrolysis transformations that would match and generate degradation products. There is evidence that the hydrolysis of esters is more likely than amide [27] which in turn is more likely than lactam hydrolysis [28] and this relationship has been represented in Zeneth using reasoning rules. There are options to allow only the most likely pathway to be shown, for example, if the relative reasoning level was set to 1, only the degradation products arising from the hydrolysis of esters would be displayed.

2.1.3 Other Processing Constraints

Dimerizations

Within the processing constraints of Zeneth, there are options to allow the query compound to react on its own or with itself and its degradation products. The user can also allow a degradation product to react with itself (but not with other degradation products) (*see* Fig. 9). A maximum monomer count can be set which limits the

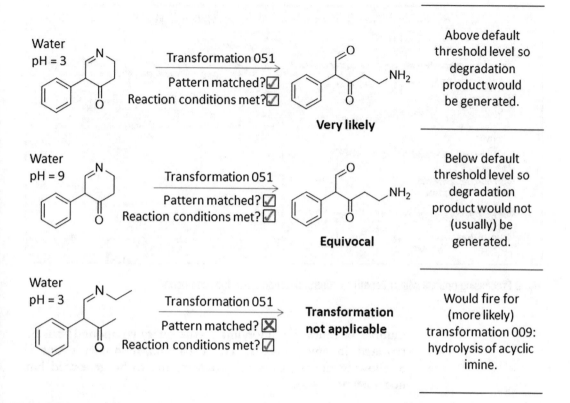

Fig. 7 Pattern matching and associated absolute reasoning for transformation 051 (hydrolysis of cyclic imine), adapted from Parenty et al. [25]

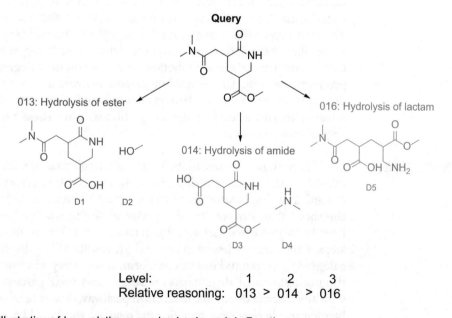

Fig. 8 Illustration of how relative reasoning levels work in Zeneth

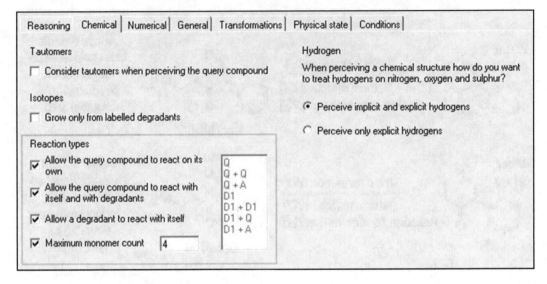

Fig. 9 Processing options within Zeneth to control reaction types that can occur

number of times the "monomer" (the query compound) can be repeated in any products. The maximum monomer count is 8, allowing dimers, trimers, tetramers, etc. to be generated but not nonamers.

2.2 Excipients and Counterions

The knowledge base contains a number of excipients (currently 61) and counterions (currently 75), which can be selected and processed with a query compound to predict potential intermolecular reactions. Common degradation products and impurities associated with these excipients and counterions are also available for selection (optional). For example, if benzyl alcohol will be present in the final formulation alongside the drug, these compounds can be run concurrently in a prediction to assess potential degradation products; see Fig. 10. Benzaldehyde and benzoic acid are known degradation products of benzyl alcohol and they can also be selected to run alongside the drug substance to assess potential degradation products.

2.3 Results Display

Once Zeneth has exhausted its library of transformations matching relevant patterns and applying reasoning and likelihood rules, it will discard any degradation products whose likelihood is below the threshold that was set and determine if all degradation products have been processed (*see* Fig. 1). When the maximum number of steps, which was set has been reached the results will be displayed as a degradation tree and in a tabular form. A summary window shows the generations of degradation products and their parents along with any intermediates in the reaction pathway, details of which can be seen by clicking on a specific intermediate (*see* Fig. 11).

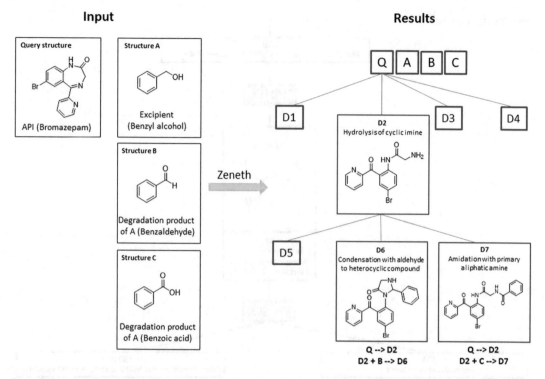

Fig. 10 Excipients and their common degradation products can be run alongside an drug substance to assess the potential of intermolecular reactions. Benzaldehyde and benzoic acid can be optionally selected alongside the main excipient

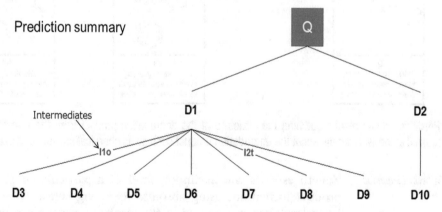

Fig. 11 Prediction summary results outlining the degradation pathway and any intermediates

A second window outlines the detail for each degradation product, including its structure, chemical formula, and mass as well as the absolute and relative reasoning that was applied to it (*see* Fig. 12). Finally a results table gives further information including formula loss and mass difference along with the ability to filter on several columns to help identify particular degradation products.

Prediction detail

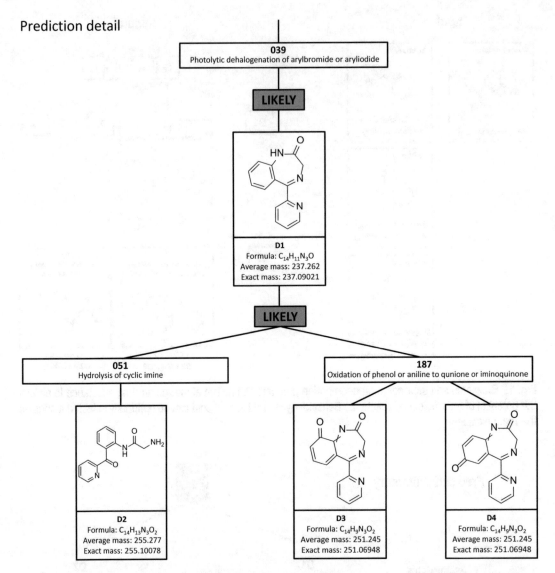

Fig. 12 Prediction detail results outlining the structure of the degradation product from the transformation which occurred along with details about the degradation product such as its chemical formula and exact mass

2.3.1 Pathway Likelihood   Zeneth assesses the likelihood level of a particular degradation product formation, using absolute reasoning rules. These likelihood levels are represented in the results tree using a color code (*see* Fig. 13a). There are then different methods to project this likelihood assessment within the program. Step likelihood is calculated solely from the absolute reasoning rules and views each degradation product in isolation, as an individual step in the pathway. Therefore, step likelihood has the potential to allow a degradation product to have a higher probability than its parent for example D1 to D6 to D12 in Fig. 13a, suggesting a very likely degradation product from an unlikely parent. This could be construed as an

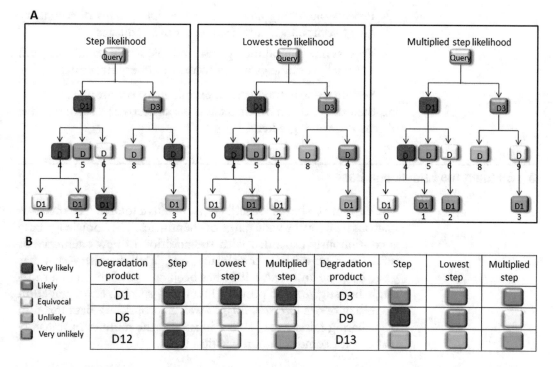

Fig. 13 (a) An illustration to demonstrate the different methods used to calculate likelihood levels in Zeneth. (b) An illustration to demonstrate how likelihood is affected depending on the method chosen

unlikely event. Pathway likelihood is calculated from the step likelihood of the steps leading to that degradation product and there are two methods available: lowest step likelihood and multiplied step likelihood.

Lowest step likelihood considers all the steps in a pathway leading to a degradation product and does not allow any degradation product to have a higher likelihood than its parent. Multiplied step likelihood obeys the same principle but converts each likelihood level into a numerical probability, multiplying the likelihood of each step to determine the resulting degradation products' likelihood level.

Multiplied step is a method aimed at predicting more realistic pathway likelihoods, allowing increased granularity. The multiplication of likelihood levels results in less weight being given to less likely pathways, which will subsequently result in fewer false-positive results being predicted (*see* Fig. 13b).

2.4 AutoZeneth

AutoZeneth is a feature within the interface of Zeneth, which in essence allows batch processing to be performed. Users have three processing options:

1. Process multiple compounds against a single set of conditions, and optionally a single group of secondary query structures.

2. Process one compound against multiple groups of secondary query compounds, and a single set of conditions.

3. Process one compound against multiple sets of conditions, and optionally a single group of secondary query structures.

Secondary structures can be excipients or counterions (including their degradation products and impurities), or a second active pharmaceutical ingredient.

3   Building the Knowledge Base

The current version of Zeneth (v7) contains a total of 446 transformations that cover a wide range of chemistries. The knowledge base is continuously expanded with the addition of new chemistry or refinement of existing transformations. The chemistry that has gone into the knowledge base has been compiled through a thorough investigation of primary literature, specialized degradation chemistry books [27, 29, 30], as well as proprietary data through data sharing initiatives. Table 1 illustrates the number of transformations for some common reaction types.

3.1   Transformation Chemistry

This section surveys some of the chemistry covered in each of the six categories in Table 1 and provides a broad overview of the science present in the knowledge base. As full details of the transformations are not discussed, R groups in the description pictures represent carbon or hydrogen, unless stated otherwise.

3.1.1   Oxidative Chemistry

Oxidation is a fairly common pathway for drug degradation and efforts to minimize this process involve storage of compounds under anaerobic conditions. The reaction can be of three general types. The first involves free radicals that are generated from

Table 1

Composition of the Zeneth knowledge base according to reaction type [version 2016.1.1]

Transformation category	Number of transformations
Oxidations	143
Hydrolyses	87
Condensations and additions	90
Isomerizations and rearrangements	56
Eliminations and fragmentations	32
Photochemical reactions	38
Total	446

compounds when exposed to light, heat, or transition metals (e.g., copper or iron that can be present as impurities). This initiation step is followed by the propagation stage, where molecular oxygen reacts with the free radical to form a peroxy radical. The peroxy radical has the capacity to remove a hydrogen atom from the compound to generate a hydroperoxide, which generates another free radical. This process continues until the free radicals are destroyed by inhibitors or other reactions that terminate the chain.

Another common oxidation process involves the direct reaction of peroxides and hydroperoxides (e.g., the N-oxidation of aliphatic tertiary amines to give amine oxides). Hydroperoxides also tend to be photolabile and, therefore, can break down to form hydroxyl and alkoxyl radicals, which then act as the oxidizing agents. Finally, organic compounds are susceptible to oxidation by the reaction with singlet oxygen, a high-energy form of molecular oxygen.

Currently, Zeneth has 143 oxidation transformations that cover a wide range of functional groups. Some of these are discussed in Table 2. The chemistry in this section continues to be extended as more knowledge becomes available.

Table 2
Examples of functional groups that undergo oxidation in the knowledge base

Transformation type	Functional group	Comments
Autoxidation	Aldehyde	These are readily oxidized to give carboxylic acids
Autoxidation	Alcohol	Primary and secondary alcohols are susceptible to oxidation to give aldehydes or ketones, respectively. Benzylic, allylic, and propargylic alcohols can similarly undergo autoxidation
Oxidation	Alkene	These can be attacked by peroxides to produce epoxides
Autoxidation	Amine	Primary or secondary amines bearing a primary or secondary alkyl group can be oxidized to give imines. Tertiary amines bearing a primary alkyl group can undergo autoxidation to give amides
Autoxidation	Ether	Ethers with an α-hydrogen can be oxidized to an alcohol and carbonyl compound. Benzylic ethers can undergo autoxidation as well as by peroxides to give the hydroperoxides which can break down further to carbonyl compounds
Autoxidation	Carboxylic acid	Carboxylic acids are susceptible to oxidative decarboxylation by autoxidation if the α-carbon is activated by further conjugation
Oxidation	Heteroaromatic	Heteroaromatic compounds can undergo a variety of oxidation reactions under the influence of peroxides and hydroperoxides or singlet oxygen

Transformations are written in a general format to encompass a greater amount of chemical space. An example is the oxidation of an alcohol to give the corresponding aldehyde or ketone (*see* Fig. 14).

3.1.2 Hydrolytic Chemistry

Drug compounds that are susceptible to hydrolytic degradation are generally derivatives of carboxylic acids, e.g., esters, amides, imides, lactones, or lactams.

Hydrolysis represents the most widely encountered mode of drug degradation mainly due to the fact that many drugss contain hydrolyzable groups along with the ubiquitous nature of the water molecule. The reaction is catalyzed by acid or base and, therefore, is pH dependent. As such Zeneth has many pH profiles that can be used to describe the likelihood of a particular hydrolytic reaction (*see* Fig. 15). Table 3 shows some of the functional groups that are covered in the knowledge base that undergo hydrolytic degradation. Other transformations in this category include the hydrolytic cleavage of alkyl and acid halides, nitriles, mono- and dithioacetals, phosphonamidic acid, phosphinamides, and thionophosphates.

3.1.3 Condensations and Additions

This section details some adduct-forming reactions in Zeneth, which have been broadly split into two types: addition and condensation (*see* Tables 4 and 5). The condensation reactions differ from the addition reactions as they involve loss of water or another small leaving group (addition followed by elimination).

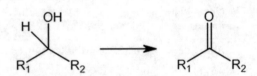

Fig. 14 Transformation 62: oxidation of alcohols

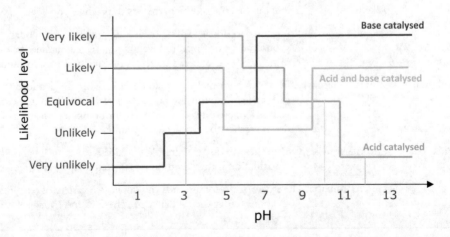

Fig. 15 Construction of pH profiles describing how pH affects the likelihood of a pH-dependent reaction

Table 3
Examples of functional groups that undergo hydrolysis in the knowledge base

Functional group	Comments
	Amines can undergo acid-catalyzed hydrolysis if one of the alkyl groups can form a stabilized carbenium ion. This is the case for tertiary alkyl groups and also for benzyl, allyl, and propargyl groups
	Acyclic carboxamides are hydrolyzed giving carboxylic acids and amines. Similarly, urea is hydrolyzed giving carbamic acids and amines
	Esters undergo acid-catalyzed hydrolysis easily if the alkyl group can form a stabilized carbenium ion. Also N-monosubstituted and N,N-disubstituted carbamate esters can hydrolyze to generate the free alcohol and an unstable carbamic acid intermediate
	The beta-lactam ring is readily hydrolyzed to give an amine and a carboxylic acid

Table 4
Examples of condensation reactions in the knowledge base

Condensation reactions	Comments
	Aldehydes and ketones can react with hydroxylamines (R_3=OH), hydrazines (R_3=NH_2), and sulfenamides (R_3=S-) to give the corresponding oximes, hydrazones, and thiooximes, respectively
	Both alcohols and amines can react with acyl halides, acid anhydrides, and mixed organic-inorganic anhydrides, imides, thioesters, N-acyl azaaromatic compounds, and N-acyl ammonium compounds to yield the corresponding esters and amides, respectively. The reaction takes place very readily, even more so in base

3.1.4 Isomerizations and Rearrangements

Isomerization is the process of conversion of the drug into a compound with the same formula, including tautomerism and stereoisomerism. The conversion of the drug from one isomer into another is still regarded as degradation, because any change in structure can result in a loss of activity or produce other undesirable

Table 5
Examples of addition reactions in the knowledge base

Addition reactions	Comments
	Alkenes that are activated by an electron-withdrawing group can undergo hydration. The reaction takes place readily in base
	Carbonyl compounds having at least one enolizable hydrogen can react with imines or carbonyl compounds in a Mannich or an aldol reaction, respectively

Table 6
Examples of isomerization and rearrangement reactions in the knowledge base

Reactions	Comments
	β, γ Compounds can undergo allylic isomerization under basic conditions to give the α,β-unsaturated (conjugated) compounds (R_1 must be an electron-withdrawing group)
	Phenyl esters can rearrange photochemically in a reaction called the photo-Fries rearrangement. Light cleaves the ester homolytically into a phenoxyl and acyl radical pair. The radicals recombine to give an acyl cyclohexadienone which rapidly tautomerize to the acylated product

effects. Table 6 illustrates some of the isomerization and rearrangement reactions covered in the Zeneth transformations knowledge base.

3.1.5 Eliminations and Fragmentations

Zeneth covers a number of different eliminations and fragmentations. Table 7 illustrates some of the examples.

3.1.6 Photochemical Reactions (Table 8)

For a compound to be photoreactive it must contain a chromophore that is able to absorb light. For pharmaceutical photostability testing, light absorption in the near UV (UV-B, 280–315, UV-A, 315–400 nm) or in the visible part of the spectrum is of concern. Chromophores such as conjugated carbon-carbon or carbon-heteroatom double bonds, or aromatic/heteroaromatic rings, all absorb strongly in this region. Conjugated aldehydes or ketones are

Table 7
Examples of elimination and fragmentation reactions in the knowledge base

Reactions	Comments
	Alcohols can be dehydrated in strongly acidic conditions (protonation of the alcohol followed by loss of water) to give the alkene
	Sulfoxides having an alkyl chain with a β-hydrogen can undergo elimination to give alkenes and sulfenic acids. Selenoxides undergo the same reaction to give alkenes and selenenic acids
	Decarboxylation of compounds, such as β-oxo, α-nitro, and α-cyano acids, generally where the alpha carbon atom of the carboxylic acid is attached to an electron-withdrawing group
	1,2,5-Thiadiazoles can undergo thermal fragmentation (via a formal retro-1,3-dipolar cycloaddition) into nitriles and nitrile sulfides. The nitrile sulfides are unstable, losing sulfur to give a second nitrile
	1,2,4-Oxadiazoles that are unsubstituted at the 5-position are susceptible to hydrolysis. The mechanism of the reaction depends on the pH

Table 8
Examples of photochemical reactions in the knowledge base

Chromophore	Comments
Alkenes Allenes Ketenes Cumulenes	In conjugation, these absorb strongly in the UV irradiation and can undergo [2+2] cycloaddition reactions to yield the corresponding cyclobutane derivatives
Aromatic rings Heteroaromatic rings	These absorb strongly in the near UV
Ketones Aldehydes	Conjugated α-hydroxyketones undergo photolysis giving two carbonyl compounds
Aromatic nitro compounds Aromatic nitrite esters Aromatic amines	These can undergo photolysis to generate aryloxyl and nitrogen oxide radicals. Diaryl amines that contain a chloro, bromo, or iodo substituent at the 2-position of one of the aromatic rings can photocyclize to give the tricyclic carbazole
Phenyl esters	These can rearrange photochemically in a reaction called the photo-Fries rearrangement

typical examples of moieties that are photolabile, especially where the conjugating group ensures that the carbonyl group will have appreciable absorption. The conjugating group can be an aromatic ring or an extended system consisting of an alkene or alkyne that itself is conjugated to a further unsaturated group.

4 Conclusions

In silico models to predict drug degradation have applications in the development of drugs by supporting both the prediction and identification of drug impurities. Zeneth is a software application with the ability to predict the potential forced degradation pathways of organic compounds under various environmental conditions. The software can also consider excipients and counterions alongside a query molecule to assess the potential for intermolecular reactions. It supports the elucidation of plausible degradation pathways and suggests a likelihood level for their formation based on a weight of evidence argument.

The main advantage of in silico approaches is that they can be used as an aid to examine raw analytical data to elucidate the structure of degradation products. It provides the less experienced chemist with in cerebro insights for interpreting the experimental data and thus to make informed decisions that can reduce the requirement for time- and resource-consuming investigations. Degradation experts can increase productivity by using the software as a tool to anticipate and understand the results at an early stage.

The program relies heavily on its chemical transformation knowledge base. This is continually enhanced by the addition of new chemistry as well as the refinement of the existing transformations. The knowledge is peer reviewed and primary literature evidence is used to create the scope, determine likelihood, and add examples where possible for each transformation. Overall the program provides an unbiased approach of forced degradation prediction via a total recall of known expert knowledge.

References

1. ICH (2003) Q1A(R2): stability testing of new drug substances and products. http://www.ich.org/products/guidelines/quality/article/quality-guidelines.html. Accessed 21 Sept 2016
2. ICH (1996) Q1B: stability testing: photostability testing of new drug substances and products. http://www.ich.org/products/guidelines/quality/article/quality-guidelines.html. Accessed 21 Sept 2016
3. ICH (2006) Q3A(R2): impurities in new drug substances. http://www.ich.org/products/

guidelines/quality/article/quality-guidelines.html. Accessed 21 Sept 2016
4. ICH (2006) Q3B(R2): impurities in new drug substances. http://www.ich.org/products/guidelines/quality/article/quality-guidelines.html. Accessed 21 Sept 2016
5. FDA 21 Code of Federal Regulations (2015) Part 211, cGMP in Manufacturing, Processing, Packaging, or Holding of Drugs and Finished Pharmaceuticals: 21 CFR 211.165(e): Testing and release for distribution; 21 CFR 211.166 (a)(3): Stability testing; FDA Guidance for

Industry, Analytical Procedures and Methods Validation for Drugs and Biologics

6. ANVISA Brazil RDC 53 (2015) Regulation on report, identification and qualification of degradation products

7. ICH M7 (2014) Assessment and control of DNA reactive (mutagenic) impurities in pharmaceuticals to limit potential carcinogenic risk

8. Ugi IK, Bauer J, Baumartner R, Fontain E, Forstmeyer D, Lohberger S (2000) Computer assistance in the design of syntheses and a new generation of computer programs for the solution of chemical problems by molecular logic. Pure Appl Chem 60:1573–1586

9. Gasteiger J, Hutchings MG, Seller H, Low P (1988) Prediction of chemical reactivity and design of organic synthesis. In: Warr WA (ed) Chemical structures: the international language of chemistry. Springer, Berlin, pp 343–359

10. Bauer J, Fontain E, Ugi I (1992) IGOR and RAIN—the first mathematically based multi-purpose problem-solving computer programs for chemistry and their use as generators of constitutional formulas. Match 27:31–47

11. Dugundji J, Ugi I (1973) An algebraic model of constitutional chemistry as a basis for chemical computer programs. Top Curr Chem 39:19–64

12. Bauer J, Herges R, Fontain E, Ugi I (1985) IGOR and computer assisted innovation in chemistry. Chimica 39:43–53

13. Fontain E, Reitsam K (1991) The generation of reaction networks with RAIN. 1. The reaction generator. J Chem Inf Comput Sci 31:96–101

14. Ott MA (2004) Cheminformatics and organic chemistry. Computer assisted synthetic analysis. In: Noordik JH (ed) Cheminformatics developments. IOS Press, Amsterdam

15. Ugi I, Bauer J, Blombeger C, Brandt J, Dietz A, Fontain E, Gruber B, von Scholley-Pfab A, Senff A, Stein N (1994) Models, concepts, theories and formal languages in chemistry and their use as a basis for computer assistance in chemistry. J Chem Inf Comput Sci 34:3–16

16. Ihlenfeldt WD, Gasteiger J (1995) Computer-assisted planning of organic syntheses: the second generation of programs. Angew Chem Int Ed 34:2613–2633

17. Szymkuc S, Gajewska EP, Klucznik T, Molga K, Dittwalk P, Startek M, Bajczyk M, Grzybowski BA (2016) Computer-assisted synthetic planning: the end of the beginning. Angew Chem Int Ed Engl 55:5904–5937

18. Corey EJ (1971) Centenary lecture. Computer-assisted analysis of complex synthetic problems. Quart Rev Chem Soc 25:455–482

19. Pensak DA, Corey EJ (1977) LHASA—logic and heuristics applied to synthetic analysis. In: Wipke WT, Howe WJ (eds) Computer assisted organic synthesis, vol 61. ACS, Washington, pp 1–32

20. Jorgensen WL, Laird ER, Gushurst AJ, Fleischer JM, Gothe SA, Helson HE, Paderes GD, Sinclair S (1990) CAMEO: a program for the logical prediction of the products of organic reactions. Pure Appl Chem 62:1921–1932

21. Hollering R, Gasteiger J, Steinhauer L, Schulz KP, Herwig A (2000) Simulation of organic reactions: From the degradation of chemicals to combinatorial synthesis. J Chem Inf Comp Sci 40:482–494

22. Gasteiger J, Jochum C (1987) EROS, a computer program for generating sequences of reactions. Top Curr Chem 74:93–126

23. Socorro IM, Taylor K, Goodman JM (2005) ROBIA: a reaction prediction program. Org Lett 7:3541–3544

24. Pole DL, Ando HY, Murphy ST (2007) Prediction of drug degradants using DELPHI: an expert system for focusing knowledge. Mol Pharmaceut 4:539–549

25. Parenty ADC, Button WG, Ott MA (2013) An expert system to predict the forced degradation of organic molecules. Mol Pharmaceut 10:2962–2974

26. Kleinman MH, Baertschi SW, Alsante KM, Reid DL, Mowery MD, Shimanovich R, Foti C, Smith WK, Reynolds DW, Nefliu M, Ott MA (2014) In silico prediction of pharmaceutical degradation pathways: a benchmarking study. Mol Pharmaceut 11:4179–4188

27. Smith MB, March J (2001) March's advanced organic chemistry: reactions, mechanisms and structure, 5th edn. Wiley, New York

28. Connors KA (1990) Chemical kinetics: the study of reaction rates in solution. Wiley-VCH, New York

29. Baertschi SW, Alsante KM, Reed RA (2011) Pharmaceutical stress testing: predicting drug degradation (drugs and the pharmaceutical sciences), vol 210, 2nd edn. Informa Healthcare, London

30. Li M (2012) Organic chemistry of drug degradation. Royal Society of Chemistry, Cambridge

Forced Degradation and Long-Term Stability Testing for Oral Drug Products: A Practical Approach

Markus Zimmer

Abstract

Forced degradation or stress testing on proto-formulation is considered as the most predictive approach towards long-term stability studies. The aim of applying stress is to identify the weaknesses of the chosen formulation identified by the use of suitable analytical test methods. Based on the experience gained from forced degradation (stress) stability studies, no new and unknown impurities should be detected during ICH (primary) stability studies at later development stages. For the primary stability testing design, matrixing and bracketing approaches can be used for testing of new drug products, if sufficiently justified. Knowing that bracketing is usually accepted by the different authorities, the design and strategy for matrixing should be discussed in advance before starting these stability studies.

Key words Bracketing, Matrixing, Forced degradation, Stress testing, Correction factor, Mass balance, Orthogonal method, Oxidation, Hydrolysis, Proto-formulation, Structure elucidation, In silico, Compatibility, Binary mixture

Abbreviations

CMC   Carboxymethyl cellulose
DoE   Design of experiment
DSC   Differential scanning calorimetry
ELSD   Evaporative light scattering detector
HPLC   High-pressure liquid chromatography
HSM   Hot-stage microscopy
LC   Liquid chromatography
m/m   Mass/mass
MS   Mass spectrometry
NMP N-methyl-2-pyrrolidone
RH   Relative humidity
SFC   Supercritical fluid chromatography
TAMC   Total aerobic microbial count
TGA   Thermogravimetric analysis
TLC   Thin layer chromatography
TYMC   Total yeast/mold count

Sanjay Bajaj and Saranjit Singh (eds.), *Methods for Stability Testing of Pharmaceuticals*, Methods in Pharmacology and Toxicology, https://doi.org/10.1007/978-1-4939-7686-7_4, © Springer Science+Business Media, LLC, part of Springer Nature 2018

UV   Ultraviolet
v/v   Volume/volume
XRPD   X-ray powder diffraction

1   Introduction of Stress Testing

Stress testing on drug substance and drug product is an essential part in order to check the suitability of the developed analytical methods regarding their stability-indicating power. The detection and structure elucidation of the formed impurities as well as the identification of associated degradation pathway are crucial to understand the weakness of the drug substance and the chosen formulation exposed to different stress environments. Finally, forced degradation studies are figuring any potential stability issues during development and industrialization phase.

Several ICH guidelines are dealing with forced degradation, forced decomposition, or stress testing, which are synonyms used for the same phenomenon: characterizing the degradation pattern of the chosen compound or formulation by identifying any increase in degradation impurities. An overview of the ICH guidelines of concern is listed below:

1. Q1A(R2) (stability testing of new drug substances and products) requires identification of degradation products, establishment of the degradation pathways, and validation of the stability-indicating power of the analytical procedures employed for assessment of drug substance stability [1].

2. Q1B (photostabilitiy testing) requires demonstration that light exposure of the drug or product would not result in an unacceptable change in quality. It suggests testing in a sequential manner, starting with the fully exposed product, and then progressing as necessary to the product in the primary packaging and subsequently to the secondary packaging [2].

3. Q1E (evaluation of stability) describes that the adequacy of the mass balance should be assessed. Especially all factors that could cause an apparent failure of mass balance need to be considered, including mechanism(s) of drug degradation [3].

4. Q2(R1) (validation of analytical procedures) gives more details about the stress environments: forced degradation should include samples stored under relevant stress conditions like light, heat, humidity, acid/base hydrolysis, and oxidation [4].

5. Q3B(R2) (impurities in the new drug product) requires that any lab studies, including stress testing, should have the aim to detect degradation products and all the results obtained should be summarized [5].

6. Q6A (specifications) requests that organic impurities arising from degradation should be monitored in the new drug product [6].

However, all these different guidelines do not clearly distinguish between stress testing for drug substance and drug product. Even if situation for the drug substance itself is already clearly described, the situation for the drug product and the associated requirements are not sufficiently addressed in these guidelines. Therefore, it can be stated that no clear practical advice is given by ICH guidelines on how to perform forced degradation or stress testing for a drug product.

This situation is in consistency with the fact that only little official requirements from the different health authorities are currently published. Since 2015, the Brazilian agency ANVISA emphasized on performing forced degradation on drug product by applying all stress conditions, which were identified as relevant to degradation of the drug substance [7]. The intention of this stress test is to check if any additional new impurities were formed in the presence of the excipients used for the formulation intended to be marketed. This approach on drug product forced degradation does not only include solid-state stress studies in the presence of the chosen excipients, but even stress in solution, if the mechanism of degradation in the product was proven to be destructive for the drug itself [8, 9].

Some other requirements have been laid down by regulatory authorities from ASEAN [10], Singapore [11] and CDSCO, India [12], but some of these guidelines are still in a draft stage [13]. Now-a-days, USFDA is also asking for specific tests determining degradation impurities for drug product under stress for any NDA application and even for clinical studies.

In any case, the aim of the forced degradation on drug product is to ensure that all relevant degradation products are generated by suitable and predictive stress conditions. Nevertheless, an overkill (i.e., too extensive stress and exhaustive impurity formation) should be avoided, because the results will not be representative for long-term storage conditions. In addition, the likelihood of potential mutagenic impurity formation should also be addressed. A suitable identification threshold should be defined and above this level the in silico mutagenicity evaluation using Derek, Leadscope, or Multi-Case should be started. If the outcome of the in silico evaluation is deemed positive, the elucidation of the corresponding structure should be initiated. Hence, the aim of preforming forced degradation on drug product is to secure the control space for quality release testing by applying a well-designed knowledge space including all potential modes of degradation, ensuring a good power of degradation prediction. This strategy is schematically presented in Fig. 1.

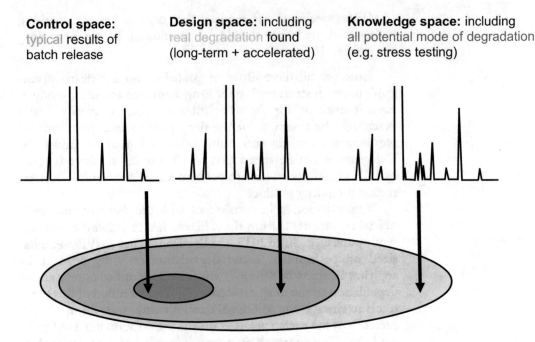

Control space: typical results of batch release

Design space: including real degradation found (long-term + accelerated)

Knowledge space: including all potential mode of degradation (e.g. stress testing)

Fig. 1 Knowledge space definition for forced degradation

Most of the recent publications deal with specific details regarding practical approaches of stressing the drug substance itself in solid state and in solution [14], with and without specific electrochemical oxidation of the molecule [15]. Quite often, these conditions are too strong (over-discriminating) and do not automatically cover all drug product relevant degradation pathways as well as all potential degradation impurities. Most of these publications use forced degradation strategies associated with the classical test conditions (i.e., heat, humidity, oxidative conditions, and light exposition). The stress tests have to be performed twice: first during early drug development and later for registration purposes before industrialization and commercialization take place [16]. In some literature, more severe or exotic stress conditions are marginally mentioned.

Drug substance-specific literatures for pharmaceuticals and biopharmaceuticals give an overview of already developed analytical methods, including the interpretation of the stress test results obtained [17, 18]. Only few of these publications address the prediction of stability of a formulated drug product with respect to long-term stability and/or associated shelf-life calculation. Exception is the quality by design models like "Accelerated Stability Assessment Program (ASAP)", which takes into account the influence of increased temperature and humidity implementing a humidity-corrected Arrhenius equation [19].

2   Stress Testing for Drug Product

The reason that stress testing drug product is important is that in most of the cases pure drug cannot be administered without any functional or nonfunctional excipients, and therefore, the drug substance will be given as a formulated mixture. The final state of the formulation can be solid (e.g., tablets, capsule, powder, transdermal systems), semisolid (e.g., transdermal systems, creams, lipophilic oral forms like soft gels, or melt-extruded formulations), a suspension state (e.g., transdermal systems, spray, oral liquids), or liquid (e.g., oral solution, syrup, inhalation, and vaccines for injection).

The direct contact of the excipients with the drug can have an important impact in terms of stability, because most of the excipients are not fully inert from a chemical or physical point of view. The impact of the excipients towards any potential excipient-drug interaction can be more or less important and temperature dependent, based on the drug substance structure, its concentration in the formulation (drug load), and the kind of interaction (e.g., catalytic versus non-catalytic) and can be influenced also by the particle size of the drug substance itself. In case the drug substance is smaller than the excipients, a "quasi liquid model" can be assumed for which the drug substance in excess is filling all the interstitial spaces between larger excipient particles [20]. Some excipients do stabilize a formulation by changing the direct physicochemical environment of the drug substance, but normally destabilization will occur. This negative stability impact can be directly caused by the different functional groups of the excipients through chemical interaction with the drug substance, or by excipient-specific impurities (e.g., peroxides), degradation products, or any other chemical residues present in the excipients, while reacting with the drug. The presence and amount of active water on the surface of excipients could also have a significant influence [21]. Depending on their structure, some excipients may enhance microbial growth, which could be a cause for physicochemical interaction or a source of destabilization of the developed formulation.

2.1   Modes of Degradation for Drug Products

Generally, the potential negative impact of excipients in terms of drug stability can be distinguished between chemical and/or physical interaction:

1. The order of chemical drug/excipient interactions leading to potential drug degradation is hydrolysis, oxidation, polymerization, and charge interaction. Other instances of degradation are Maillard reaction, e.g., caused by lactose or any other "sugar" like impurities from carboxymethyl cellulose (CMC) producing free radicals. In addition, dehydration, hydrolysis, epimerization, cyclization, and transesterification can also

occur in the presence of silicon dioxide (Aerosil™) that acts as a Lewis base [22].

2. Any physicochemical interaction can be further divided into those leading to visible and/or non-directly/less visible changes or delayed responses. The visible interactions mean change of appearance, precipitation or crystallization of the drug, change in color or disintegration, slowdown of dissolution kinetic, and all kind of organoleptic changes like generation of unpleasant smell. Non-directly visible, less or delayed detectable, or only indirectly measurable interaction could be caused by any change in polymorphic form, amorphization, and change in salt or complexation, which results in a more or less significant loss of bioavailability or change in dissolution profile, which is often used as a correlating in vitro test.

The most commonly encountered mode of interaction is hydrolysis, which happens due to ubiquitous presence of free water. The functional groups prone to hydrolysis are esters, amides, lactones, or lactams [23]. In aqueous solution, the degradation potency of water can be demonstrated by using ^{18}O-labelled water and UPLC-MDS detection. This combination allows detection of the newly formed hydrolytic drug substance impurities [24]. Unfortunately, this ^{18}O-labelled water strategy cannot be applied for most of the drug products because many excipients already contain an important percentage of water, which is either more or less chemically "fixed" or freely available (surface or adsorbed water). The percentage of water in commonly used excipients is summarized in Table 1.

The degree of crystallinity/hygroscopicity of excipients could also have a significant impact on the stability of the drug. The more amorphous the excipient, the more water can be absorbed, which could either destabilize the drug by increasing the free (active) water content in the formulation or stabilize the drug by forming a complex with the water present, which helps in avoiding any further hydrate formation of the drug. This is especially important

Table 1
Total water content of commonly used excipients

Excipient	Total water content (%)
Crospovidone	Up to 60
Dibasic calcium phosphate, dihydrate	~20
Magnesium stearate	Up to 15
Gelatin (capsule shell)	10–15
Cellulose (e.g., MC, HPC, HPMC)	Up to ~10

for those drugs, which are sensitive for this kind of hydrate formation.

The second mode of decomposition for drug product is oxidation, especially critical in the presence of aldehydes, alcohols, phenols, alkaloids, as well as unsaturated fats or oils in the formulation. Oxidation leads to free radicals as an induction process, which can be immediate or sometimes delayed and which is catalyzed by important oxygen levels, traces of heavy metal ions (almost found in all excipients), or light. The free radicals react with oxygen forming peroxy radicals, which in turn interact with oxidizable compounds, generating additional free radicals to fuel further reactions, also called propagation.

Oxidation can also be directly caused by peroxides, which could be found as traces in excipients (e.g., polyethylene glycol (PEG)). Free radical, acting in a single-electron transfer, could also come from a Maillard reaction with sugar or "sugar-like" compounds.

Degradation pathways like charge interaction or polymerization are less common mechanisms. In case of a charge interaction, soluble and ionizable excipients can generate counterions that interact with ionizable drug leading to the formation of insoluble drug-excipient products. Physically, this can be a rapid interaction and easily detectable in liquid systems (e.g., sodium alginate or carboxymethyl cellulose (CMC) proves negatively charged anions, which interact with positively charged drug). The effect may also be less detectable in vitro, if this interaction occurs in vivo by administrating solid oral dosage forms, following ingestion and hydration in the gastrointestinal (GI) tract.

The shift of functional groups in the molecule or intermolecular cyclization could lead to dimeric and higher molecular weight species promoted by excipients, if they either have requisite functional groups present for these kinds of interactions or contain residues that catalyze this process or are being susceptible to change themselves providing additional possibilities for the generation of "species" participating in this "breakdown" process.

2.2 Different Approaches for Drug Product Stress Testing

Different approaches are known for drug product forced degradation/stress testing:

1. Literature search in order to avoid known critical compounds such as magnesium stearate/sodium croscarmellose and lactose. The commonly available knowledge of published data can be used to avoid any "classical" interaction, right from the beginning of the drug product development.

2. In silico approach using different software, those dealing with interaction of drugs with excipients, can be used to check the potential formation of first- and second-order degradation impurities in the presence of different excipients. A software (e.g., Zeneth/Lhasa Ltd.) is built on the knowledge shared by

the pharma companies on a nonprofit basis in order to define the likelihood of degradation based on practical experiments. Another software (e.g., ASAP, FreeThink Technologies) uses the stress stability results obtained from increased humidity and temperature experiments in order to predict the long-term stability profile (*see* Chap. 3). The isoconversion, relative humidity (RH) impact, and statistical evaluation are used as basic principles for this assessment [19, 25].

3. Fast solid-state screening methods are differential scanning calorimetry (DSC), isothermal microcalorimetry, hot-stage microscopy (HSM), powder X-ray diffraction (XRPD), solid-state NMR (ssNMR), or Fourier transformed infrared spectroscopy (FT-IR). These methods do not give any detailed information about the mechanism or interaction/degradation (root cause), but they can give a first hint towards any physico-chemical interaction [26, 27]. Some of the most commonly used techniques are briefly presented below:

- DSC compares the curves obtained from binary (1:1, m/m) physical mixtures of the individual excipients with the pure drug. Significant shift of the melting point or the appearance of new endo/exothermic peaks or any variation in the corresponding enthalpies could indicate an interaction or incompatibility, but a further characterization is not possible. Therefore, the interpretation of these results could be misleading in terms of root cause definition.

- Isothermal microcalorimetry allows detection of the rate of absorbed heat and heating flow signals in the range of μW. The thermal activity of the drug substance and the excipients are measured individually, and then the output of the blend is compared to the non-interaction curve constructed from the individual components.

- HSM allows monitoring efficiently the solid-state interaction like possible dissolution of one compound into another that could be erroneously interpreted as incompatibility by DSC methods.

- Vibrational spectroscopy (Fourier transformed infrared, Raman, FT-IR) is sensitive to the structure and the relative environment of the organic compounds. Effects like desalting hydrate formation, dehydration, polymorphic changes, or transformation into amorphous forms can be easily detected.

- XRPD measurement can help to detect incompatibilities, which occur during manufacturing processes like compression and wet granulation in terms of change in crystallinity and polymorphic form.

- Solid-state (ss) NMR allows detecting any drug-excipient interaction by measuring the chemical shift due to the change of the electron density at the interaction carbon atom. Molecular mobility of water can also be detected, which is directly correlated to the drug substance stability.

4. One-to-one binary compatibility testing, analyzed by using HPLC methods, often performed at 1:1 ratio (m/m), is used to exclude those excipients showing an obvious phenomenon of noncompatibility. This very resource- and time-consuming approach does not often address the real ratio between drug substance and excipients in the final formulation and, therefore, the results obtained can be misinterpreted. Very frequently, the real formulation does not behave like the binary mixtures in terms of degradation.

5. Another aspect is factorial design of experiment (DoE) with statistical evaluation of several potential mixtures of a standard drug product. The relatively complex results obtained are statistically analyzed and could give a ranking or a selection of the most promising combination of drug substance and excipients in terms of compatibility, even if the interpretation of these results is often quite difficult.

6. Preliminary proto-formulation testing allows elucidating the interaction of several excipients with the drug substance itself in a finished formulation in terms of any compatibility issues. This approach is considered as the most predictive one. The composition of formulations is not arbitrarily chosen as for binary or multi-compatibility experiments and, therefore, these results are deemed more representative for the long-term storage stability behavior of drug product, even if the final composition could be somewhat different. During the manufacturing process, these proto-formulations are exposed to certain manufacturing process steps (e.g., milling, sieving, mixing, granulation, and compression), which could have a direct impact in terms of physicochemical transformation. Changes in temperature, pressure, relative humidity (RH), and close interaction to the direct excipient environment could initiate changes like chemical degradation and amorphization or change in polymorphic form, even if the manufacturing parameters are not fully representative for the final (commercial) formulation [28]. The main issue of this approach is the risk to have any extraction or solubility issue during the sample preparation for analysis, which could lead to an incomplete recovery of the drug and further risk of formation of any impurities. For this reason, the verification of the mass balance is deemed crucial.

2.3   Test Material

To test a drug product under stress, four different kinds of exposure could be relevant for solid oral formulation to elucidate any potential instability:

- Temperature.
- Humidity.
- Oxidative environment.
- Light exposition.

For forced degradation, batch stability samples should be tested without any primary packaging material in order to allow the environment to interact directly with the samples. For practical reasons, the sample preparation after stressing and before analyzing has to be standardized. Five test formulation units (e.g., tablets or capsules) are placed together in a wide-neck glass bottle and all of them are analyzed together as a composite sample at each stability time point and for each storage condition. The samples are prepared in duplicate ($n = 2$), which allows analysis of two samples of five units (each) for each stability time point.

Depending on the type of oral formulation and taking into account the sensitivity of the drug substance itself, the temperature and humidity conditions chosen for the stress could be different. First, a temperature above 70 °C is not recommended due to the risk of forming secondary degradation products, which are no longer representative of the degradation pattern expected for long-term storage conditions. Therefore, 70 °C and 70 °C/80% RH should be selected as standard stress conditions for oral drug products, if the drug substance shows a melting point above 130 °C.

For gelatin capsules or formulation containing temperature-sensitive drug substance (melting point below 130 °C), it might be useful to reduce the chosen temperature to about 50 °C (dry) and 50 °C (humid) while maintaining high relative humidity of about 80% RH. In some cases, liquefaction could occur during stress testing, which is not an issue for the further analysis. Whatever physical state is obtained after stressing (e.g., liquefaction, sintering, cake formation), all five specimens are solubilized together before analyzing. The preparation of the samples in duplicate will guarantee the reproducibility of the results by analyzing two individually prepared samples for each storage condition and each stability time point.

Depending on the temperature chosen, 7 or 15 days may be sufficient for stressing (*see* Table 2). The aim of the forced degradation is to reach degradation levels of up to about 10–15%. Higher degradation does not reflect the reality expected for long-term storage. Even if this level is not reached, there may not be need to apply more drastic conditions, provided that the results are easy to interpret for the long-term stability prediction. More than 15% of

Table 2
Storage conditions for forced degradation on drug product

Storage condition	Testing interval (days)			
Tablets				
70 °C/80% RH (open)	(3)	7	15	(30)
70 °C (closed)	(3)	7	15	(30)
70 °C (NMP, closed)	(1)	3	(7)	
Gelatin capsules or temperature sensitive drug products				
50 °C/80% RH (open)		(7)	15	30
50 °C (closed)		(7)	15	30
50 °C (NMP, closed)	(3)	7	(15)	
Photostability according to ICH				
For example SUN-Test (ICH option 1)	(1)	3		

Note: () - optional testing interval, only analyzed if scientifically needed or not sufficient degradation obtained
A relative humidity of 80% RH can be easily obtained by using a desiccator filled with a saturated salt solution of KCl (solubility of KCl at 50 °C: 42.6 g/100 g of water and at 80 °C: 51.1 g/100 g of water)

impurities are considered as critical due to the risk of obtaining secondary degradation products. In some cases, the required level can already be reached after 3 days of stress. To understand the kinetics of degradation in the drug product, at least two independent time points are recommended for each condition. If the level of degradation after 15 or 30 days of stress is too important, the obtained secondary impurities can be easily distinguished from the corresponding primary degradation impurities by comparing these results with those obtained at earlier time points. Nevertheless, even secondary degradation products may help to better understand the overall degradation pathway of the compound identifying the main weaknesses of the chemical structure.

Oxidative conditions with several modes of oxidation could be applied by using N-methyl-2-pyrrolidine (NMP). For this test design, five test samples/specimens have to be put into a large, glass bottle and then about 2–5mL of NMP has to be added before closing the vial. The size of the vials is considered as crucial to ensure a sufficient airspace which will allow oxidizing the present formulation. The ratio of filling versus free air space should be at least 1:5 (v/v). In case that film-coated tablets are used, these tablets have to be broken into two parts or crushed into larger particles in order to be better exposed to NMP which acts as oxidizing solvent. In case that capsules are used, the capsules have to be opened and the contents have to be put together with the shells into the container. Three days might be sufficient for this mode of oxidation in slurry at elevated temperature (at least 50 °C, but more pronounced at 70 °C). A double mode of action is ensured by NMP, i.e., oxidation by radical and peroxide production [29].

Photostability stress testing should be done by applying three times ICH Q1B conditions [2]. If this exposure is too strong, a shorter exposure time of about 1 day with an overall illumination of about 1.2 million lux h and a near-ultraviolet energy of a minimum of 200 Watt h/m^2 with a spectral distribution of 320–400 nm should be sufficient. To start photostability testing, the oral formulations should be used "as is" without any grinding or mechanical reworking. Hard-gelatin capsules should be tested first "as is" without opening and second by emptying the content of the capsules into a petri dish. The testing of the intact capsule elucidates the protective properties of the capsules' shell versus the present amount of water bound towards degradation. Testing the content of capsule without shell maximizes the exposure of the granulated formulation to the light. A dark control covered by aluminum foil has to be examined systematically in parallel in order to exclude any temperature (warming) effects.

2.4 Analytical Methods

For all forced degradation experiments discussed above, the analytical tests to be applied are listed in Table 3. Visual evaluation (e.g., coloration or changes in solid state) could give initial hints regarding any chemical issues. Moreover, first change could indicate any incompatibility or degradation (e.g., Maillard reaction), which may not be visible or quantifiable at the beginning of degradation process by the analytical methods applied.

For the verification of assay and related impurities by high-pressure liquid chromatography (HPLC), a second, different (using a different column or gradient) or orthogonal method (e.g., SFC, TLC, or IC) should be applied in order to check that all formed impurities are detected and adequately reported. In addition, a universal mode of detection (e.g., mass spectrometric (MS) or MS/MS) or a second mode of detection (charged aerosol (Corona™), light scattering (e.g., evaporating light scattering detector (ELSD)) or fluorometric detection in parallel to the classical UV/diode array detection could be used in order to ensure that all impurities, even with a low or no UV response, can be detected in a systemic manner. If MS detection is used, it has to be ensured that the mode (e.g., electro spray or ionization) of activation is working for all impurities present in a complex matrix formulation. In order to ensure that the sample is completely solubilized during preparation, the most suitable extraction solvent has to be selected first. In case that potential impurities do not have the same solubility as the drug itself, several mixtures or several solvents have to be tested towards matrix effect and recovery issues. The excipients commonly used are not soluble in organic solvents and therefore

Table 3
Analytical testing for forced degradation studies on drug product

Test item	Description
Description (visual)	Change in color or aspect could be helpful to detect minor chemical changes
Assay (LC)	To be determined using an external reference standard. In addition, the mass balance should be verified by taking into account the impurity level obtained
Related impurities (LC)	The aim of the forced degradation is to lead to about 10–15% degradation
Chiral impurities (chiral LC or SFC)	Required in case that the compound is chiral and a conversion could be obtained in solid state
Water content (Karl Fischer [KF])	The amount of absorbed water can help to interpret the mode of degradation or the formation of a (mono/poly)-hydrated form microcoulometry should be used instead of KF in case of low water amounts ($<0.5\%$ (m/m))
Dissolution (UV or LC)	Verifying the dissolution rate in case the individual specimens are still intact (i.e., they can be used individually using USP2 (paddle) and not aggregated together under humid stress storage conditions)
Polymorphism (XRPD/Raman) TGA Differential scanning calorimetry (DSC)	In case that the compound has several polymorphic forms or hydrates and a conversion could occur into another form or salt

some kind of solubility issues or precipitation could occur which cannot be easily detected during sample preparation. In addition, the separation of the non-solubilized solid residuals should be done preferably by centrifugation instead of filtration, because filtration can favor any adsorption of the drug substance or impurities on the filtration membrane. If the most suitable solvent or solvent mixture has been selected for the sample preparation, it has to be ensured that no negative impact could occur on any chromatographic parameters (e.g., degradation on column, peak doubling, peak tailing or fronting) during sample analysis.

In case that the signal from an impurity is dependent on the UV response, a correction factor has to be introduced in the calculation of these impurities in order to guarantee a sufficient mass balance. The first approximate correction factor could be established by comparing the UV spectra at the chosen wavelength or by varying the wavelength using a diode array detector or using a UV-independent detection mode (e.g., charged aerosol detector), even if some complementary detection modes are often not linear over a large range of absorption. At levels of 1.0% (area-%) or higher for a new formed impurity, a structure elucidation should be initiated (MS and MS/MS). As a generic rule, a total standard variability of about 5% for the mass balance can be considered as uncritical depending on the number and level of impurities obtained. At levels of 5% or higher, the relevance and applicability of the ICH M7 guideline should be considered towards mutagenicity evaluation, which has to be discussed on a case-by-case basis and depending on their probability of formation under long-term storage conditions. These impurities should be checked in silico (e.g., Derek, MultiCase, Leadscope) and later tested in in vitro mutagenicity models (e.g., Ames 2 or Ames) after their isolation or synthesis, if the outcome of the in silico evaluation is positive [30].

Normal-phase, chiral liquid chromatography (LC) or supercritical fluid chromatography (SFC) methods could additionally be used in order to check any potential changes in terms of enantiomer ratio, if chemically deemed possible. These methods are recommended to be applied at least at the last stress stability time point in order to generate data to answer any potential questions from the health authorities, even if these questions might chemically not always be justified.

The verification of the water content (e.g., free, adsorbed, or hydrate) can give some important information about any potential risk towards physicochemical instability, if the compound is deemed sensitive to hydrolytic degradation. The type of water uptake can be easily followed either by Karl Fischer (total water) or microcoulometry (surface and total water depending on the titration curve obtained). Differential scanning calorimetry (DSC) or thermogravimetric analysis (TGA) is more selective because it can distinguish between all types of water by successive water losses. In addition, DVS experiments can characterize the sorption and desorption hysteresis of the formulation. This provides information about specific humidity ranges that could potentially induce polymorphic transition. The verification of the physical form depends on the concentration of the drug substance in the final drug product. Drug substance loads of less than 10% (m/m) might be difficult to explore in terms of physical changes within the drug product depending upon the selectivity of the methods applied (e.g., X-ray powder diffraction (XRPD), Raman).

3   Objective of Long-Term Stability Studies

The aim of the primary stability studies is to confirm the degradation profile expected for these storage conditions - based on the experience gained during drug product development and taking into account the results derived from the forced degradation stabilities - and to estimate the shelf-life to be claimed for registration with the support of statistics (if appropriate). Primary stability studies are typically scheduled for duration of 3–5 years under long-term conditions, preferably at 30 °C/65% RH. Storage at 30 °C/75% RH could be an option for a worldwide submission (i.e., including zone IVb countries), if sufficiently stable.

In case of any non-expected stability issues, more conservative storage conditions (25 °C/60% RH) should be added to the protocol as optional testing points or reserve samples in order to switch during the ongoing stability study, if needed. Refrigerated conditions (5 °C) should always be added as a reference that is tested only if needed or requested by certain agencies (e.g., Canada, Japan). To define and justify a broad storage label such as 2–30 °C, samples stored at that condition may be tested for that purpose at least annually.

Long-term testing should be accompanied by photostability testing, which is recommended to be performed as near as possible to the initial test point. For this test, an overall illumination of at least 1.2 million lux hours and an integrated near-ultraviolet energy of not less than 200 Watt h/m^2 should be ensured and the oral formulations should be used as is without any grinding or mechanical reworking. A dark control covered by aluminum foil has to be included systematically in order to exclude any temperature (warming) effects. In the case where the bulk formulation is confirmed to be light sensitive, the test has to be performed using the primary packaging material. The intended clinical or marketing secondary packaging has only to be tested in case the primary packaging fails to sufficiently protect the drug product justifying the labelling for light protection.

3.1   Test Material

The batches under stability testing for regulatory submission must be representative of the commercial formulation, packaging, and processes used. In case of differences that are not negligible, the first three commercial batches should be put on stability to prove their comparability.

3.2   Packaging

Batch stability samples should be packaged in the final primary packaging (e.g., blister Al/PVC, Al/PVDC, Al/PCTFE (Aclar®) or Al/Al or HPDE/glass bottles) with different size, volume, and filling based on the intended commercialization strategy. The selection of the blister material in terms of water vapor transition rate should be based on the results gathered during stress testing studies. In case of bottles, the container storage orientation has to be defined prior to the start of the stability study in order to allow (or not) interaction with the container closure system (e.g., storage upright versus storage inverted). The secondary packaging definition is mandatory for photostability testing if primary packaging material does sufficiently protect the drug product from light degradation.

Table 4
Typical study design for studies on drug product intended to be marketed worldwide

Storage condition	Testing interval (months)										
	0	3	6	9	12	18	24	30	36	48	60
Long-term											
5 °C ± 3 °C (refrigeration)			x				x	(x)	x	(x)	(x)
30 °C ± 2 °C/65% RH ± 5% RH	x	x	x	(x)	x	x	x	(x)	x	(x)	(x)
or 30 °C ± 2 °C/75% RH ± 5% RH (zone IVb)		x	x	(x)	x	x	x	(x)	x	(x)	(x)
Intermediate											
25 °C ± 2 °C/60% RH ± 5% RH	(Reserve samples only, analyzed in case of instability issues at 30 °C/65% RH)										
Accelerated											
40 °C ± 2 °C/75% RH ± 5% RH		x	x								
Photostability											
For example SUN-Test (ICH option 1)	x				1 day						

Note: () - optional testing interval

3.3 Storage Conditions

Common long-term, intermediate, as well as accelerated storage conditions following ICH Q1A(R2) guideline for a worldwide submission are listed in Table 4 [1]. A sufficient amount of additional reserve samples may be stored for each storage condition without being routinely tested, but being pulled and investigated only on demand in case of any analytical investigation needs (e.g., in case of unexpected results). The quantity of the reserve samples should allow performing at least 2 times full testing for long-term storage and at least 1 full testing for accelerated storage.

As soon as the samples are pulled from the stability chambers for analyzing, they have to be stored at defined storage conditions until testing, typically the used long-term storage conditions, protected from light and moisture for all storage samples.

4 Bracketing and Matrixing Design for Stability Testing

ICH Q1D recommends that matrixing and bracketing can be applied, if sufficiently justified, to the testing of new drug substances and products, but provides no further guidance on that subject [31]. A reduced stability design can be a suitable alternative to a full testing design, when multiple design factors are involved. Any reduced design should have the ability to adequately predict the retest period or shelf-life. During the course of a reduced designed stability study, a chance to resort to full testing or to a less reduced design can be considered, if a justification is provided and the principle of full design and reduced design is followed. However, proper adjustments should be made to the statistical analysis, where applicable, to account for the increase in sample size as a result of the change. Once the design is changed, full testing or less reduced testing should be carried out through the remaining time points of the stability study.

4.1 Bracketing Approach

Bracketing design may be an option to reduce the stability testing effort for each test interval, if more than one strength and/or packaging configuration of a homothetic or very close to market formulation is followed on stability. In this case, not all of the strengths will be submitted to the authorities; only the extremes of certain design factors (e.g., strength, container size, or filling) are tested and reported at all time points as in a full design (*see* Table 5). The design assumes that the stability of any intermediate level is represented by the stability of the extremes tested. If the stability of the extremes (dosages or packaging sizes/volumes) is shown to be different, the intermediates should be considered no more stable than the least stable extreme.

For the intermediate-strength samples, which are not deemed to be tested, it is recommended to store at least three or four times the amount needed for full testing in case of any issues for the extreme dosage strengths. The testing of the interim samples is launched in exceptional cases only, e.g., if one of the extremes has shown a significant change (i.e., a confirmed out-of-specification result) or a trend to fail staying within its specifications for the full target shelf-life or if testing the interim strength(s) is requested by a regulatory agency.

In the case where there are several packaging sizes, more sophisticated designs could be applied (*see* Table 6). This bracketing approach is commonly accepted by most of the authorities without any further request and saves about 50% of laboratory resources in total.

Table 5
Bracketing approach for drug product stability using three strengths and one packaging

Strength on stability (homothetic or close to market formulation)	Test design
Lowest	Storage and full testing
Middle	Storage and no routine testing
Highest	Storage and full testing

Table 6
Example for bracketing (three strengths, three packaging sizes)

Strength		Low			Middle			High		
Batch		First	Second	Third	First	Second	Third	First	Second	Third
Container/closure (volume)	Low	X	X	X				X	X	X
	Middle									
	High	X	X	X				X	X	X

4.2 Matrixing Approach

Following ICH Q1D [31], matrixing is the design of a stability schedule such that a selected subset of total number of possible samples for all factor combinations would be tested at a specific time point. At a subsequent time point, another subset of samples for all factor combinations would be tested. The design assumes that stability of each subset of samples tested represents the stability of all samples at a given time point (*see* Table 7). Matrixing could be applied if a homothetic or very close to market formulation is followed on stability. In any case, the use of matrixing approach has to be discussed with the health authorities before starting, typically at the end of Phase IIb meetings (EoP2b).

Matrixing design requires a statistical support with balanced protocols allowing to evaluate a fraction of all possible combinations of factors (e.g., strengths, packaging) of a drug at each intermediate time point, thereby significantly reducing the required resources and equipment run-time. In a design where time points are matrixed, all selected factor combinations should be tested at the initial and final time points. If full long-term date is not available for review before approval, all selected combinations should be tested at 12 months or at the last time point prior to submission. When a secondary packaging system contributes to the stability of the drug product, matrixing can be performed across the packaging systems. Each storage condition should be treated separately under its own matrixing design. Matrixing should not be performed across test attributes. Factors that can be matrixed are the following:

1. Different strengths with identical formulations
   (a) With different fill plug sizes for capsules.
   (b) With varying amounts of the same granulation for tablets.
   (c) Same process and equipment.
2. Container sizes and/or filling sizes in the same container closure system.
3. Intermediate time points.

Table 7
Matrixing approach according to ICH Q1D

Number of combinations of factors, excluding time points	Amount of supportive date available		
	Substantial (e.g., significant body of data on production batches for supplemental changes)	Moderate (e.g., sufficient amount of data on clinical batches for original NDA approval)	Little or not (e.g., little or no data on clinical batches for original NDA approval)
Large (e.g., 3 * 3 * 3)	Fractional (e.g., 1/2)	Fractional (e.g., 5/8)	Full (matrixing not suitable)
Moderate (e.g., 3 * 3 * 3)	Fractional (e.g., 5/8)	Fractional (e.g., 3/4)	Full (matrixing not suitable)
Very small (e.g., 3 * 3 * 3)	Fractional (e.g., 3/4)	Full (matrixing not suitable)	Full (matrixing not suitable)

Factors that can be matrixed, if justified based on supporting data:

1. Different strengths with differing relative amounts of drug substance and excipients.

2. Different container closure systems.

3. Orientations of container during storage.

4. Drug substance manufacturing sites.

5. Drug product manufacturing sites.

Factors that should not be matrixed:

1. Initial and final time points.

2. Test parameters.

3. Dosage forms.

4. Storage conditions.

A statistical justification could be based on an evaluation of the proposed matrixing design with respect to its power to detect differences among factors in the degradation rates or its precision in shelf-life estimation. The stability data obtained under a matrixing protocol should respect three steps in statistical analysis:

1. Individual linear regressions are applied to the three batches to test the significance of the slopes.

2. Covariance analysis tests the poolability of the data: (a) If the test for equality of the slopes leads to $p < 0.25$, then the batch is treated individually. (b) If the test for equality of the slopes leads to $p > 0.25$ and the test for equality of the intercepts leads

to $p < 0.25$, the calculations are done for each batch but the common slope is used. (c) If the test for equality of the slopes leads to $p > 0.25$ and the test for equality of the intercepts leads to $p > 0.25$, the data are pooled.

3. Shelf-life, calculated on the individual data or pooled data as a function of the covariance analysis results, is based on the 95% one-sided confidence curves. The expiration dating period is the point where the 95% one-sided confidence interval for the mean intersects the specification limit. In case of one analysis per batch, the overall expiration dating period will depend on the minimum time a batch may be expected to remain within acceptable limits.

All the calculations use individual independent measurements. In case of less than two quantifiable values per batch, at least for two batches, the compound is considered as stable without any statistical analysis. Otherwise, if values below the limit of quantification are not available, they are estimated by half the time of quantification. However, matrixing following ICH Q1D can be done:

- Only on time points (complete design with 5/8 approach, *see* Table 8)
- On time points while the strength is bracketed (3/4 matrix and bracketing design, *see* Table 9)
- On time points and factors (*see* Table 10)

Table 8
Complete matrixing design with 5/8 time points

Batch Strength	First batch Low	Middle	High	Second batch Low	Middle	High	Third batch Low	Middle	High
Container/closure	1 2 3	1 2 3	1 2 3	1 2 3	1 2 3	1 2 3	1 2 3	1 2 3	1 2 3
Schedule	1 2 3	2 3 1	3 1 2	2 3 1	3 1 2	1 2 3	3 1 2	1 2 3	2 3 1

Time point (months)	0	3	6	9	12	18	24
1		X	X		X		X	X
2		X		X	X	X	X
3		X		X	X	X	X

Table 9
Bracketing design and 3/4 matrixing (overall size: 1/2)

Batch Strength	First batch — Low			First batch — Middle			First batch — High			Second batch — Low			Second batch — Middle			Second batch — High			Third batch — Low			Third batch — Middle			Third batch — High		
Container/closure	1	2	3	1	2	3	1	2	3	1	2	3	1	2	3	1	2	3	1	2	3	1	2	3	1	2	3
Schedule	1	2	3				3	1	2	2	3	1				1	2	3	3	1	2				2	3	1

Time point (months)	0	3	6	9	12	18	24	36
1	X	X		X	X	X		X
2	X	X	X		X		X	X
3	X		X	X	X		X	X

Table 10
Matrixing on time points and factors

Strength Container size	Low — A	B	C	Middle — A	B	C	High — A	B	C
Batch 1	1	2		2		1		1	2
Batch 2		3	1	3	1		1		3
Batch 3	3		2		2	3	2	3	

Time point (months)	0	3	6	9	12	18	24	36
1	X		X	X	X	X	X	X
2	X	X		X	X		X	X
3	X	X	X		X	X		X

5 Analytical Testing

The stability-indicating test items listed in Table 11 have to be performed at each stability time point. All analytical methods are required to be sufficiently validated according to ICH guidelines. Analytical results have to be compared to the current acceptance criteria given that these limits were defined for the quality of the test material.

Table 11
Analytical testing for worldwide ICH stability studies

Test item	Comments
Description (visual)	Change in color or aspect could be helpful to detect minor chemical changes
Assay (LC)	To be determined using an external reference standard
Related impurities (LC)	Verify the impurity profile compared to that of the stress studies
Dissolution (UV or LC)	Verify the impact of the storage condition towards the dissolution behavior
Disintegration	Could replace dissolution testing for BCS1 compounds or done additionally
Chiral impurities (chiral LC or SFC)	To be done in case that the compound is chiral and a conversion could be possible in solid state
Water content (KF or microcoulometry)	In case that the presence of active (free) water could negatively influence the chemical or physical stability
Physical form (XRPD)	In case that the compound has several polymorphic forms and a conversion into another form or salt might be possible in solid state
Microbiological contamination (TAMC, TYMC, *E. coli*)	To be tested at least at the end of the stability study

Note: *LC* - liquid chromatography, *SFC* - supercritical fluid chromatography, *XPRD* - X-ray powder diffraction, *TAMC* - total aerobic microbial count, *TYMC* - total yeast/mold count

---

6 Conclusion

Excipients are often not inert from the physicochemical point of view. A lot of potential test designs for stressing drug substance/excipient mixtures are currently in practice by the pharmaceutical companies. In order to be as predictive as possible towards long-term stability study outcomes, the focus should be on proto-formulations testing under "soft" stress conditions. During these studies, suitable chemical and physical test conditions should be applied to identify the weaknesses of the chosen formulation. The verification of the mass balance including a first approximate verification of any correction factor for new impurities detected is an integral part for this first drug product assessment. In addition, any potential matrix effect in terms of recovery issues during sample preparation or lack of method selectivity should be addressed. The design of the (primary) stability design for drug product should be based on the knowledge gained from stress testing experiments as well as during clinical formulation development covering a period of 36 or 60 months of investigation. Preferably 30 °C/65% RH or

30 °C/75% RH should be chosen as long-term storage condition, depending on the stability of the formulation towards humidity.

In any case, at least 12 months' real-time stability data should be provided during submission in order to claim a sufficient shelf-life for marketing purposes. Based on the experience from forced degradation stabilities (stress tests), no new and unknown impurities should be detected during ICH stability studies. The batches under stability testing for submission must be representative of the commercial formulation, packaging, and processes used. Matrixing and bracketing approaches can be applied, if sufficiently justified, to the testing of new drug substances and products. Knowing that bracketing is usually accepted, the design and strategy for matrixing, which depend upon the different intended formulations, packaging sizes, and statistical software used for evaluation, should be discussed in advance with the authorities before starting these stability studies. Use of any in silico prediction shelf-life calculation (e.g., ASAP) utilizing stress test results could be helpful during the discussion with the health authorities if this is a concern, in terms of stability design and shelf-life claiming.

References

1. ICH Harmonised Tripartite Guideline Q1A (R2) Stability testing of new drug substances and products, step 4 version (2003). http://www.ich.org/home.html

2. ICH Harmonised Tripartite Guideline Q1B, Photostability testing of new drug substances and products, step 4 version (1996) http://www.ich.org/home.html

3. ICH Harmonised Tripartite Guideline Q1E, Evaluation for stability data, step 4 version (2003, February). http://www.ich.org/home.html

4. ICH Harmonised Tripartite Guideline Q2 (R1), Validation of analytical procedures: text and methodology, step 4 version (2005). http://www.ich.org/home.html

5. ICH Harmonised Tripartite Guideline Q3B (R2), Impurities in new drug products, step 4 version (2006). http://www.ich.org/home.html

6. ICH Harmonised Tripartite Guideline Q6A, Specifications: test procedures and acceptance criteria for new drug substances and new drug products: chemical substances, step 4 version (1999). http://www.ich.org/home.html

7. Brazilian Health Surveillance Agency (ANVISA) Resolution RDC n° 53/2015. http://www.portal.anvisa.gov.br

8. Tattersall P, Asawasiripong S, Takenaka I, Castoro JA (2016) Impact from the recent issuance of ANVISA resolution RDC-53/2015 on pharmaceutical small molecule forced degradation study requirements. American Pharmaceutical Review

9. Janzen H (2016) Forced degradation studies—comparison between ICH, EMA, FDA and WHO guidelines and ANVISA's resolution RDC 53/2015, Master of Drug Regulatory Affairs, Faculty of Mathematics and Science, University of Bonn/Germany

10. ASEAN (2012) Guideline on stability of drug product, Philippines

11. HAS (2011) Guidance on medicinal product registration in Singapore, Singapore

12. CDSCO (2010) Draft guidance on approval of clinical trials and new drugs. New Delhi, India

13. Singh S, Junwal M, Modhe G, Tiwari H, Kurmi M, Parashar N, Sidduri P (2013) Forced degradation studies to assess the stability of drugs and products. Trends Anal Chem 49:71–88

14. Blessy M, Patel RD, Prajapati PN, Agrawal YK (2014) Development of forced degradation and stability-indicating studies of drugs—a review. J Pharm Anal 4(3):159–165

15. Torres S, Brown R, Zelesky T, Scrivens G, Szucs R, Hawkins JM, Taylor MR (2016) Electrochemical oxidation coupled with liquid chromatography and mass spectrometry to study the oxidative stability of active

pharmaceutical ingredients in solution: a comparison of off-line and on-line approaches. J Pharm Biomed Anal 131:71–79

16. Alsante KM, Ando A, Brown R, Ensing J, Hatajik TD, Kong W, Tsuda Y (2007) The role of degradant profiling in active pharmaceutical ingredients and drug products. Adv Drug Deliv Rev 59:29–37

17. Jain D, Basniwal PK (2013) Forced degradation and impurity profiling: recent trends in analytical perspectives. J Pharm Biomed Anal 86:11–35

18. Tamizi E, Jouyban A (2016) Forced degradation studies of biopharmaceuticals: selection of stress conditions. Eur J Pharm Biopharm 98:26–46

19. Watermann KC (2011) The application of the accelerated stability assessment program (ASAP) to Quality by Design (QbD) for drug product stability. AAPS J 12(3):932–937

20. Waterman KC, Gerst P, Dai Z (2012) A generalized relation for solid-state drug stability as a function of excipient dilution: temperature-independent behavior. J Pharm Sci 101(11):4170–4177

21. Bharate SS, Bharate SB, Bajaj AN (2010) Interaction and incompatibilities of pharmaceutical excipients with active pharmaceutical ingredients: a comprehensive review. J Excip Food Chem 1(3):3–26

22. Wu Y, Dali A, Gupta A, Raghavan K (2009) Understanding drug-excipient compatibility: oxidation of compound A in a solid dosage form. Pharm Dev Technol 14(5):556–564

23. Airaksinen S (2005) Role of excipients in moisture sorption and physical stability of solid pharmaceutical formulations. Academic Dissertation, Faculty of Pharmacy, Helsinki

24. Ludvigsson JW, Andersson T, Kjellberg V (2016) A new method to identify hydrolytic degradants in drug substances with UPLC-MS using ^{18}O-labelled water. J Pharm Biomed Anal 122:9–15

25. Parenty AD, Button WG, Ott MA (2013) An expert system to predict the forced degradation of organic molecules. Mol Pharm 10(8):2962–2974

26. Schmitt EA, Peck K, Sun Y, Geoffroy JM (2001) Rapid, practical and predictive excipients compatibility screening using isothermal microcalorimetry. Thermochim Acta 380:175–183

27. Patel JP, Ahir K, Patel V, Manami L, Patel C (2015) Drug excipient compatibility studies: first step for dosage form development. J Pharm Innov 4(5):14–20

28. Shulka R, Singh R, Arfi S, Tiwari R, Tiwari G, Pranaywal (2016) Degradation and its forced effect: a trenchant tool for stability studies. Int J Univers Pharm Life Sci 7(4):4987–4995

29. Reynolds DW, Galvani M, Hicks SR et al (2012) The use of N-methylpyrrolidone as cosolvent and oxidant in Pharmaceutical stress testing. J Pharm Sci 101(2):761–776

30. ICH M7 (2014) Assessment and control of DNA reactive (mutagenic) impurities in pharmaceuticals to limit potential carcinogenic risk, step 4. http://www.ich.org/home.html

31. ICH Q1D (2002) Bracketing and matrixing designs for stability testing of new drug substances and drug product, step 4. http://www.ich.org/home.html

Chapter 5

A Model Approach for Developing Stability-Indicating Analytical Methods

Peter Persich, Mario Hellings, Shalu Jhajra, Pradeep Phalke, and Koen Vanhoutte

Abstract

Analytical methods play a key role in the pharmaceutical development of drugs. The method development process continuously evolves in parallel with the evolution of the drug and its products. Additionally, the likelihood of approval is strongly dependent on the development phase of the drug candidates. Therefore, it makes sense to differentiate the analytical method development and validation strategy between early and late development. In this chapter, we elucidate a strategy to develop liquid chromatography methods that are fit-for-purpose in early development and robust in late development.

Key words Liquid chromatography, Stability-indicating, Analytical method development, Analytical method validation, Early development, Late development, Forced degradation study, Method screening, Sample preparation, Gage R&R

1 Introduction

In the pharmaceutical development of drugs, analytical method development, validation, and transfer play a key role and can have a large contribution in efficiency improvement, cost, and time reduction of the overall development process. These method-related activities are strongly linked to each other, i.e., changes required in the method in turn might require supplemental validation or transfer activities [1].

Analytical method development is a continuous process that progresses in parallel with the evolution of the drug products [1]. Inherently, the method development process is impacted by changes in the synthetic route of the drug substance, changes in the formulation, and/or changes in the manufacturing process of the drug product. On top of it, high product attrition rates are commonly observed in the pharmaceutical industries engaged in innovative and or/new chemical entity product development. A recent study of clinical development success rates between 2006 and 2015

Sanjay Bajaj and Saranjit Singh (eds.), *Methods for Stability Testing of Pharmaceuticals*, Methods in Pharmacology and Toxicology, https://doi.org/10.1007/978-1-4939-7686-7_5, © Springer Science+Business Media, LLC, part of Springer Nature 2018

revealed that the overall likelihood of Phase 1 drug candidates to reach final approval was only 9.6%. Of the four development phases (Phase I, Phase II, Phase III, and regulatory filing), the drug development transition of Phase II to Phase III encountered the lowest success rate [2]. Consequently, it makes sense to differentiate between early development (ED) and late development (LD) phases with their individual requirements and objectives. In a simplified picture, ED strategies have to enable a generalized and fast throughput of drug candidates to gain a timely proof of therapeutic concept. In contrast to that, the goal in LD is robustness and practicability. The latter often requires the implementation of case-specific processes and control strategies. All these observations lead to the need for fit-for-purpose method development/validation/ transfer strategies, which ensure that laboratory resources are optimally deployed, while the methods still meet the individual goals required at each stage of drug development [1, 3]. A glimpse of method development/validation strategies is can be found in Fig. 1.

In early phase, the first analytical methods focus on the determination of potency of the drug substance and also the drug product to ensure correct dose delivery in the clinic. These methods should be stability-indicating, being able to identify key impurities as well as degradation products, thus ensuring a consistent safety profile. At last, the methods should help to evaluate drug characteristics, such as crystal form, drug release, and content uniformity because these properties are key to ensuring the bioavailability. As

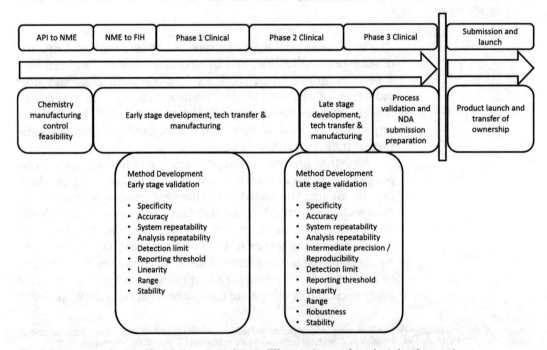

Fig. 1 Method development/validation strategies at different stages of product development

drug development progresses, the analytical methods are refined and expanded, based on increased drug substance and drug product knowledge. In the later phases of drug development, when drug substance and drug product processes are locked and need to be transferred to global manufacturing facilities, analytical methods need to be cost effective, easily executable, and robust such that they perform consistently, irrespective of where they are implemented [1, 3].

In this chapter we elucidate a strategy that is fit-for-purpose during ED and has a strong focus on robustness in LD. Due to its unrivaled specificity, universality, and conclusiveness, we focus this chapter on the development of liquid chromatographic (LC) methods, which is the main technique employed in analytical control strategies.

2   Early Stage Method Development

2.1   General Considerations

The development of stability-indicating analytical methods poses a particular challenge for projects in the ED. As outlined above, there are good reasons to consider the ED to cover all preclinical and early clinical phases until Phase 2b. Independently from the complexity of each individual project, there are four main points of attention when developing a stability-indicating method in ED:

1. Naturally, at this early stage only very little is known about the expected impurity or degradation profile of a drug candidate as no comprehensive stability studies or batch records are available.

2. Changes and improvements of the synthetic route, chemical reaction conditions, purification steps, formulations, and manufacturing process are rather common in ED. All these changes may have an impact on the impurity profile and stability performance of the drug candidate.

3. As the focus in preclinical and early clinical phases is on patient safety, a reasonably comprehensive understanding of expected impurities and degradation products is a must despite above-mentioned uncertainties.

4. Improvements made in subsequent phases of development strongly depend on findings in ED, hence relying on a steep learning curve.

Despite these considerations, it is a fact that the majority of drug candidates will fail during preclinical and ED. Hence, time, effort, and resources spent for the development of an ED analytical method have always to be weighed against the need for a high-throughput efficiency. As a solution to this dilemma, it is recommended to not aim for a "perfect" method for a particular drug candidate, but rather work towards a method being "fit-for-purpose" in the ED phase. It is worth to purposefully establish a general systematic approach and process flow for the development of an ED method. Following of this approach enables a standardized, speedy, and resource-friendly process for each individual case.

2.2 General Process to Develop an ED Method

Before discussing the approach of developing an assay/purity method for ED projects, one should reflect on the general features and requirements of such a "fit-for-purpose" method. Although some of these requirements hold true for LD methods as well, the following are the main features to focus on in the case of an ED method:

Stability-indicating: An ED method should be able to detect any known, but also unforeseen deviations, from the target product profile. This means that in the best case, all degradation products and synthesis-related impurities are well detectable and do not co-elute with the drug substance peak. This allows the method to be called "stability-indicating". Furthermore, in most cases this method is also supposed to be used for setting of specifications or kinetic model-based predictions of the shelf-life like accelerated stability assessment program (ASAP) [4] (*see* Chap. 10). For this reason, it should be a goal as well that major degradation products and impurities are not just separated from the drug substance peak, but also from each other, to be able to correctly quantify them. It is emphasized to focus on those degradation products having a high probability of being shelf-life limiting. A co-elution of other (minor) degradation products and impurities can be regarded as acceptable as long as it is well documented in the method description.

Compatible with mass spectrometry (MS): Compatibility of the method with MS accounts for the little degree of knowledge during ED and will enable a steep learning curve regarding the nature and criticality of newly observed degradation products and impurities. Any expected changes in synthesis and manufacturing process may give rise to unexpected and unknown impurities or degradation products in the drug substance or the drug product, requiring their identification. The option to run the ED method, if required, on an LC-MS instrument will not only help to gain further understanding of process parameters, but also assists in meeting regulatory expectations regarding the safety of the product. To enable compatibility with MS, the ED method should avoid nonvolatile components in the mobile phase, such as phosphate buffers.

Simple and standardized: For the vast majority of ED projects, it is the main goal to get an answer on the critical questions regarding compound safety, clinical efficacy, or therapeutic proof of concept.

That is why a high-throughput efficacy of drug candidates in the ED phase is required to get these questions answered as soon as possible. Therefore, analytical methods in the ED phase should be as simple, straightforward, and standardized as possible. Such an approach enables quick method development, transfer, training, and laboratory implementation.

Amongst the above, the feature "stability-indicating" is certainly the most important one. To be able to systematically develop stability-indicating methods, the execution of a forced degradation study of the drug substance is inevitable. This should, therefore, be the first activity performed prior to the actual method development. As a forced degradation study is designed to investigate the intrinsic stability of the drug substance, its outcome usually does not depend on the source of the drug substance, as irrespective of the source, the molecule will undergo degradation in the same way. So this study can be performed on a readily accessible laboratory scale or medicinal chemistry batch of the drug substance. It is beyond the scope of this chapter to describe the execution of a forced degradation study and excellent reviews can be found elsewhere [5]. However, this study should cover at least the most relevant degradation pathways (hydrolytic, oxidative, thermal, and light) and also evaluate the stability in organic solvents in order to identify a suitable dilution solvent for the ED method. In order to maximize the chance to detect all relevant degradation products from a forced degradation study, some general rules should be followed when analyzing the stress samples:

1. Use of a powerful chromatographic method with a good separation capability and a wide chromatographic gradient, maximizing the chance of detecting a broad range of possible polar and nonpolar compounds.

2. Collection of chromatographic data of stressed samples over a wide range of detection wavelengths using a photodiode array (PDA) detector.

3. Use of at least one other orthogonal detection technique like a benchtop mass detector (e.g., single quadrupole) for degradation products with a poor UV response.

Following of these rules will make sure that all relevant degradation products for a forced degradation study are detected and none of them gets missed either by not eluting from the column or by co-eluting with the drug. Other approaches, like 2D-LC, would be possible as well, but require dedicated instruments and much more time of development and hence are less useful for ED projects with their constrained timelines and resources.

It is recommended to identify the major degradation products under each condition and to elucidate the structure by MS. For the development of a stability-indicating method a decision on

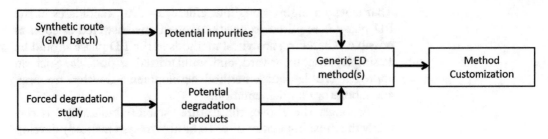

Fig. 2 Process flow to develop an ED method

potential degradation products has to be made. A critical evaluation of the forced degradation data is required in order to identify those degradation products that have a high probability to be observed under stability testing conditions. Although the degradation profile is very compound specific, 3–5 major degradation products from a forced degradation study, considered as potential degradation products, should be sufficient in most cases. Figure 2 shows the process flow to develop an ED method.

As the final method is supposed to monitor not just the degradation products, but synthesis-related impurities as well, an assessment of those potential impurities is needed. This might be difficult, since the final synthetic route (e.g., for the first GMP batch) has to be known. Even if this route is known, typically not enough data are available to assess the criticality and purging effects of synthetic precursors. Also, the formation of side reactions is often not fully understood at this stage. Therefore, in most cases a purely paper-based assessment on potential impurities needs to be performed. It is scientifically sound to assume that firstly the precursors of the last synthetic steps and secondly actual impurities detected in the final drug substance batch are likely potential impurities for later batches as well. Also in case of potential impurities, it is recommended to aim for 3–5 compounds to be considered for method development.

This above-described assessment of potential degradation products and impurities is a prerequisite for method development activities in ED and it should be a good practice to perform this assessment on a standard basis. Different approaches are possible to proceed with all this information towards a suitable final method. It is the opinion of the authors that performing a comprehensive screening of all possible chromatographic parameters (e.g., columns, mobile phases, flow rates, column temperature amongst others) is not a suitable strategy in the ED phase. It is rather better to preselect a limited number of robust and versatile generic methods with a predefined set of parameters. These generic methods can be considered as fixed working platforms for the development of all ED methods. Only if the resolution of preselected impurities and degradation products is considered to be not sufficient (e.g., by not meeting a predefined goal of USP resolution Rs >2), a purposeful variation of the gradient as the sole parameter should be performed, as amongst all parameters the chromatographic gradient has the highest impact on the resolution of two peaks. It is understood that this approach may not be reasonable to deliver a suitable method in sporadic cases. In particular, cases of drug substances with unusual physicochemical properties (e.g., nucleotides) may require the use of very specific chromatographic conditions. Nevertheless, it should be the goal to purposefully preselect the generic methods in a way being applicable for the vast majority of the drugs.

2.3   ED Methods and Customization

It is obvious that this approach is only superior towards a comprehensive screening of parameters if the number of preselected generic methods is low. This consequently means that the generic methods should be as robust and broadly applicable as possible. The two herein shown generic methods (*see* Table 1) are rather examples of Waters®-based U(H)PLC systems, but respective variants are equally possible.

Table 1
Two generic ED methods

System	Waters UPLC H-Class
Mobile phase A (*Method A*)	10 mM NH$_4$Ac in water/acetonitrile (95/5) pH 7.0
Mobile phase A (*Method B*)	10 mM NH$_4$Ac in water/acetonitrile (95/5) + 0.1% TFA pH 2.5
Mobile phase B	Acetonitrile
Column	BEH C18, 150 mm * 2.1 mm * 1.7 μm
Flow rate	0.3 mL/min
Colum oven temperature	45 °C
Sample concentration	As appropriate based on peak response
Injection volume	≥2 μL
Detection	λ_{max} of the drug

Gradient program		
Time	**% Mobile Phase A**	**% Mobile Phase B**
0	100	0
10	5	95
13	5	95
14	100	0
17	100	0

Both generic methods differ only in the composition of the aqueous mobile phase. If wanted, as an additional variation, a different second column might be possible as well (e.g., using HSS T3 150 mm*2.1 mm*1.8 μm). However, it is not recommended to increase the number of generic methods beyond that, as this approach would lose its benefit compared to comprehensive screening.

In case of the generic methods in Table 1, the neutral method (Method A) is preferred as compared to the acidic (Method B) due to a better MS response in negative ion mode in the absence of TFA. Hence, the drug substance and relevant degradation products and impurities are first injected with generic Method A (*see* Fig. 3). Acceptance criteria to go ahead with a particular method are a good peak shape, a good UV response, and a good MS response. If it becomes obvious that these criteria are not met by this particular method, another generic method should be tried. Only if all generic methods fail, a comprehensive screening as standardly done in LD should be followed (*see* Sect. 3.1.2). Once an adequate method is selected, a customization of the gradient is performed. The reason for performing this customization is twofold: first, the main peak should get an adequate retention, and the second, drug and relevant impurities and degradation products must be baseline separated. An adequate retention of the drug would be in the range of 40–80% of the chromatographic runtime. This is required to ensure that compounds, which are more or less polar than the drug, are separated and detectable. This value can be achieved by implementing a flatter or steeper gradient compared to the generic gradient.

To enable the method meeting the most important acceptance criterion (separation of the drug peak from defined impurity and degradation product peaks), the gradient will be further modified in case of co-elution. Different approaches can be followed here, but the most promising is the implementation of a flatter gradient in the region of co-elution by adding additional steps to the chromatographic run, increasing the total runtime, or starting the chromatographic method with a short isocratic run to resolve early co-eluting peaks (e.g., of two major degradation products). In this way, an adequate purity of the drug peak is ensured. It is recommended to use MS detector to evaluate peak purity. Once all these acceptance criteria are met, the chromatographic parameters can be regarded as final.

The example in Fig. 4 illustrates this approach by first checking good peak shape, UV, and mass response of the drug in the generic method (A). The same is done for selected degradation products and impurities (B), and in the absence of co-elution (C) the chromatographic part of the method can be regarded as final and fit-for-purpose in ED.

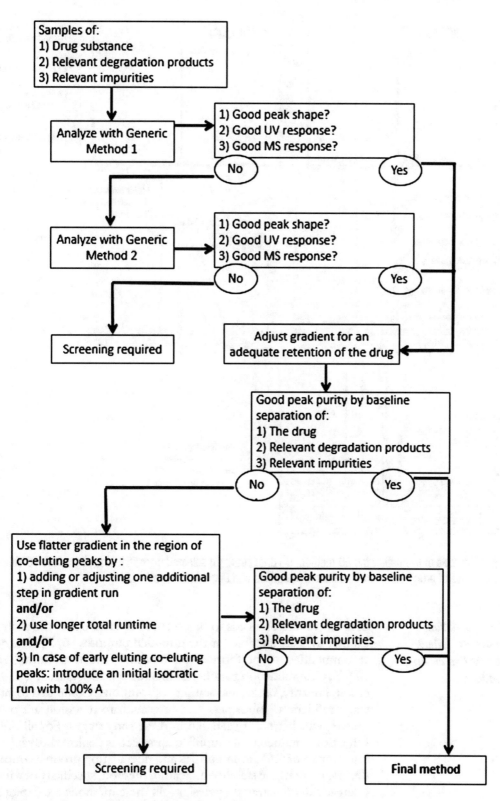

Fig. 3 Process flow to customize the generic methods

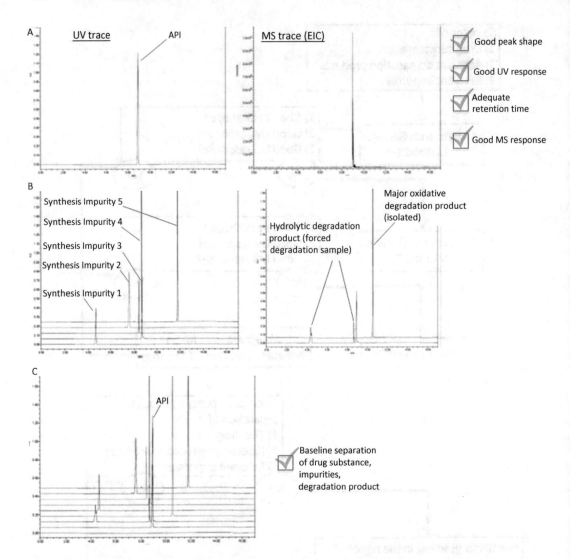

Fig. 4 Example of evaluating the ED method: (**A**) drug peak; (**B**) selected impurities and degradation products; (**C**) overlays of drug peak with all selected impurities and degradation products

2.4 Validation of the ED Method and Its Use for Drug Product

Method validation needs to be executed to ensure that the analytical methods are suitable for the intended purposes [6, 7]. It is not recommended to perform a full method validation during the ED. Typical validation parameters include specificity, accuracy, precision, linearity, range, and stability of solutions. Compared to late-stage validation, robustness and intermediate precision are parameters, which are not validated in these early stages. For all other validation parameters, a simplified approach is deployed. By injecting samples of relevant impurities and degradation products during development of the stability-indicating method, specificity of which is already demonstrated by design. As these methods are deployed as well for assay and purity assessments, a combined validation approach is performed. For drug assay, accuracy will be assessed using a minimum of three independent determinations over a minimum of three concentration levels (80%–100%–120%) covering the specified range, and even weighing separately at each concentration level. For purity, accuracy is assessed using a minimum of three determinations over a minimum of three concentration levels (reporting threshold being one of them), covering the specified range where one stock solution with dilution over three levels is sufficient. In combined assay/purity methods, this results in a linearity assessment of six concentration levels covering the specified range. In early phase, only system precision and analysis repeatability are assessed, while intermediate precision is evaluated only during late-stage validation. System precision is determined from five or six replicate injections of the same reference solution dependent on the RSD requirement (respectively, $\leq$2% or >2%). Analysis repeatability is assessed using a minimum of three independent determinations and can be combined with the accuracy tests.

Although the above approach describes the development of a stability-indicating assay/purity method for the drug substance, the so selected chromatographic conditions should be appropriate for corresponding drug product as well. Typically, only the sample preparation needs to be revised, while the other chromatographic conditions can remain the same. This obviously strongly depends on the actual formulation and dosage form and the same principles apply as in LD (*see* Sect. 3). In general, the use of a largely standardized assay/purity method for the drug product is encouraged for the same reason as for the drug substance method. Regarding validation for drug product, specificity is demonstrated by spiking with placebo, while additionally filtration/extraction studies might be required if the sample matrix is difficult to dissolve.

3   Late-Phase Method Development

Candidate molecules that are proven to be clinically successful in the early phase, move to the next, i.e., the late phase of the product development starting from clinical phase 2b. The available knowledge about the molecule such as its physicochemical characteristics, degradation pathway, impurity profile, and analytical methods used in the early phase forms the basis for development activities of analytical methods for the late phase.

As discussed in the previous section, the analytical methods used in the ED are considered to be "fit for purpose". Changes in the route of synthesis of the drug substance or qualitative/quantitative changes in the excipients may have an impact on the analytical methods when development progresses from early phase to late phase. As their capabilities are not fully evaluated at this stage, the early-phase methods may or may not be applicable as such for testing the product in the LD.

This section focuses on the development of LC methods for analysis of products in LD.

3.1 Approach for LC Method Development for LD

In contrast to ED, the process of method development in LD considers many more parameters, such as the nature of the sample, type of equipment, columns, mobile-phase composition, and operating parameters of the method.

LD method development is a systematic, scientific, risk-based, holistic, and proactive approach that begins with predefined objectives. In a broad sense, method development in LD can be classified into four phases: "initial phase", "screening and optimization phase", "sample preparation phase", and "risk assessment and evaluation phase". A schematic representation of the method development along with the involved activities is shown in Fig. 5. LC method development consists of two important aspects: firstly, the development of the chromatographic part of the analytical method defining the chromatographic parameters, and secondly the development of a sample preparation procedure, being part of the analytical method. During method development, these two processes can be handled separately.

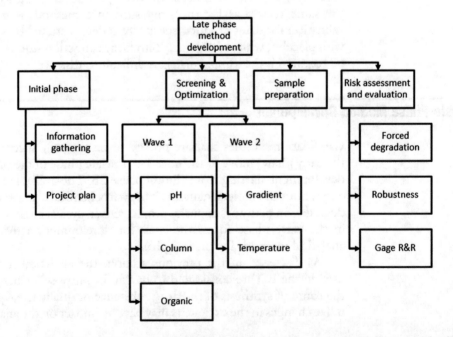

Fig. 5 A schematic representation of the late-phase method development along with the involved activities

3.1.1   Initial Phase

The "initial phase" is the foundation phase that mainly focuses on gathering information related to the product and the creation of a project plan. The basic information gathered for the drug substance and drug product includes, but is not limited to:

1. *Physicochemical properties of the drug substance*: Physical and chemical properties, solubility at various pH/solvents, molecular structure/formula, pKa/pKb, etc.

2. *Other characteristics related to drug substance*: Impurity profiling, degradation pathways, UV absorption spectrum, compatibility with other drug substances (in case of fixed-dose combinations), pH stability, photosensitivity, hygroscopicity, primary and secondary packaging type, etc.

3. *Experience from ED method development*: Experiments, findings, and corresponding conclusions made during ED method development are referenced from the development report.

4. *Characteristics of drug product*: Proposed formulation composition, excipients and their properties, any information on drug-excipient compatibility, *etc.*

The project plan includes the intended use of the analytical method as well as the analytical method requirements. If a method is intended to be used for assay/purity testing of a drug substance/product, the following information will guide the developer to have an appropriate method in place:

- An assessment of the existing early-phase method and its performance characteristics. This is to evaluate whether a further optimization of the early-phase generic method would be sufficient to be compliant with the late-phase requirements or a complete new method development is required.

- Expected changes in the specifications: Many times, during late phase, the drug product specifications are dynamic and may undergo changes, such as the specified limits for the impurities/degradation product that are tightened during the LD. Anticipation of such changes helps in deriving a validation plan that would accommodate all such possible changes.

- Technical information regarding hardware and chromatographic data system software capabilities: This is to ensure that the method requirements are aligned with the instrument qualification package.

- The method performance requirements and associated validation ranges.

- For LC impurity methods, the method should be able to separate impurities as follows:

(a) For specified impurities: All impurities must be separated from each other and the principal analyte.

(b) For unspecified potential impurities: These impurities must be separated from the principal analyte. The method should also be able to separate process impurities of the drug substance. If not, a sound scientific rationale should be provided.

3.1.2 Screening and Optimization Phase

Computer-organized screening and method optimization systems enable a fast and thorough assessment of different chromatographic parameters and allow the developers to rapidly determine the best possible chromatographic conditions linked with the analytical method requirements [8–10]. These systems typically consist of an automated software package in conjunction with one or more chromatographic systems. These software packages are based on statistical design of experiments taking into account effects of individual experimental variables along with combined effects of selected variables. As such, method screening using these software packages is faster and more efficient as compared to traditional method development using one factor at a time (OFAT). An OFAT approach can miss the combined effect of several experimental factors on the chromatography. Commercially available examples of automated screening and optimization software packages include Fusion®, Autochrom®, Chromsword®, etc.

From a chromatographic system perspective, any LC system can be used. However, UHPLC systems are viewed as more useful as these consume less solvents, have a better resolution, and have shorter run time as compared to HPLC systems, thus providing a lean approach to the method development. The chromatographic systems should be equipped with quaternary solvent managers and multiple column switching valves integrated in a thermostated column compartment. This is to allow the screening of multiple buffers as well as different stationary phases. Additionally, these chromatographic systems preferably are attached to multiple detectors such as PDA and mass spectrometry (MS) allowing peak tracking and evaluation of peak purity and co-elution. These automated systems commonly are set up for two waves of screening and optimization as shown in Fig. 5.

A selection of representative samples and knowledge of product specifications are critical inputs to these screening and optimization systems, as these factors do have an impact on the outcome of method screening process. Selected samples should contain all specified but also unspecified process impurities and degradation products from drug substance and drug product. Impurity spiking can be done at a suitable level, e.g., at the respective specification limit, if impurities are missing from the sample.

During the first wave, the key primary parameters to be included are pH, column stationary phase, and organic solvents as these factors have significant impact on method selectivity. Volatile buffers are usually preferred as these are MS compatible. Selection of pH can be from acidic to basic pH, 2.5, 4.8, 7.0, and 9.0, as they can help separate impurities with differing pKa values. Columns selected for screening are expected to differ widely in terms of selectivity and polarity. Acetonitrile, methanol, and their binary mixtures are the organic solvents of choice for reversed-phase LC, as these solvents are capable of separating a wide range of impurities with good peak resolution and symmetry. During the second wave, adapting the column oven temperature, mobile-phase gradient, and/or flow rate can be considered.

The final outcome of the computer-organized screening and method optimization system is a suggestion of the best possible chromatographic conditions delivering the predefined requirements regarding separation power. The best overall answer suggested by the software package is always verified to avoid any possible errors. Additionally, the outcome enables the method developer to choose a method of alternative selectivity: e.g., with a different stationary phase and chromatographic conditions. This method can be used as an orthogonal method to challenge the specificity of the primary method.

Figure 6 shows a typical ACD/Autochrom workflow from selecting a starting method, its optimization, eventually leading to the final method [8].

2D-LC is one of the new interesting upcoming technologies in chromatographic method development. 2D-LC is a multidimensional technique where the injected sample can be separated through two major types of separation, either by specific peak selection (heart cutting) or by fully passing the entire sample over both dimensions (comprehensive). These systems can be deployed in several manners to assist in the chromatographic method development:

- By running an orthogonal method in the second dimension, the specificity of the primary method in the first dimension can be assessed.

- By running the primary method in both dimensions, an assessment for "on-column reactions" can be made. This is important to assure that only process-related impurities and drug substance/drug product-related degradation products are considered.

- Whenever the primary method is not MS compatible and new peaks need to be investigated/identified, the second dimension can be run with a MS-compatible method, enabling peak identification.

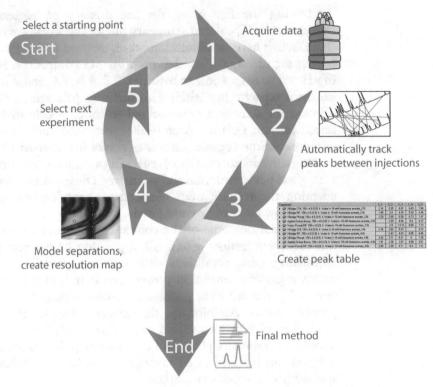

Fig. 6 A typical ACD/Autochrom workflow from selecting a starting method, its optimization, and leading to the final method [8]

3.1.3 Development of the Sample Preparation Procedure

Sample preparation is one of the most critical steps in method development for drug products and can later, if not thoroughly underbuilt, cause multiple issues in function of method robustness and performance. Sample preparation of drug product typically focuses on two processes: first, the disintegration or dispersion of the dosage form and secondly the dissolution or solubilization of the drug. To develop an effective and robust sample preparation procedure, the first step is to review the available drug substance and drug product information collected during the ED. The information helps to decide in the selection of diluent to extract and dissolve drug and to determine how to disperse the dosage form.

When selecting the disintegration/dispersion conditions, the following can be considered:

1. Addition of a suitable diluent such as water or an aqueous buffer, which causes the dosage form to disintegrate followed by a period of shaking or stirring. When shaking is critical, hand shaking is typically avoided as this potentially leads to robustness issues when executed by different analysts worldwide. Therefore, in such cases it is advised to deploy automated

shaking devices, with a clear set of predefined shaking parameters (e.g., type, time, volume, bottle orientation, amplitude).

2. Deploy mechanical means such as manual or automated grinding.

3. Sonication should be avoided due to inconsistency in sonic wave intensity, excessive sample heating, and potential sonication-induced degradation.

In function of method robustness, it is key to evaluate the different options for disintegration/dispersion and to optimize the agitation parameters.

For selecting the dissolving/extraction diluents, the following can be considered:

1. pH adjustments.

2. Different organic solvents and levels of the solvent: The level of organic solvent used can vary between 0 and 100%. Methanol, acetonitrile, ethanol, and propanol are the most commonly used organic solvents as they are compatible with LC and typically provide good extraction of the drug. It is recommended to use at least a minimum of organic solvent even if the drug is water soluble to aid in solubilizing potential unknown impurities and degradation products. Additionally, 100% organic solvent should be avoided in sample diluents, if feasible, to prevent elevated RSD values on injection repeatability. In case high levels of organic solvents are used, syringe draw speed must be evaluated for different brands of UHPLC and specified accordingly in the test method.

3. Adapting the ionic strength as this can influence the effectiveness of the extraction of the drug.

4. Addition of additives, e.g., surfactants to break up drug-excipient interactions: The final sample diluent shall be as compatible as possible with the mobile phase to ensure good peak shapes. To execute the diluent screening, it is advised to deploy a design of experiment (DoE) approach, as outlined in the literature [11].

Other recommendations in function of sample preparation are as follows:

5. Sample homogeneity: Where possible, a composite of 20 units of product under analysis should be made for assay/purity testing. The contents of 20 capsules should be used. Whole-tablet sample preparations may be possible for those containing low amount of actives, but should still target 20 units. For other dosage forms, such as creams, liquids, and oral solutions, homogeneous samples should be prepared as much as possible. Exceptions are where sample stratification may be meaningful,

such as top, middle, and bottom tube sections of cream products for stability testing.

6. Removal of insoluble components left over after the disintegration/dispersion and dissolving/extraction phase. This can be achieved by filtration, centrifugation, or solid-phase extraction. Filtration is preferred as the other options are more difficult to standardize.

7. Small volumetric pipettes (e.g., ≤2.0 mL) should be avoided as even a small variation shows a large influence on quantitative results.

8. Volumetric flasks should be between 25 and 500 mL made of Class A borosilicate glass. If amber flasks are required for light protection, preferably externally coated flasks should be used.

9. Weighed reference standard amounts for drug substance and drug product should be ≥75 mg. Lower amounts are acceptable using a suitable balance in case limited reference material is available.

10. The number of manipulation steps and active time of involved analyst need to be kept minimal.

11. Parallel dilutions are preferred over serial dilutions (dilutions are made directly from initial stock solutions with the lowest number of dilution steps).

12. Preferred solution stability for sample and standard preparations is at least 7 days. Considerations to solvent and storage conditions should be given to obtain desired solution stability.

13. An assessment of the hygroscopic behavior of the reference material, the sample, and all the different formulations (also the crushed tablets where applicable). For it, dynamic vapor sorption curves for all different cases should be available. This information can be crucial in understanding the potential impact and control of the grinding and weighing part of the sample preparation procedure.

14. Autosampler vials, caps, and septa should be evaluated for any potential sample evaporation or interaction. Amber autosampler vials may contain traces of elements that catalyze some degradation reactions and should be used with caution only as needed or preferably externally coated vials should be used.

At the end, the entire sample preparation procedure should be tested and validated to confirm that it works as expected and completely extracts the drug from the dosage form.

3.1.4 Risk Assessment and Evaluation

The development process of any new analytical method must include a "risk assessment", which is the proactive evaluation of the success rate of the method when it is routinely applied for its intended purpose. An anticipation of future possible failures can be done through certain studies such as the forced degradation and robustness testing, which are parts of the method validation exercise. It is also advisable to perform a "Ring Test or Gage R&R" wherein the method is evaluated by the "probable customers", such as the quality control laboratories of the manufacturing units where the product is intended to be manufactured, tested, and released. A "customer feedback" can prove important in finalizing the method parameters.

3.1.5 Forced Degradation Study to Establish Stability-Indicating Nature of Method

Forced degradation is a study wherein the drug product is subjected to various environmental stress conditions (*see* Table 2). The purpose of forced degradation study is to understand the degradation pathway of the drug substance in the drug product and to evaluate the stability-indicating nature of the analytical method. A stability-indicating method is expected to quantify active and degradation products, which may form during the shelf-life of a drug product. A representative comparison diagram of forced degradation condition is shown in Fig. 7. A prior knowledge of the

Table 2

Recommended experimental conditions for drug substance and drug product stress testing

Reaction	Stress condition	Duration for drug substance	Duration for drug product
Acid/base hydrolysis	Solution or suspension in dilute acid, for example 0.1 N HCl, and dilute base, for example 0.1 N NaOH at 60 °C or room temperature	0, 1, 3, 7 days	
Oxidation	Solution or suspension in diluted peroxide solution, for example, 0.3% or 3% H_2O_2 at room temperature		
	Exposure of drug substance to solutions of radical chain initiators such as AAPH (4,4′-azobis (2-amidinopropane) dihydrochloride) or transition metals such as 0.3 mM Cu(II)Cl_2 and 0.2 mM Fe (II)$Cl_2 + O_2$ at 60 °C		
Photostability	For drug substance, solution or suspension in sealed vial exposed to light source as defined in ICH ($1\times$ to $2\times$) at $\leq$30 °C (optional)	Duration depends on light chamber model and settings	
	Expose drug substance or drug product in an open dish to light source as defined in ICH ($1\times$ to $2\times$) at $\leq$30 °C		
Thermal[a]	Sealed vial at 70–80 °C or sealed vial at 40–60 °C	1–6 weeks 2 weeks	2 weeks 8 weeks
Thermal[a]/ humidity	Open dish at 70–80 °C, >65% RH or open dish at 40–60 °C, >65% RH	1–6 weeks 2 weeks	2 weeks 8 weeks

Note: [a]Higher temperature stressing is suggested for the rapid generation of degradation products. Lower stressing temperatures may be used

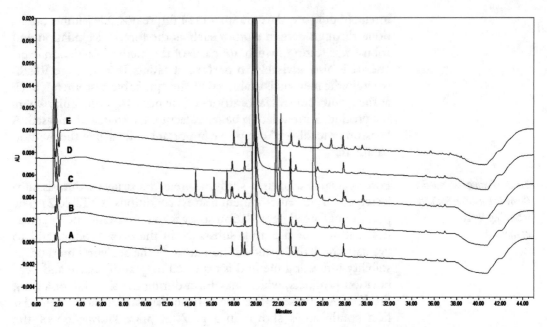

Fig. 7 Forced degradation chromatogram—(**a**) acid degradation, (**b**) base degradation, (**c**) oxidation degradation, (**d**) thermal degradation, and (**e**) photolytic degradation

sensitivity and degradation pattern of the molecule and a similar study performed on the drug substance play a key role in deciding the stress conditions to which the drug product needs to be exposed. Forced degradation studies, similar to those typically performed in ED, can be used as guidance for the selection of appropriate stress conditions. The stability-indicating nature of the method has to be challenged by an orthogonal method of a different selectivity. Alternative detection techniques such as LC-MS and/or 2-dimensional chromatography shall be used for orthogonality. Forced degraded samples finally need to be evaluated for peak purity and mass balance.

3.1.6 Robustness

The purpose of robustness testing is to indicate the factors that can significantly influence the outcome of the studied responses [12, 14]. This gives an idea of the potential problems that might occur when the method is repeated at different conditions. Therefore, these problems can be anticipated by controlling the significant factors, for example, by including a "precautionary statement" in the method description. The external variables (different laboratories, analysts, instruments, sample lots, experiment days, and operating conditions such as temperature) and internal variables (e.g., pH, buffer concentration, mobile-phase flow rate, mobile-phase composition, chromatographic column, sample preparation procedure) are the risks to any analytical method, which must be assessed prior to finalization of the method. This helps during transfer of the developed method to different testing laboratories/ sites and provides an indication of its reliability during normal use. LC chromatographic parameters considered in robustness testing include the following:

1. HPLC or UHPLC column (at least two different lots of packing material).
2. Column temperature ($\pm 10\%$).
3. pH (± 0.2 units).
4. Flow rate ($\pm 10\%$).
5. Buffer concentration ($\pm 10\%$).
6. Initial mobile-phase ratio (A/B) and/or solvent composition ($\pm 1\%$ absolute, each component varied accordingly).
7. Injection volume ($\pm 20\%$ absolute).
8. Gradient slope ($\pm 5\%$ relative).
9. Wavelength (target ± 2 nm).
10. HPLC/UHPLC equipment (at least two different instruments, different manufacturers or models preferred, if available).
11. Solvent brand and purity may be considered.

The initial values of drug substance assay and specified/validated impurities or other components, as needed, are compared with values obtained on changing the way of sample preparation, by varying parameters such as:

1. Type of organic solvent used for extraction.
2. Type and pH of buffer used for extraction.
3. Percentage of organic solvent in extraction solvent.
4. Sample and matrix concentrations.
5. Mixing and equilibration times and speed (force).
6. Grinding of tablets (manual, coffee grinder, Retsch mill) while accounting for possible effects such as hygroscopy.
7. Type of mixing (shaker, e.g., horizontal (tree), orbital, sonication).
8. Centrifuge time and RPM.
9. Sequence of dilution steps.
10. Filter type.

3.1.7   Gage R&R

Gage R&R, which stands for gage repeatability and reproducibility, is a statistical tool that measures the amount of variation in the measurement system arising from the measurement device and the people taking the measurement. The purpose is to determine the

contribution of total variation from differences within each opera-
tor, between operators, and between laboratories [13, 14].

The measurement variation (Gage R&R) includes several factors such as laboratory, analyst, instruments, equipment, and materials. Several laboratories have to be selected to participate in the
Gage R&R study. Within each laboratory, preferably two analysts
shall be involved.

Selection of different batches for a Gage R&R study is one of
the important aspects. Various batches must be selected to represent the range for which variability needs to be assessed.

4   Conclusion

A fit-for-purpose phase-dependent method development, validation, and transfer strategy is proposed. This is to ensure a fast
throughput of drug candidates in ED while dealing with high
product attrition rates and the rapid evolution of the drug product
in these early phases. In ED, this translates to a general systematic
approach starting from two standardized methods for assay/purity,
with a simplified validation excluding robustness and intermediate
precision. These methods, which need to be stability-indicating and
able to identify key impurities as well as degradation products, are
based on a U(H)PLC platform with UV and MS detection. In LD,
when the drug substance and drug product processes are locked,
the focus of our approach shifts towards robustness and practicability of the assay/purity methods. Computer-organized screening
and optimization systems are deployed to determine the best possible chromatographic conditions (e.g., pH, column stationary
phase, organic solvents, column temperature, flow rate) linked
with the analytical method requirements. By using design of experiments, different options for disintegration/dispersion and dissol-
ving/ extraction are explored, leading to an effective and robust
sample preparation procedure. Finally, robustness tests and Gage
R&R studies are executed, to understand the variability of the
assay/purity method and to ensure that the method can be executed in routine operation in the manufacturing sites. There is lot
more to share on the overall method development and ways to
success but to remain in scope of this chapter the authors think
that above high-level guidance will help the developer to come up
with a robust stability-indicating method in a shorter time and
contribute to establish a quality measurement control on key attributes of product.

Acknowledgements

The authors want to thank the colleagues from "Janssen" who provided insight and expertise that contributed to the approaches outlined in this chapter. They also want to express their gratitude to Dr. Saranjit Singh and Dr. Sanjay Bajaj for providing the opportunity to write this chapter.

References

1. Lee RW, Goldman L (2012) The central role of analytic method development and validation in pharmaceutical development. Life Science Connect. Guest Column

2. Clinical Development Success Rates (2006–2015) A study published by Biotechnology Innovation Organization, Biomedtracker and AMPLION

3. Boudreau SP, McElvain JS, Martin LD, Dowling T, Fields SM (2004) Method validation by phase of development: An acceptable analytical practice. Pharm Technol

4. Waterman KC (2011) The application of the Accelerated Stability Assessment Program (ASAP) to Quality by Design (QbD) for drug product stability. AAPS PharmSciTech 12 (3):932

5. Baertschi SW, Jansen PJ, Alsante KM (2011) Stress testing: a predictive tool. In: Pharmaceutical stress testing—predicting drug degradation, 2nd edn. Informa Healthcare, London

6. FDA (2000) Guidance for industry—Analytical procedures and method validation, chemistry, manufacturing, and controls documentation, Center for Drug Evaluation and Research (CDER) and Center for Biologics Evaluation and Research (CBER), August 2000

7. International Conference on Harmonization (2005) Quality Guidelines Q2(R1), Validation of Analytical Procedures, Text and Methodology

8. Sneyers R, Peeters J, Malanchin V, Cimpan G, Vazhentsev A (2013) Computer Organised Screening and Method Optimisation System—Phase 2 [COSMOS 2]. Janssen Pharmaceutical Companies of Johnson & Johnson, Beerse, Belgium and Advance Chemistry Development, Inc. (ACD/Labs), Toronto, Canada

9. Steiner F, Brunner A, Mcleod F, Galushko S. Automated method development utilizing software-based optimization and direct instrument control. Dionex Corporation, Germering, Germany and ChromSword, Mühtal, Germany

10. Jayaraman K, Alexander AJ, Hu Y, Tomasella FP (2011) A stepwise strategy employing automated screening and DryLab modeling for the development of robust methods for challenging high performance liquid chromatography separations: a case study. Anal Chim Acta 696:116–124

11. Nickerson B (2011) Sample preparation of solid oral dosage forms. In: Nickerson B (ed) Sample preparation of pharmaceutical dosage forms. Springer

12. Burns DT, Danzer K, Townshend A (2009) A tutorial discussion of the use of the terms "Robust" and "Rugged" and the associated characteristics of "Robustness" and "Ruggedness" as used in description of analytical procedures. J Assoc Public Anal (Online) 37:40–60

13. Dejaegher B, Jimidar M, Cockaerts P, Smeyers-Verbeke J, Vander Heyden Y (2006) Improving method capability of a drug substance HPLC assay. J Pharm Biomed Anal 42(2):155–170

14. Vander Heyden Y, Nijhuis A, Smeyers-Verbeke J, Vandeginste BG, Massart DL (2001) Guidance for robustness/ruggedness tests in method validation. J Pharm Biomed Anal 24(5–6):723–753

Chapter 6

Protocols for Characterization of Degradation Products with Special Emphasis on Mutagenic Degradation Impurities

Steven Hostyn, Peter Persich, Shalu Jhajra, and Koen Vanhoutte

Abstract

Delivering safe products to ensure patient safety is key for the pharmaceutical industry. Therefore, thorough control strategies need to be put in place during the development and manufacturing of pharmaceutical products to avoid potential health threats. During the last decennium, regulatory authorities have put more emphasis on assessing and controlling mutagenic impurities, which has resulted in the compilation of ICH M7 guideline. In this chapter, we present possible approaches on how to comply with ICH M7 requirements, with a focus on degradation products that are formed in the final drug product upon its storage during shelf-life. In this chapter, we describe systematic strategies to proactively select and identify the degradation products that might be considered relevant for safety assessment in accordance with ICH M7.

Key words Degradation products, Mutagenic degradation impurities, ICH M7, Threshold of toxicological concern, Forced degradation studies, Excipient compatibility, Stability, Characterization protocols

1 Introduction

Throughout the entire process of pharmaceutical development and even after the market launch, patient safety is amongst the most important parameters for pharmaceutical companies. In the finalized drug product, which is meant to be administered to the patients, possible health threats may arise from the following:

1. The drug: The safety of the drug is extensively assessed in preclinical and clinical trials during development and by monitoring for adverse effects after marketing (pharmacovigilance).

2. Excipients: In the vast majority of cases, excipients are used that are generally recognized as safe (GRAS) [1] or those that have been assessed to be safe based on preclinical investigations.

3. Impurities: Any component of the drug product that is not the drug substance, excipient or water. Generally, these are

Sanjay Bajaj and Saranjit Singh (eds.), *Methods for Stability Testing of Pharmaceuticals*, Methods in Pharmacology and Toxicology, https://doi.org/10.1007/978-1-4939-7686-7_6, © Springer Science+Business Media, LLC, part of Springer Nature 2018

controlled at levels that have been qualified preclinically, and are considered to be safe.

It is clear that amongst these three, assessing and predicting the effect of impurities is very difficult as their presence in the finalized drug product, despite being undesired, is often unforeseeable. Hence, the implementation of thorough control strategies is one of the greatest challenges in the pharmaceutical development process.

Impurities can originate during drug substance synthesis, drug product manufacturing, degradation of the drug substance, drug-excipient interaction(s) and even all other possible types of interactions during storage, viz., drug-drug (in fixed-dose combinations, FDCs), drug-packaging material, drug-impurity from excipients, etc. These can be observed at the time of the execution of adequate stability studies as described by guidelines ICH Q1A [2] and Q1B [3]. Further guidelines that provide harmonized information on reporting, identification, and qualification of impurities, both synthesis related and degradation products, are ICH Q3A [4] and ICH Q3B [5]. ICH Q6A [6] covers their control through appropriate specifications.

During the last decennium, regulatory authorities have put more emphasis especially on assessing and controlling mutagenic impurities in pharmaceutical products, leading to a number of regional [7, 8] and ultimately a superseding ICH guideline M7 in June 2014 [9]. In this context, mutagenicity refers to the induction of permanent transmissible changes in the structure of the genetic material of cells or organisms. These changes (mutations) may involve a single gene or a block of genes. On the other hand, genotoxicity, is a broader term which refers to the ability of a compound to interact with DNA and/or the cellular apparatus that regulates the fidelity of the genome, such as the spindle apparatus and topoisomerase enzymes. The latter term also includes damage that may not necessarily be transmissible to the next generation of cells. Genotoxic damage in somatic cells may lead to development of cancer. Carcinogens (i.e., those compounds that may cause cancer) can be mutagenic or can have another mode of action. Conversely, not all mutagens are carcinogens. Regulatory authorities have focused especially on mutagenic carcinogens as these may not have a threshold mechanism of action. Other types of genotoxicants that are non-mutagenic typically have threshold mechanisms, and usually do not pose carcinogenic risk in humans at the level ordinarily present as impurities.

Although not representing a legal or regulatory obligation, rather referred to as "current thinking", ICH M7 closes a gap in the assessment of impurities in drug substances and drug products referred in ICH Q3A and Q3B as "unusually toxic" impurities requiring "lower thresholds". Mutagenic impurities may be harmful at levels much lower than those covered in control strategies for impurities according to ICH Q3A and Q3B. Furthermore, and in contrast to these guidelines, the scope of ICH M7 applies also to compounds in clinical development. Although some exceptions are listed (e.g., products intended for advanced cancer) and alternative approaches to control mutagenic impurities are claimed to be equally possible, it is clear that ICH M7 demands the proactive establishment of additional global control strategies by pharmaceutical companies.

It is the scope of this chapter to present possible approaches on how to comply with ICH M7 focusing on degradation products formed in the final drug product during storage conditions. Particularly, systematic strategies to proactively select and identify those degradation products considered relevant for safety assessment, as outlined in ICH M7, are described herein.

2   Implications of ICH M7 for Degradation Products

The threshold of toxicological concern (TTC) concept was developed to define an acceptable intake for any unstudied chemical that poses a negligible risk of carcinogenicity or other toxic effects. The methods upon which the TTC is based are generally considered to be very conservative, since they involve a simple linear extrapolation from the dose giving a 50% tumor incidence (TD_{50}) to 1 in 10^6 incidences, using TD_{50} data for the most sensitive species and most sensitive site of tumor induction.

For the application of TTC values in the assessment of acceptable limits of mutagens, a value of 1.5 µg/day corresponding to a theoretical 10^{-5} excess lifetime risk of cancer is considered justified. This should be put into the context of a natural chance of more than 1 in 3 for development of the cancer. Generally, mutagens should not be present in levels above the TTC in the final drug product, when considering lifetime exposure. For highly mutagenic substances (the so-called cohort of concern), limits even below the TTC may be appropriate. Since in many cases lifelong exposure may not be realistic, in ICH M7 so-called acceptable intakes (AI) were defined, i.e., limits to be applied based on the duration of exposure (divided into classes of <1 month, <1 year, <10 years, or ≥10 years).

In order to be able to establish adequate control strategies for mutagenic degradation products, it is of great importance for pharmaceutical companies to have a structured and model-based, protocol for mutagenicity assessment. For this reason, it is useful to differentiate between actual and potential degradation products. Actual degradation products are those above the identification threshold as described in guidelines ICH Q3A and Q3B, and are found in long-term stability samples. As outlined above, these

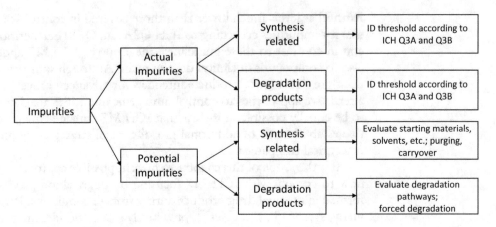

Fig. 1 Classification of impurities and how to assess for mutagenicity

guidelines do not apply for substances in the development phase. Nevertheless, degradation products that are formed in clinical batches above the mentioned identification thresholds should be considered for mutagenicity assessment, according to ICH M7. It is understood that for many drug candidates, appropriate AI values would result in impurity levels that are in the range of ppm levels and thus significantly lower than the recommended identification thresholds. In this case, usual analytical techniques to control chemical purity of the drug product do not suffice for the detection of all hazardous and potentially mutagenic degradation products. Therefore, the concept of "potential impurities" is applied (*see* Fig. 1). For these potential impurities/degradation products, the most important factor in deciding whether assessments are required is the probability of presence in the drug substance or product at significant levels, i.e., actual levels that would be above acceptable safety limits. For synthesis-related potential impurities, this can be achieved by reviewing the used starting materials, reagents, as well as known side products and evaluating their risk of carryover into the final drug substance and purging effects. Hence, for these compounds it is generally known what to look for in the final product and, where required, adequate analytical methods can readily be developed to quantify them down to ppm levels. The situation is different for potential degradation products, which are expected to be formed in the drug product, but are not yet confirmed by long-term stability studies. Thus, based on pure theoretical evaluation, it is usually not possible to foresee the formation of potential degradation products being formed in quantities around the relevant AI. Consequently, if any degradation products are formed above identification threshold of ICH Q3A and Q3B in long-term conditions, ICH M7 states: "Knowledge of relevant degradation pathways can be used to help guide decisions on the selection of potential degradation products to be evaluated for mutagenicity, e.g., from degradation chemistry principles, relevant stress testing studies, and development stability studies". This means that beyond accelerated stress conditions (e.g., 40 °C/75% RH, 6 months) and respective photostress studies (ICH Q1B), additionally adequate stress testing or forced degradation studies (FDS) have to be performed to establish potential degradation products that have a high probability of formation in the drug substance or drug product, at levels above the relevant AI. Although very specific in many other aspects, ICH M7 provides no further guidance on the nature of these studies. Clearly, the design of forced degradation studies needs to be chosen thoughtfully. On the one hand, these studies must be designed in a way not to miss the relevant potential degradation products. On the other hand, excessive stress testing may generate inadequately many irrelevant degradation products for an assessment of mutagenicity. It is this subtle balance that poses a particular challenge, for which possible strategies need to be in place.

Relevant impurities (i.e., actual identified impurities/degradation products and potential ones anticipated to be above relevant AI limits) need to be assessed for potential mutagenicity. This is usually a stepwise approach; an initial literature study may provide data regarding the known mutagenic potential of an impurity. Obviously, this is only possible if compound specific data are available. If this is not the case, quantitative structure-activity relationship (QSAR) assessment focusing on bacterial mutagenicity predictions should be performed using at least two complementary methodologies. These steps are mandatory and lead either to a classification as class 4/5 (non-mutagenic) or class 3 (potentially mutagenic) (*see* Table 1). The actual status of a class 3 potential mutagen can be confirmed (becoming class 3) or overruled (becoming class 4 or 5) by actually performing a bacterial mutagenicity assay (e.g., AMES). For this test, sufficient quantities of the pure degradant need to be available. As indicated before, this test is

Table 1
Classification and proposed actions for impurities after assessment of mutagenicity

Class	Definition	Proposed limit or action
1	Known mutagenic carcinogens	Compound-specific limit
2	Confirmed mutagens according to bacterial mutagenicity test (e.g., Ames)	Appropriate TTC
3	Alerting structure according to QSAR; different than that of the drug	Appropriate TTC or refute with bacterial mutagenicity test (e.g., Ames)
4	Alerting structure according to QSAR; same as that of the drug	Treat as non-mutagenic
5	No alerting structure according to QSAR	Treat as non-mutagenic

not mandatory, however, a class 3 potential mutagenic impurity should in that case always be treated as being mutagenic. As a matter of fact, by performing an AMES test, there is still a high likelihood that an initial class 3 impurity would prove to be non-mutagenic. It is beyond the scope of this chapter to describe the details of these studies and reviews can be found elsewhere [10].

As degradation products formed in a FDS are always potential by definition, the relevance of the particular degradation pathways, therefore, needs to be confirmed. For this confirmation, samples of the drug product exposed to accelerated conditions (e.g., 40 °C/ 75% RH, 6 months) can be screened for the presence of the particular degradation products. The use of other kinetic models is in agreement with ICH M7 and may have the advantage to prove this relevance in an even shorter timeframe. Only if a particular degradation product is confirmed to be present in relevant samples, should safety assessments be performed and adequate control strategies need to be established. Various options are possible to ensure that a specific degradation product does not exceed its relevant AI limit. Mitigation and control strategies strongly depend on the nature of the degradation product and must be assessed on a case-by-case basis. Amongst others, protection against environmental influences like humidity or other measures to inhibit degradation processes are viable strategies in many cases.

3   Overview of Strategies in the Pharmaceutical Industry

While ICH M7 provides sufficient guidance on how to assess the potential mutagenicity of identified and relevant degradation products, it leaves a challenge in how to decide which potential degradation products are relevant and, therefore, requires further safety assessment and possibly control. In order to establish a systematic approach, there are two aspects that are required to be focused upon.

The first is the general methodology for FDS that is employed to evaluate the intrinsic stability of the drug substance. The experimental design of stress studies has not been described in detail in any guideline and thus is handled differently by each company. Obviously, this has a major impact on the observed potential degradation products. Although recommendations on the performance of FDS have been published [11], the setup, extent, and scope can differ a lot between companies.

Second, no rules for identification thresholds exist for these FDS. Again, a lot of variability exists in current practices of pharmaceutical companies surrounding the question, as to which of the (sometimes numerous) degradation products from a FDS are to be identified and characterized as to consider them for an assessment of mutagenicity.

/* not used */

3.1   Approaches to Conduct Forced Degradation Studies

In a benchmarking study of 2003, FDS performed by different pharmaceutical companies were compared [12]. As an outcome of this study, it was found that the majority of companies performed stress studies in the preclinical phase and usually repeated it at a later stage. This overview revealed that 70% of companies were identifying major degradation products formed in samples on 5–20% degradation of the drug substance. For analysis, mainly LC-diode array (65% of studies) or LC/UV (30% of cases) was used. Despite the differences in these studies, the vast majority of them were targeted to reveal the intrinsic stability of the drug candidate by covering all relevant degradation pathways. Hence, 95% of companies were performing acid/base, oxidative, photostress, and thermal/humidity stress testing on the drug substance. For the drug product, 90% of companies performed thermal/humidity and photostress studies, but only 65% performed oxidative and only 60% acid/base stress experiments.

In 2005, the Impurity Profiling Group (IPG), being a consortium of several pharmaceutical companies and Utrecht University, tried to harmonize stress testing approaches for drug substances and drug products [13]. It was the main goal "to investigate relevant stress conditions and comparison to degradation profiles obtained under accelerated/long-term real time stability conditions". However, it was recognized that the definition of fixed stress testing conditions being applicable for all drug candidates is not possible as these turned out to be too harsh for some molecules while inadequately mild for some others. In 29% of cases, fixed conditions lead to no degradation while the same conditions gave excessive degradation in 24% of cases out of which 14% even did not give a single relevant degradation product. Only in 13% of cases predefined fixed conditions were adequate to correctly predict at least one or all actual degradation products.

It can be concluded that it makes more sense to allow a range of applicable stress conditions to obtain a good predictability of degradation pathways rather than predefining fixed conditions. As a guiding principle, degradation should be in the range of 5–15%. Stress testing should not last longer than 3 months for solid-state experiments, 14 days for stress testing in solution, and particularly not more than 24 h for oxidative stress testing. More specifically, a minimum of proposed conditions for a FDS are as follows:

1. In solid, 40 °C/75% RH open dish for 3 months or 5–15% degradation (whatever is reached first).

2. In solid, 50–60 °C/ambient RH open dish for 3 months or 5–15% degradation (whatever is reached first).

3. Photostability according to ICH.

4. In solution, pH 2 at ambient temperature for 2 weeks or 5–15% degradation (whatever is reached first).

5. In solution, pH 7 at ambient temperature for 2 weeks or 5–15% degradation (whatever is reached first).

6. In solution, pH 10–12 at ambient temperature for 2 weeks or 5–15% degradation (whatever is reached first).

7. In solution, 0.1–2% H_2O_2 at neutral pH at ambient temperature and neutral pH for 24 h or 5–15% degradation (whatever is reached first).

However, it is the authors' opinion that these minimum recommendations do not suffice to reveal all relevant degradation pathways in all the cases and a more extended protocol is required for this purpose (*see* Sect. 4.3).

3.2 Proposed Identification Strategies for Degradation Products

The question as to what potential degradation products need to be identified is a critical one, as a fully identified structure does trigger an assessment of mutagenicity with all consequences, as described in ICH M7. While in a typical forced degradation study, numerous degradation products might be formed, there is no industry-wide accepted approach on which of those can be considered relevant and hence require structural identification. In this context, Dow et al. presented in 2013 a commentary on the strategy implemented at Eli Lilly [14], which was followed by a more general discussion in 2015 on "strategies to address mutagenic impurities from degradation in drug substances and drug products" [15]. Although not expressing a regulatory requirement, the latter article is a cross-industry contribution representing the most recent interpretation and recommendation of viable options on the practical implementation of ICH M7 regarding potential degradation products. Three different strategies are described on how to use FDS results to select degradation products for identification:

(a) One scenario is the use of FDS samples solely to support analytical method development activities and to make sure that the potential degradation products are detectable. Only if they are formed above identification thresholds in accelerated or long-term ICH stability studies, a structural elucidation is performed.

(b) The second scenario is based on a proposal of Alsante et al. [16] to define acceptance criteria for peaks in FDS samples to be a "major degradation product" and hence to be identified. This approach requires to only consider FDS samples with a realistic degree of decomposition (<20%) (*see* Fig. 2). If this criterion is met, peaks to be identified should be present in samples where the largest peak is >10% of the total degradation. This is to avoid identification of myriad degradation products formed at similar levels by means of a non-selective degradation process. As the last criterion, other peaks than the largest should be >25% of the largest peak(s) to make sure that only relevant degradation products are covered, and those

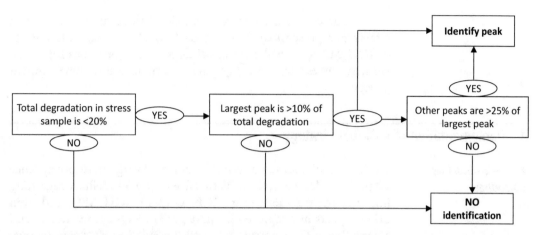

Fig. 2 Proposed decision tree to select degradation products from stressed samples for structural identification

formed in minor amounts are excluded. Such a decision tree leads to a high chance to identify only those degradation products being relevant and also having a certain probability to be formed under accelerated and long-term conditions as well.

(c) The last scenario describes the use of kinetic models to reliably predict the formation of degradation products observed under severe conditions in short-term experiments, when extrapolating to a long-term situation. This approach is often software based and includes the exposure of drug substances or drug products to conditions of higher temperature and humidity than those referred to as accelerated conditions. Only when the level formed exceeds a defined threshold, a structural identification is performed. It is beyond the scope of this chapter to describe the nature of these models (e.g., ASAP Prime©) [17] in detail, as the same is covered elsewhere (*see* Chap. 10).

It is worth mentioning that a further approach to derive structural proposals for potential degradation products is based on the use of in silico predictions of degradation profiles. Some of these commercial software have the unquestioned advantage to provide numerous structural proposals for potential degradation products and to guide the process of understanding degradation pathways of a drug [18]. However, despite the fact that the prediction accuracy of these applications is increasing continuously, they still have the tendency to overpredict and to provide too many irrelevant degradation products. Therefore, it is proposed that these systems can be used to gain knowledge regarding the potential degradation pathways, but not in hypothetical predictions for triggering a mutagenicity assessment, unless predicted degradation products have also been observed in experimental studies.

In our opinion, a combination of all three above-mentioned strategies represents the best approach to address the requirements of ICH M7 to consider potential degradation products for mutagenicity assessment during the pharmaceutical development process.

4 Implementation of a Global Strategy

4.1 Identification Categories

We have implemented a global impurity management policy since 2014 in order to comply with all existing guidelines regarding impurity management (e.g., ICH Q3A-D, ICH M7), and even other aspects not captured in these guidances (e.g., leachables and extractables). Concerning potential degradation products, as outlined above, it was critical to answer the question of which potential degradation product is to be identified and subject to mutagenicity assessment. This selection had to be addressed in a systematic manner, following a rule-based approach. The latter was expected to balance on the one hand the requirement (as per ICH M7) that a structural confirmation of a degradation product triggers an assessment of mutagenicity, and on the other hand a strong need to have some structural understanding of potential degradation products (and synthesis-related impurities), even if they turn out to be irrelevant at the end. This need was derived from the wish to gain a profound understanding of chemical manufacturing processes and to get a holistic picture of what might potentially be formed as degradation products even at very low levels.

A proper balance between the two above-mentioned needs was done to ensure that safety assessments were performed on those identified potential degradation products that were relevant for patients, i.e., which would occur at relevant levels in the drug substance or product under realistic conditions. For this reason, two different identification categories were defined:

(a) *Fully identified structures*, whose identity was confirmed using appropriate analytical techniques, i.e., at least by ^{1}H NMR.

(b) *Tentatively identified structures*, with a structure proposal generally based on mass spectrometry, but the exact identity was not confirmed. All structures derived solely from mass spectrometry are always tentative by definition, regardless of the level of confidence in the correctness of the proposed structures.

Before deciding to perform full identification of a tentative structure, we consider whether the tentative structure is also a metabolite and as such already toxicologically qualified. Actual drug substance degradation products that have been fully identified are assessed for potential mutagenicity and if necessary adequate control strategies are implemented, as required by ICH M7.

For a full identification by NMR, it is normally required to isolate the degradation products from a more complex mixture (e.g., a stressed or stability sample). For this reason, the degradation product has to be present in sufficient amounts, and therefore an adequate sample quantity is made available to apply separation and purification via semi-preparative chromatography [19]. Another viable strategy followed to fully identify a tentative structure is the chemical synthesis of a reference compound having a definite structure by design. Its identity with the tentatively identified structure is proven by co-injection in two orthogonal chromatographic methods.

This concept of tentative structures is regarded very useful as these proposals can be used to enhance the formulation/chemical process understanding (e.g., degradation pathways), but are not assessed for potential mutagenicity, as their structure is not definitively confirmed.

4.2 Actual Degradation Products

Although an identification strategy for actual degradation products in the drug substance or the drug product is also part of our global impurity management policy, it is basically identical with requirements as mentioned in ICH Q3A and Q3B. As these guidelines are very specific on which degradation products require (full) identification, and which do not, here the concept of tentative structures is not made use of.

4.2.1 Degradation Products in the Drug Substance

Actual drug substance degradation products are defined by us as those that are observed above the ICH Q3A reporting threshold during storage of the drug substance in the proposed long-term storage conditions in primary and secondary packaging. A degradation product exceeding the ICH Q3A identification threshold or a the one that falls under the category "trending" triggers full identification (*see* Table 2). Trending refers to a trend or tendency of the degradation products indicating the likelihood that at a certain time point the official (ICH Q3A) identification thresholds will be surpassed. A degradation product observed between the ICH Q3A identification and reporting threshold and showing trending will, therefore, trigger full identification, which is more conservative than the ICH M7 guideline. Following situations can be considered examples of trending:

(a) When comparing subsequent GMP batches, if the level of a synthetic impurity shows a rising trend, it is likely that in next batches the identification threshold would be exceeded.

(b) In (initial) GMP batches, if the levels for an impurity are already near the identification threshold, the possibility of an excursion above the identification threshold is likely in subsequent batches, considering normal variability between the batch levels.

Table 2
Identification thresholds for degradation products/impurities in the drug substance

Daily DS dose (mg/day)	Degradation product level	Identification
<2000	<0.05%	No
	0.05–0.10%, no trending	No
	0.05–0.10% AND trending	Full
	>0.10% or 1 mg/day[a]	Full
>2000	<0.03%	No
	0.03–0.05%, no trending	No
	0.03–0.05% AND trending	Full
	>0.05%	Full

Note: [a]Whichever is lower

4.2.2 Degradation Products in the Drug Product

We consider actual degradation products in the drug product as those impurities that arise from degradation of the drug substance or its reaction products with constituents of the drug product, including immediate container closure system. The definition, in particular, includes those degradation products that are observed above the ICH Q3B reporting threshold during storage of the drug product in the proposed long-term storage conditions and primary and secondary packaging, and also include those impurities that arise during the manufacturing of the drug product. For actual degradation products in the drug product, structures will be identified when they are above the ICH Q3B qualification threshold, which varies depending on the dose (*see* Table 3).

4.3 Potential Degradation Products

For potential degradation products, the criteria for tentative or full identification vary with the type of study, taking into account the different levels of stress and time:

(1) Forced degradation and excipient compatibility studies.

(2) Accelerated Stability Assessment Program (ASAP) studies.

(3) Temperature excursion studies.

(4) Probe/screening stability ICH GMP stability studies.

4.3.1 Forced Degradation and Excipient Compatibility Studies

FDS of the drug substance can help identify the likely degradation products, which can in turn help establish the degradation pathways and the intrinsic stability of the molecule, and developing and validating suitable analytical procedures. FDS include the effect of temperature above that for accelerated testing, humidity, oxidation,

Table 3
Identification thresholds for degradation products/impurities in the drug product

Daily DS dose (mg/day)	Degradation product level	Identification
<1	<1.0% or <5 μg TDI[a]	No
	>1.0% or >5 μg TDI[a]	Full
1–10	<0.5% or <20 μg TDI[a]	No
	>0.5% or >5 μg TDI[a]	Full
>10–2000	<0.2% or <200 μg TDI[a]	No
	>0.2% or >200 μg TDI[a]	Full
>2000	<0.10%	No
	>0.10%	Full

Note: *TDI* - Total daily intake of the degradation product
[a]Whichever is lower

Table 4
Proposed conditions for a FDS to cover majority of relevant degradation pathways

Hydrolysis (aqueous suspension)	Oxidation (aqueous suspension)	Light (solid and aqueous suspension)	Common impurities (aqueous suspension)	Thermal (solid)
0.1 N HCl, 60 °C	0.3% H_2O_2, 20 °C	3×ICH light	Formaldehyde	70 °C/75% RH
0.1 N NaOH, 60 °C	AAPH (radical initiator), 40 °C		Cu(II), Fe(II) salts	70 °C/0% RH
Water, 60 °C				80 °C/50% RH
0, 1, 3, 7 days	0, 1, 3, 7 days		0, 1, 3, 7 days	7 days

hydrolysis, and photolysis. The extent and scope of this study, as performed by us exceed the before-mentioned basic recommendations (*see* Sect. 3.1), and are shown in Table 4.

Excipient compatibility studies on the other hand are those that study the potential interaction between excipient and the drug and its influence on the drug product stability. Excipient compatibility studies are done by exposing samples only to elevated temperatures and relative humidity, but not to other stress media (e.g., acid, base, peroxides) and the same is true for drug products.

Identification (tentative or full) in this type of studies is initiated when the following conditions are fulfilled:

1. Total degradation does not exceed 25%: The experiment will be repeated with milder stress conditions if degradation is >25%

since results are considered nonvalid. In this case no identification is performed.

2. Total degradation is less than 25% and the largest peak is above 10% of total degradation.

   (a) For the major degradation products: i.e., the largest peak (>10% of total degradation) and those peaks that are at least 25% of the largest peak:

      • Individual degradation product levels are above 1%: full identification.

      • Individual degradation product levels are less than 1%: tentative identification.

   (b) For the other degradation products:

      • Individual degradant levels are above 0.1%: tentative identification.

      • Individual degradant levels are less than 0.1%: no identification.

3. Total degradation is less than 25% and there is no largest peak (i.e., a single degradant above 10% of total degradation):

   (a) Individual degradant levels are above 0.1%: tentative identification.

   (b) Individual degradant levels are less than 0.1%: no identification.

It can be seen that these criteria for a full identification are in line with those described by Alsante and Baertschi (*see* Sect. 3.2). Only, the additional requirement for individual degradation products to exceed 1% was added for reasons of practicability: Degradation products, when present at lower levels, are simply very hard to accumulate to quantities that suffice for an isolation and characterization.

Previous studies have shown that, in exceptional cases, it may not always be feasible or meaningful to establish a tentative structure, even if required according to the aforementioned thresholds. This is mainly applicable in the case of non-selective degradation under a certain stress condition resulting in a multitude of degradation products at relatively low levels. In this situation, a case-by-case approach is followed and based on the specific conditions, decisions are made regarding which degradation products are meaningful to be identified tentatively.

4.3.2 Accelerated Stability Assessment Program (ASAP) Studies

ASAP is a predictive in silico tool [20] that takes degradation data from accelerated temperature and humidity conditions and uses kinetic modelling to predict the degradation behavior at room temperature (i.e., 25 °C/60% RH). This tool provides an increased understanding of degradation and a greater confidence of shelf-life

Table 5
Identification criteria for levels predicted at the end of shelf-life by ASAP

Daily DS dose (mg/day)	Degradation product level	Identification
<1	<0.20%	No
	0.20–1.0%	Tentative
	>1.0%	Full
1–10	<0.10%	No
	0.10–0.50%	Tentative
	>0.50%	Full
>10–2000	<0.05%	No
	0.05–0.20%	Tentative
	>0.20%	Full
>2000	<0.05%	No
	0.05–0.10%	Tentative
	>0.10%	Full

estimations (*see* Chap. 10). In this case (full or tentative) identification of degradation products will take place when they are predicted to be present with a probability of >95% under the intended storage condition and packaging configuration. For ASAP studies performed on drug products, relevant levels have been defined based on the daily drug substance dose (*see* Table 5).

Predictions are made for the end of shelf-life at long-term storage condition (2 or 3 years at 25 °C/60% RH and 30 °C/75% RH and 6 months at 40 °C/75% RH). For potential degradation products in the drug substance, as predicted by ASAP, similar identification criteria are used as for actual degradation products in the drug substance.

4.3.3 Temperature Excursion Studies

Temperature excursion studies as required by ICH Q1A are intended to study the effect of short-term temperature deviations outside the label storage conditions, as they can occur, e.g., during shipment. Since in these studies stress conditions are applied, i.e., temperatures above 40 °C/75% RH, the criteria for FDS and excipient compatibility studies are used. However, if potential degradation products are detected above the set identification limit, instead of initiating identification, transportation instructions are updated to avoid product exposure to those conditions.

4.3.4 Probe/Screening Stability Studies	Probe and screening stability studies are often performed on several prototype drug products to support the selection of the final drug product composition [21]. Usually, they are treated to ICH long-term stability studies. Results and conclusions from these studies apply for the specific clinical trial they are intended for, i.e., the selected formulation and packaging configuration for a clinical trial. If no stability improvement is possibly done by reformulating or changing the packaging configuration, identification will be triggered by the criteria for ASAP studies with DP (*see* Table 5) in case of clinical phase IIB trials or beyond, and by the criteria in Table 6 in case of clinical phase I or clinical phase IIA trials.
4.4 Case Study	A FDS was performed on the drug substance to probe its stability under hydrolytic, oxidative, thermolytic, and photolytic conditions. Using the water-soluble radical initiator AAPH (2,2-'-azobis(2-amidinopropane) dihydrochloride) at 40 °C, almost 5% degradation of the drug substance was observed after 7 days (*see* Table 7).
	For identification, the criteria for potential degradation products in a forced degradation study apply. After 7 days, 4.83% degradation was observed and thus the condition can be considered

Table 6
Identification criteria set 3 for potential degradation products, probe/screening stability

Degradation product level	Identification
<0.10%	No
0.10–0.30%	Tentative
>0.30%	Full

Table 7
Identification criteria set 3 for potential degradation products, probe/screening stability

Condition	Time	RRT 0.70	RRT 0.76	RRT 0.78	RRT 0.81	RRT 0.84	RRT 0.85	RRT 0.92	Drug level
Reference									99.97
AAPH, 40 °C	0 days					0.05			99.87
AAPH, 40 °C	1 day	0.15			0.55	0.36	0.38	0.05	98.38
AAPH, 40 °C	3 days	0.27	0.09	0.08	0.66	0.75	0.28	0.11	97.20
AAPH, 40 °C	7 days	0.39	0.15	0.18	0.73	1.21	0.18	0.17	95.14

Note: Reporting threshold - 0.05% (area%)

as valid (<25% degradation). Moreover, a largest peak, larger than 10% of the total degradation, can be found eluting at RRT 0.84. The largest peak has an area% larger than 1%; therefore, the criteria are met for full identification. The area% levels for RRT 0.70 and RRT 0.81 are above 25% of largest peak RRT 0.84 (>0.30%) and are thus considered as major degradation products, but individual degradation product levels are between 0.1 and 1%. Therefore, for these degradation products tentative identification applies. For the remaining minor degradation products at RRT 0.76, 0.78, 0.85, and 0.92, tentative identification applies.

All aforementioned degradation products were tentatively identified using mass spectrometric techniques and using the tentative structures, the corresponding degradation pathways were elucidated.

Comparison with metabolite study data showed that RRT 0.84 was not a metabolite. Therefore, this degradation product was isolated on a semi-preparative scale and characterized using 1D-NMR and 2D-NMR techniques. The tentative structure was confirmed.

In silico QSAR analysis using Derek Nexus (Lhasa Limited) and Genotox Expert Alerts suite (Leadscope) resulted in a positive alert for the latter. In order to further assess the potential mutagenicity of RRT 0.84, a larger quantity of the degradation product was synthesized. Ames testing did not confirm the mutagenicity alert.

5 Conclusions

A systematic and rule-based approach to comply with global guidelines on impurity management has been established in our company. As the presence of mutagens has a major impact on patient safety, requiring thorough control strategies and mitigations, guidance was developed in-house on how to select relevant impurities and degradation products during pharmaceutical development for this assessment. The main feature of the established approach is the definition of two identification categories: (i) fully identified structures to be used for safety assessments and (ii) tentative structures to be used only for scientific and process understanding. This twofold strategy of structural identification was validated on the basis of previously marketed products to ensure that all relevant actual degradation products were indeed identified. Although identification thresholds are clearly defined to provide sufficient guidance, the policy should also allow sufficient flexibility to follow a more conservative approach. Good reasons may exist to fully identify an initial tentative structure in case of specific quality concerns. Such a decision is very compound or project specific and made only on a case-by-case basis.

It is understood that the field of assessing potential mutagenicity is very dynamic and future changes of guidelines or regulatory expectations may require an adjustment of the presented approach. However, it is the author's understanding that the described strategy represents an appropriate, proactive, and scientifically sound way to address patient safety during pharmaceutical development.

Acknowledgements

The authors want to thank the colleagues from "Janssen" who provided insight and expertise that contributed to the approaches outlined in this chapter. Special gratitude goes to Steven Spanhaak in providing crucial input resulting in the global impurity management policy of "Janssen". The authors also want to thank Dr. Saranjit Singh and Dr. Sanjay Bajaj for providing the opportunity to write this chapter.

References

1. Brusick DJ (2009) A perspective on testing of existing pharmaceutical excipients for genotoxic impurities. Regul Toxicol Pharmacol 55:200–204

2. ICH (2003) Guidance for industry: Q1A (R2) stability testing of new drug substances and products

3. ICH (1996) Guidance for industry: Q1B stability testing: photostability testing of new drug substances and products

4. ICH (2008) Guidance for industry: Q3A (R2) impurities in new drug substances

5. ICH (2006) Guidance for industry: Q3B (R2) impurities in new drug products

6. ICH (1999) Guidance for industry: Q6A (R4) specifications: test procedures and acceptance criteria for new drug substances and drug products: chemical substances.

7. EMEA committee for medicinal products for human use (CHMP) (2006) Guideline on the limits of genotoxic impurities (EMEA/CHMP/QWP/251344/2006)

8. FDA (2008 draft) Guidance for industry on: genotoxic and carcinogenic impurities in drug substances and products: Recommended approaches

9. ICH (2014) Guidance for Industry: M7 assessment and control of DNA reactive (mutagenic) impurities in pharmaceuticals to limit potential carcinogenic risk

10. Cassano A et al (2014) Evaluation of QSAR models for the prediction of Ames genotoxicity: a retrospective exercise on the chemical substances registered under the EU REACH regulation. J Environ Carcinog Ecotoxicol Rev 32:273–298

11. (a) Baertschi SW et al (2011) Stress testing: a predictive tool. In: Pharmaceutical stress testing—predicting drug degradation, 2nd edn. Informa Healthcare, London. (b) Singh S et al (2000) PharmTech 24:1–14. (c) Blessy et al (2014) J Pharm Anal 4:159–165

12. Alsante KM et al (2003) A stress testing benchmarking study. Pharm Tech 27:60–72

13. Klick S et al (2005) Toward a generic approach for stress testing of drug substances and drug products. Pharm Tech 29:48

14. Dow K et al (2013) The assessment of impurities for genotoxic potential and subsequent control in drug substance and drug product. J Pharm Sci 102:1404–1418

15. Kleinmann MH et al (2015) Strategies to address mutagenic impurities derived from degradation in drug substances and drug products. Org Process Res Dev 19:1447–1457

16. Alsante KM et al (2007) The role of degradant profiling in active pharmaceutical ingredients and drug products. Adv Drug Deliv Rev 59:29–37

17. Waterman KC, Adami RC (2005) Accelerated aging: prediction of chemical stability of pharmaceuticals. Int J Pharm 293:101–125

18. Kleinman MH et al (2014) In silico prediction of pharmaceutical degradation pathways: a benchmarking study. Mol Pharm 11:4179–4188

19. Foti K et al (2013) The role of analytical chemistry in drug-stability studies. Trends Anal Chem 49:89–99

20. Waterman KC et al (2007) Improved protocol and data analysis for accelerated shelf-life estimation of solid dosage forms. Pharm Res 24:780–790

21. Cha J et al (2011) Stability evaluations in handbook of modern pharmaceutical analysis, 2nd edn. Elsevier, Amsterdam, pp 460–505

Chapter 7

Stability Studies: Facility and Systems

Ashish Gogia and Sumathi V. Rao

Abstract

Efficient stability management system coupled with a well-organized stability testing facility is the mainstay of a successful stability program in the pharmaceutical industry. This chapter seeks to outline the infrastructure, testing requirements, and comprehensive systems to evaluate the stability performance and provides understanding of current regulations and practices in the industry.

Key words Stability facility, Stability management system, Stability protocol, OOS/OOT investigation, LIMS, SOP

1 Introduction

Stability of a drug substance or drug product refers to their ability to remain within established shelf-life specifications of identity, strength, quality, and purity till the specified period of time. Stability testing is the mechanism to obtain stability information and demonstrate that the said drug substance/drug product will meet the predefined acceptance criteria all through the defined storage period.

Stability studies shall be performed by following an approved stability protocol in a specially designed and approved facility. This chapter focuses on the requirements, and the systems followed, in general, in the pharmaceutical industry for establishing and running a successful stability study program.

2 Stability Study Facility

To set up and operate a functional stability study facility, some basic requirements are a separate housing, required number of optimally sized stability chambers, trained manpower, standard operating procedures (SOPs) for each activity, sample testing laboratory equipped with required number of test instruments, etc. Although these requirements appear to be very basic, they involve some key

Sanjay Bajaj and Saranjit Singh (eds.), *Methods for Stability Testing of Pharmaceuticals, Methods in Pharmacology and Toxicology,*
https://doi.org/10.1007/978-1-4939-7686-7_7, © Springer Science+Business Media, LLC, part of Springer Nature 2018

considerations, because failure to follow one or more of them can have significant impact on functioning of the facility, and therefore success of a stability program. The following are few of the essentials:

1. Stability facility shall be an approved laboratory set-up for handling, storage, and testing of stability samples.

2. Availability of qualified personnel, who are trained in all activities involved in stability facility operations, including documentation, data handling, and result interpretation. It may be reasonable to add that the staff shall be familiarized with SOPs of all kinds in the laboratory, including operation/calibration of analytical instruments, good laboratory practices (GLP), etc.

3. Equipped with equipment and instruments required to handle and analyze the stability samples, which include weighing balance, pH meter, sonicator, centrifuge, hot-air oven, disintegration test apparatus (DT), friability, hardness tester, Karl Fischer (KF) auto-titrator, dissolution apparatus, HPTLC/HPLC systems, etc. Instrument/equipment requirement depends upon the type of dosage forms and number of samples to be tested in a facility at any given time.

4. Availability of networking and laboratory information management system (LIMS) along with stability laboratory management model and, if possible, shelf-life prediction software like ASAP (*see* Chapter 10).

3 Stability Sample Storage Chambers

A successful stability study requires that the samples are exposed to precise and controlled storage conditions. This requires that the stability chambers are designed, installed, and operated as per the defined requirements and specifications. For acquiring the chambers meeting the company requirements, the major steps involved are the development of user requirement specifications (URS) and finalizing the design qualification document.

3.1 User Requirement Specifications for Stability Sample Storage Equipment

User requirement specification (URS) sheet is an authorized and documented evidence in an organization, which defines the requirement for the intended usage of the system, equipment, or utility in a certain facility (*see* Table 1). When any new equipment/ instrument, like stability chambers, is required to be purchased in a facility, the concerned department prepares an URS and the same is approved by engineering and quality assurance (QA) departments. The approved URS is forwarded to the selected vendor. URS for a stability chamber consists of (but is not limited to) the following details:

Table 1
Contents of a typical URS

S. no.	Contents
1	Purpose of URS
2	Scope of URS
3	Process/operational requirement Purpose of the equipment/system/instrument Process description Type of material handling Operational control requirement
4	Equipment/instrument requirement Specification of material construction Type of finish (absence of sharp edges) Functional specification requirement Required utility/available utilities GMP requirement (user level/rights, password protection, connectivity, data storage facility, and software compatibility) Safety requirement Maintenance requirement Documentation requirement (data and security) Risk assessment—using failure mode effect analysis (FMEA)

1. Capacity and size of chamber (s).

2. Number of racks and trays.

3. Required accuracy of temperature and humidity.

4. Heating and refrigeration units in chambers for regular use and the standby mode.

5. Decision on stand-alone or walk-in types.

6. Automated control systems (programmable logic controller (PLC) and/or touchscreen).

7. Door access systems (with biometric control/password or lock and key system).

8. Mobile alert systems, with defined number of users.

9. Temperature/humidity/water-level cutoff system and other safety requirements, including for overshooting/undershooting of set conditions.

10. Computer hardware and stability data management software, meeting 21 CFR part 11 [1] requirements.

11. Qualification protocols, unless in-house protocol is available.

12. Optional and spares.

3.2 Design Qualification Documentation

As per the customer URS, a design qualification document for stability chambers is prepared in consultation with the selected vendor. It contains minimally the following:

1. Stability chamber diagram.
2. Parts of the stability chamber.
3. Parts specification.
4. Quantity of each part with their certificates.
5. Working principle of each and every part, handling instructions, and utility requirement.
6. System maintenance procedure along with troubleshooting, and standard operating procedure for operating the stability chambers, and operating manual for each part.

3.3 Systematic Assessment of Installation Requirements and Risks

Stability chambers, especially the walk-ins, occupy large space (for which sufficient housing area needs to be planned in advance), consume huge electric power, generate good amount of heat owing to continuous operations of boilers and compressors (requiring environmental controls in the installation area), and need water supply and drainage systems. Therefore, a systematic assessment of preinstallation essentials and risks connected with operation and functioning of the stability storage equipment needs to be done in advance.

The overall impact on the surroundings and difficulty in compliance to current good manufacturing practice (cGMP) requirements shall also be a part of design qualification of the facility. As the stability chambers are non-stop continuous working equipment, the design has to be such that the risk to products is minimum at any given time. The risk assessment has to be done in respect of direct impact on the products, indirect product impact, and no direct product impact. The durability of control and display devices, alarms, safety systems, data loggers, computerized data storage, and/or acquisition systems shall be emphasized in the URS and the design qualification document.

3.4 Installation Qualification (IQ) Protocol

Installation qualification provides a documented evidence that ensures that the installation of that equipment is as per the predefined specifications (URS) and design. Installation qualification protocol consists of (but not limited to) the following:

1. Names of all components to be installed, including mechanical, electrical, hydronics, and other utilities.
2. Sensors with predefined specifications along with test certificates.

A representative checklist for IQ of stability chambers has been given in Table 2.

Table 2
Checklist for installation qualification (IQ)

S. no.	Checkpoints	Observation		
		Yes	No	N/A
Preinstallation				
1	Verification for damage, if any			
2	Verification/availability of all component parts			
3	Identify and verify the serial numbers			
4	Verify that the documentation is provided by the vendor (protocol and manual)			
During installation				
1	Review all calibration certificates			
2	Verify supply voltages			
Post-installation				
1	Verify installation is done as specified			

3.5 Operational Qualification Documents

Operational qualification (OQ) defines verification of operation of system components against system design documents, and checks functional requirements for mechanical, electrical, and all other instrument components. This qualification defines verification of the following in a stability chamber:

1. Temperature and humidity controlling operation of PLC with touchscreen display (HMI) (*see* Fig. 1).

2. Verification of safety devices of the system, like safety cutoff action for temperature overshoot and undershoot, safety cutoff action for humidity overshoot and undershoot, safety cutoff action of the temperature safety thermostat, and safety thermostat in humidity system.

3. Verification of automatic changeover of refrigeration system.

4. Main power failure changeover.

5. Door open study.

6. SMS alert system.

A representative checklist for OQ of stability chambers has been given in Table 3.

3.6 Performance Qualification Checklist

Performance qualification (PQ) defines the periodical verification of efficient working of all systems of stability chambers including

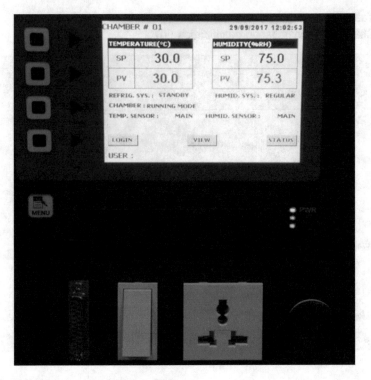

Fig. 1 Human machine interface (HMI)

Table 3
Checklist for operational qualification (OQ)

S. no.	Checkpoints	Observation		
		Yes	No	N/A
1	Verification of stability chamber details			
2	Verification of operation, calibration, cleaning, and maintenance of stability system			
3	Verification of operation of safety devices of system			
4	Verification of the printer interface facility of printer interface unit			
5	Verification of training records			
6	Verification of operation of all parts, controls, gauges, and other components			

accuracy and uniformity of the temperature and humidity. The activity involves the following:

1. Accuracy of temperature and humidity of the master sensor.
2. Uniformity of temperature and humidity attained in regular and standby modes in empty chambers and also in 80% sample-loaded chambers.

Table 4
Checklist for performance qualification (PQ)

S. no.	Checkpoints	Observation		
		Yes	No	N/A
1	Verify the accuracy of the temperature and humidity			
2	Verify the uniformity of the temperature and humidity			

A representative checklist for PQ of stability chambers has been given in Table 4.

3.7 Organizing for Requalification

Requalification shall be defined as equipment, facilities, utilities, and systems to be evaluated at an appropriate frequency to confirm that they remain in a state of control in the form of scheduled qualification/calibration. Where requalification is necessary and performed at a specific time period, the period shall be justified, and the criteria for evaluation defined. The possibility of small changes over time shall be assessed. Routine requalification of facility, equipment, utilities, and system should be considered based on the outcome of risk management principles, which include factors such as calibration, verification, and maintenance data. Criteria for requalification are:

1. Replacement of critical components of the equipment that can impact the performance.

2. Major breakdown or modification of the equipment.

3. Change in location of the equipment.

4   Software Qualification

There is an increasing inability to separate the hardware and software parts of the modern instruments. In many instances, the software is needed to qualify the instrument, and the instrument operation is essential when validating the software. Therefore, to avoid overlapping and potential duplication, software validation and instrument qualification can be integrated into a single activity.

Software used for instruments can be classified into four groups: firmware, instrument control software, data acquisition software, and processing software.

Stability control system software is essential for managing the operation of stability chambers and also for data management. The software should comply with 21 CFR Part 11, 21 CFR 211.68, and EU annexure 11 [1, 2] requirements to prevent data integrity issues. The following are the suggested key features:

1. Operating system (e.g., Microsoft Windows).
2. Document software (e.g., Adobe Acrobat Reader).
3. Full administration rights to be given.
4. Operating system update must be kept off.
5. Power-saving mode of the PC must be kept off.

Minimum requirements for hardware in which the software is installed are:

1. 22 GHz or higher processor, 4 GB or higher RAM, adequate system memory.
2. USB port, CD-ROM.
3. IP address required for each HMI to communicate to the chamber.

4.1 Installation Qualification of Software

Installation qualification (IQ) defines the successful installation of operating system and stability software that acquires data from the stability chamber, and stores and displays it. The important aspects in the IQ are:

1. Verifying that the operating system is compatible with the processor, RAM, etc.
2. That all files required to run the stability software are present.
3. That all documents required to train system personnel are available and approved.

During IQ, the emphasis is on confirmation that each instruction provided to the system and the expected results eventually matches with the actual results. The difference between the expected and the actual results should be considered as a deviation, which should be resolved before validation certificate is signed.

4.2 Operational Qualification of Software

Operation qualification (OQ) in this context defines the verification of the following details like:

1. Access control verification, which verifies the log-in with user name, change password, new password, password validity, and number of password attempts with wrong password.
2. Data security, backup, and storage verification, which verify the data creation, control for the user for data modification, data deletion, and data storage, and procedure for auto backup and manual backup.
3. Audit trail features that allow the generation of system-based chronological report linked to the specific user and the chamber for verifying date and time log modifications.

4.3 Performance Qualification of Software

Performance qualification (PQ) is the documented verification that the equipment or system operates consistently and gives reproducibility within the defined specifications and parameters for prolonged periods. A representative list of reports generated by stability software includes the following:

1. Chamber environmental control report - Complete report of main sensor of the chambers: It requires the user to fill up the date range, time, chamber ID, and print interval. This report contains the record of the temperature and humidity maintained in a chamber over the period.

2. Chamber alarm report - Records complete report regarding the activities of the alarms for various chambers.

3. Data logger report - Continuously records the temperature and humidity values at specified intervals.

4. Data logger alarm report - Provides report of excursion of temperature and humidity over the period of study that had set the alarm on.

5. Event alarm report - Complete report of all events that had been the reason of alarm (e.g., UPS changeover, power shutdown and resumption).

6. Audit trail report (chamber-wise) - Complete report of all activities performed on the chamber.

7. Audit trail report (user-wise) - Complete report of all activities performed by each user.

8. Mean kinetic temperature (MKT) report - Report of average temperature and MKT for a date range and the chamber ID.

9. SMS alert report - Details of SMS sent to the users with their identification and the time at which the message was sent along with the record of acknowledgement message, if provided.

10. Door access report - Details of the time at which the door was opened and closed, and by which user.

These reports can be searched according to the date and time entered and can be downloaded (e.g., in PDF format).

5 Standard Operating Procedure for Stability Chambers

A typical SOP with respect to stability chamber consists of the following different sections:

1. Purpose: This section indicates the purpose of the SOP, whether operation or calibration of stability/walk-in stability chambers.

2. Scope: This section indicates the operation procedure for exact equipment make, model, capacity, and stability storage condition.

3. Responsibility: This section explains who is responsible and accountable for maintenance, cleanliness, operating the chambers, recording the data, maintaining the logbook for each and every chamber separately, charging and withdrawal of stability samples from chamber, and preventive maintenance activity.

4. Accountability: Head, stability and head, QA.

5. Procedure:

   (a) Ensure that chamber outside area and the surroundings are clean and free from dust.

   (b) Verify that the main switch of the chamber, followed by the switches, wherever required, is in "ON" position, e.g., of heater(s), compressor(s), and boiler(s).

   (c) Ensure that the temperature human machine interface (HMI) controller and RH HMI controller have been set for temperature and relative humidity conditions as per the protocol for each of the chambers, like:

   40 °C ± 2 °C & 75% ± 5% RH (range: 38–42 °C & 70–80% RH).

   25 °C ± 2 °C & 60% ± 5% RH (range: 23–27 °C & 55–65% RH).

   30 °C ± 2 °C & 65% ± 5% RH (range: 28–32 °C & 60–70% RH).

   30 °C ± 2 °C & 75% ± 5% RH (range: 28–32 °C & 70–80% RH).

5.1 Settings of the PLC for Monitoring Stability Chambers

1. Ensure that the PLC is on and HMI screen is displayed.

2. HMI initial screen (*see* Fig. 1) shows the date, time, temperature in °C and in % RH, chamber mode, system mode (e.g., regular mode/standby mode), USER, LOGIN, VIEW, STATUS icons, and event alarm. All information related to chamber is available by operating the above-mentioned icons.

3. HMI screen operates with individual log-in user ID and password.

4. HMI screen should display related information by operating each and every icon with individual user ID and password.

5. User shall activate the event alarm either through HMI, which is having individual user ID and password by pressing "ALARM" icon or software by pressing "Accept" icon.

5.2 Stability Chamber Operation Through Software

1. Switch on the computer and log-in with user name and password allocated to the individual users. Log-in window will appear on the screen on the left bottom side with option to enter the user name and password.

2. After log-in, a display screen will open with two rows of icons. On the upper row, there is a menu bar that has icons representing current status, configuration, reports, help, and logout.

3. On the next row of the display screen, the menu bar has icons like current status, status details, data log table, data log graph, chamber graph, door access, audit trail, event alarm, MKT report, GSM report, and chamber report. By clicking on the current status, the equipment ID(s) will display and by selecting the equipment ID the current status of temperature and humidity is accessed.

4. Click on "Reports" icon, and the following reports will display under the navigation: chamber report, chamber alarm report, data logger report, data logger alarm report, event alarm report, audit trail report (chamber-wise), audit trail report (user-wise), audit trail common report, MKT report, SMS report, door access report, etc.

5. Select the details, respectively, "From Date" and "To Date" and "From Time" and "To Time" (e.g., Select 01/06/2017 00.00 to 01/06/2017 23:59), equipment ID, and print interval (e.g., 30 min) and then click on "View report" menu for data logger report display, with temperature and humidity data in a PDF format.

6. By selecting the "Data logger Report" icon under the "Navigation" the display will appear with "From Date" and "To Date" and "From Time" and "To Time", equipment ID, print interval, view report, and reset.

7. Ensure that all data are acquired or downloaded on a daily basis for all the chambers through the respective software.

8. To check data alarm log, click the "Data logger Alarm Report". Then select particular chamber "From Date" and "To Date" and "From Time" and "To Time" (e.g., Select 01/06/2017 00.00 to 01/06/2017 23:59) equipment ID, and print interval (e.g., 30 min) and then click on "View report" menu for data logger alarm report in PDF format. It will display temperature and humidity data, which are not within the limit.

9. To check event alarm log, go to "Event Alarm Report" icon and click on it. Then select particular chamber "From Date" and "To Date" and "From Time" and "To Time" (e.g., select 01/06/2017 00.00 to 01/06/2017 23:59) and equipment ID, and then click on "View Report" menu for event alarm report in PDF format.

5.3 Procedure for Charging and Withdrawal of Stability Samples

1. For charging/incubating, samples need to be labeled properly with the respective condition.

2. For entering into the walk-in stability chamber, log in with respective user ID and password, and press the "confirm" icon to open the door.

3. Press the light switch "ON/OFF" (given in front of walk-in stability chambers) to put "ON" the light lamp inside the chamber.

4. Unlock and pull to open the chamber door, enter inside, and immediately close the door. Load or unload from the tray, where the sample has to be placed or removed according to monthly plan.

5. After exit from the chamber, close the chamber door and lock the door immediately and press "ON/OFF" light switch to "OFF".

5.4 Instructions for Charging and Withdrawing the Samples

1. Sample has to be placed in the confirmed area with stability labels having incubating date and stability test condition. Withdraw the samples as per the protocol frequency of withdrawal date.

2. Ensure that all the samples are properly arranged inside the chamber, about 2 cm away from the inner walls and between each package, for the proper circulation of air and humidity.

3. Samples should be placed/withdrawn from the sample tray according to the date and month.

4. The chamber door should be closed immediately after entering and exiting from the chamber to maintain temperature and humidity within the range.

5. The logbook should be recorded for withdrawing or charging of the samples.

5.5 Annexure

Nil

5.6 Abbreviations

SOP   Standard operating procedure
QA   Quality assurance
RH   Relative humidity
ID   Identification

5.7 References for Storage Conditions

ICH guidelines
MHRA guidelines

6   Mapping of Stability Chambers

6.1   Calibration and Performance Verification

The calibration and performance verification activities are generally performed once in 6 months by approved external agency. This chamber calibration activity is performed by placing data logger/external calibrator sensors inside the chamber near the master sensor for 1 h, recording temperature and humidity every 10 min. Validation activity is performed by placing data logger/external calibrator sensors inside the chamber at different locations for 24 h and recording temperature and humidity every 10 min. Figure 2 presents a sample temperature and humidity sensor distribution diagram.

The acceptance criteria for calibration of stability chambers/walk-in humidity chambers are control of temperature and humidity within specified limits of $\pm$ 0. 5 °C and $\pm$ 2.0% RH. The acceptance criteria for validation of stability chambers/walk-in humidity chambers are temperature and humidity controlled within specified limits of $\pm$ 2.0 °C and $\pm$ 5.0% RH.

6.2   Preventive Maintenance Activity of Stability Chambers

Planned preventive maintenance (PPM) activity with PLC shall be performed every month by the engineering department personnel. In this PPM, the following checks are recommended to be performed, though the given list may not be exhaustive and other checks may be required to be performed, depending upon the specifications of the stability chamber:

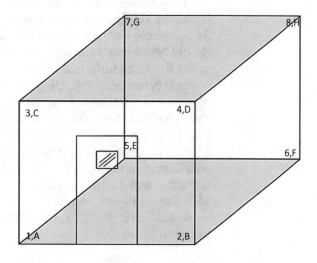

Internal Sensors location noted as: 1, 2, 3, 4, 5, 6, 7, 8.

External Sensors location noted as: A, B, C, D, E, F, G, H.

Fig. 2 Temperature and humidity sensor distribution diagram

1. Electrical switchgear - Check for electrical connections of control circuit, contactors, and wires for loose connections. Clean panel boards with vacuum cleaner.

2. Air blower - Check the airflow in blower, fan motor bearings, seating, and proper mounting.

3. Boiler tanks - Clean the boiler tank and accessories, clean the makeup water tank, and arrest all leakages.

4. Heaters - Check the boiler and dry heaters thoroughly, including the connections.

5. Solid - State relays and timers - Check for input signal voltage, output power supply, and proper functioning.

6. Cooling coil and steam coil - Check for any blockage, sludge formation, or algae on the surface of cooling fans and clean the cooling coil by using vacuum cleaner, air blower, and water jet pump.

7. Condenser/chiller unit - Check compressor, fan, condenser coil, and air blower.

8. Internal surface - Check the chamber and arrest any water leakages, and clean or buff if any corrosion is found.

9. PLC inputs and outputs - Check for all PLC input and output wires for loose connections, and tighten, if required. Check physical condition and functioning of all channels for temperature/RH, check water level, door limit, and safety thermostat for proper functioning. Check PLC outputs for blower, cooling unit, dry heater, and boiler heater functioning.

It is recommended that the temperature and humidity data should be verified through software/equipment daily, i.e., once in 24 h. Soft copy of report should be saved; first page of the soft copy should be reviewed through the printout by the respective supervisors for minimum, maximum, and average reading as per the acceptance criteria; and filing should be done. Any discrepancy observed in set temperature and humidity continuously for more than 1 h should be addressed through investigation for excursion of temperature or humidity report. Alarm and SMS systems are usually set to automatically report any discrepancy observed in set temperature and humidity. Alarm hooter, fixed in the chamber, should sound in the stability chamber and security room, and SMS should be sent to mobile phones of authorized persons. The working of emergency phones, if installed inside the walk-in chamber, shall be verified.

7   Handling of Stability Samples and Futuristic Approach

Sufficient number of samples should be subjected to stability studies as per the written and approved stability study protocol. The exact number of stability samples should be calculated depending on the types of study to be conducted and the number of tests to be performed at each interval as well as the total number of intervals. Also, the number of control samples needs to be counted alongside. This information about stability samples should be included in the stability protocol. Selection of batches for stability studies should be done on predetermined batches. The batches for new products should include the first three prospective process validation batches or batches, in which any major process change has taken place that may have a significant impact on the stability of the product.

Further, the following considerations are important with respect to handling of the samples:

1. Where a large pack (cartons of unusually bigger size or bulk packs (HDPE container) having large container size) is to be placed, the sample should be packed in smaller sized simulated containers and cartons, as appropriate.

2. If a drug product is available in more than one primary pack, then three batches should be selected out of each of the primary packs. In case a drug product is packed in 30, 100, 250, and 500 mL HDPE bottles with child-resistant closer (CRC) caps, then only the maximum and minimum packs should be kept for the stability studies as per bracketing and matrixing, provided that the same vendor and same material of construction are used. However, if in some cases the HDPE bottles are fitted with HDPE caps and some with metal caps, these should be considered as different packs.

3. The concept of bracketing and matrixing [3] should also be introduced if the drug product is available in more than one strength and in different package sizes. Use of bracketing and matrixing needs appropriate justification, which can be asked by regulatory authority.

4. Stability samples once received should be verified for the quantity and stored under controlled temperature.

5. The samples should be incubated within 7 days from the date of receipt.

6. Stability samples should be charged for stability study within 30 days after completion of packing and batch release.

7. If the stability study is delayed for more than 30 days after batch release, the sample should be retested for initial results (T_0), the same should be used as initial data, and immediately the same should be loaded for stability study without any delay.

8. Stability studies on three batches should be performed for change in any mode of pack, e.g., shift from HDPE bottles to Alu–PVC blisters, glass bottles to HDPE bottles or containers, Alu-Alu blisters to Alu-PVC blisters, or Alu-PVC/PVDC blisters.

9. In general, one batch for the change in batch size and change in equipment should be subjected to long-term and accelerated stability study. When multiple strengths are available, change in the source of drug substance should call for stability of one batch, while the lowest and the highest strengths should be covered as a routine stability study with a new drug substance.

10. Stability studies need not be repeated for the following variations in the finished products:

    (a) Tightening of the existing specifications.

    (b) An additional pack size for tablets or capsules with same primary packing material.

    (c) Change in the source of conventional excipients.

For registration purposes, test samples of products containing fairly stable active ingredients are taken from two different production batches; in contrast, samples should be taken from three batches of products containing easily degradable active ingredients or substances on which limited stability data are available. The batches to be sampled should be representative of the manufacturing process, whether pilot plant or full production scale. Wherever possible, the batches to be tested should be manufactured from different batches of active ingredients. In ongoing studies, current production batches should be sampled in accordance with a predetermined schedule. Detailed information on the batches should be included in the test records, namely the packaging of the drug product, batch number, date of manufacture, batch size, etc.

7.1 Labeling of Stability Samples

Labels affixed on the samples should have the following details:

1. Date in, date out, period, and storage conditions.

2. These samples should be identified with an appropriate label of "storage conditions" with different colored labels for each condition, e.g., green: 25 °C - 60% RH; light blue: 30 °C - 65% RH; dark blue: 30 °C - 75% RH; red: 40 °C - 75% RH; and black: 2 °C - 8 °C.

7.2 Testing Frequency

In the development phase and for studies in support of an application for registration, a reasonable frequency of testing of products containing relatively stable active ingredients is suggested to be:

1. Accelerated studies: 0, 3, and 6 months or as per requirements.

2. Intermediate studies: 0, 6, 9, and 12 months or as per requirements.

3. Long-term studies: 0, 3, 6, 9, 12, 18, 24, 36, 48, and 60 months or as per requirement.

4. Ongoing studies: Samples may be tested at 6-month intervals for the confirmation of the provisional shelf-life, or every 12 months for well-established products.

8 Challenges in Stability Testing

Test results are considered to be positive when neither significant degradation nor changes in the physical, chemical, and, if relevant, biological and microbiological properties of the product have been observed, and the product remains within its specification. A significant change under accelerated storage condition is considered to have occurred if:

1. The assay value shows a 5% decrease as compared with the initial assay value of a batch.

2. Any specified degradation product is present in amounts greater than its specification limit.

3. The pH limits for the product are no longer met.

4. The specification limits for the dissolution of 12 capsules or tablets are no longer met.

5. The specifications for appearance and physical properties (e.g., color, phase separation, caking, hardness) are no longer met.

If any change is observed, it should be documented as out-of-specification (OOS), out-of-trend (OOT) laboratory incident or deviation. Storage under test conditions of high relative humidity is particularly important for solid dosage forms in semipermeable packaging. For products in primary containers designed to provide a barrier to water vapor, storage conditions of high relative humidity are not necessary. As a rule, accelerated studies are less suitable for semisolid and heterogeneous formulations, e.g., emulsions, where intermediate testing is resorted to. In long-term studies, the experimental storage conditions should be as close to the projected actual storage conditions in the distribution system as practicable.

Thorough investigation is carried out in case any deviation is reported in stability results. In a pharmaceutical organization, OOS/OOT investigations are performed following standard protocols and checklists. The objective of such investigation is to find out the root cause of the deviation and establish that the result is an OOS/OOT and not a human error. Various approaches have been used historically for the identification of OOT using nonstatistical approaches (*see* Table 5). Detailed investigations are done in different phases at laboratory level on persons involved in analysis of, instruments, and procedures to conclude the reason for OOS/OOT result (*see* Table 6). OOT is triggered based on the product history as well as internal guidelines. However, other

Table 5
Checklist for OOT identification

S. no.	Checkpoints	Observation Yes	No
1	Three consecutive results are outside the results	☐	☐
2	The difference between consecutive results is outside of half the difference between the prior result and the specification	☐	☐
3	The result is outside 5% of initial result	☐	☐
4	The result is outside 3% of previous result	☐	☐
5	The result is outside 5% of the mean of all previous results	☐	☐

Table 6
OOS/OOT laboratory investigation checklist

S. no.	Phase 1 laboratory investigation Parameters to be checked	Yes/No/NA	Remarks
A	*Sample preparation*		
1.	Was the sample prepared by trained personnel?		
2.	Was the balance calibrated?		
3.	Were the weight print and the correct transcription of weight in the calculation of the test result done?		
4.	Was clean, dried, and appropriate glassware used for sample preparation (for example, amber-colored glassware)?		
5.	Any obvious evidence of glassware contamination (visual)?		
6.	Was sample prepared freshly?		
7.	Were the samples completely transferred?		
8.	Was there a spillage while transferring the sample?		
9.	Was the correct test procedure used?		
10.	Was the sample appropriately processed as per the applicable test procedure, e.g., mechanical shaking, sonication, heating/warming/cooling, protection from light, and dispersion, performed as per the approved method?		
11.	Were the sample dilutions correctly performed as per the method of analysis? Were correctly calibrated pipettes used?		
12.	Whether the reagents/chemicals used were of recommended grade and prepared as per the analytical method?		
13.	Were the calculations used to convert raw data values verified?		

(continued)

Table 6
(continued)

S. no.	Phase 1 laboratory investigation Parameters to be checked	Yes/No/NA	Remarks
14.	Was a validated calculator used?		
15.	Was correct/valid solvent/reagents/diluents used for sample preparation?		
16.	Was the sequence of addition of solvent/reagent/diluent as per the approved method of analysis?		
17.	Were the samples filtered/centrifuged/membrane filtered properly before introduction into instrument or analysis by classical method? Was proper code of filter used for sample filtration?		
18.	Were appropriately rinsed vials used for sample transfer in auto-sampler? Were vials appropriately labeled?		
19.	Were the samples correctly transferred to auto-sampler devices and correctly labeled for traceability?		
20.	Were samples appropriately stored in between the tests/days during analysis?		
21.	Others, if any _____		
B	*Testing*		
1.	Was the analysis done by a qualified analyst?		
2.	Was a similar incidence recorded for the same analyst?		
3.	Were samples/standards correctly prepared for each test as per specification?		
4.	Was correct/valid standard (as applicable) used for testing the sample?		
5.	Were sample/standard preparations stored under appropriate conditions (time, temperature, pressure) before and during analysis?		
6.	Was there any evidence that the standards and reagent were not properly labeled?		
7.	Were standards and reagents/test kits/media/mobile phase used within their expiration dates?		
8.	Was there evidence that the standards and reagents have degraded?		
9.	Was there evidence that the reagents, standards, and other materials used for test were contaminated?		
10.	Was analysis performed on calibrated instruments?		
11.	Was there any evidence of malfunction of the allied equipment?		
12.	Was correct instrument/equipment used?		
13.	Did the mobile-phase composition and preparation of samples, diluents, and filters used during analysis meet applicable test procedures?		

(continued)

Table 6
(continued)

S. no.	Phase 1 laboratory investigation	Yes/No/NA	Remarks
	Parameters to be checked		
14.	Was there any possible contamination from syringe or auto-sampler carryover?		
15.	Were instrument parameters set as per the specification?		
16.	Were the details and the sequence specified in the method of analysis followed?		
17.	Was the chromatographic response from the instrument as expected, based on previous experience for the same product?		
18.	Was the sequence of samples on instrument correct?		
19.	Was the system suitability criteria met?		
20.	Were the correct column/testing accessories used as per specification?		
21.	Did an electrical surge/decrease occur when the instrument was operating?		
22.	Others, if any_____		
C	*Data evaluation*		
1.	Was correct/approved and valid report format used?		
2.	Were all the relevant entries in analytical worksheet filled with correct transcription of raw data?		
3.	Were correct calculations done as per the testing method of analysis?		
4.	Was the interpretation of results of test done correctly?		
5.	Was the data collation from instrument in sequential order?		
6.	Were correct and validated Excel sheets used for calculations?		
7.	Was correct standard purity used in calculation?		
8.	Was correct formula used during calculation on Empower/LIMS software?		
9.	Others, if any _____		
D	*Data evaluation/review*		
1.	Was each test in worksheet/specification checked for correlation?		
2.	Are all signatures/dates/raw data/printouts from the instrument/equipment available with report?		
3.	Are all applicable charts/spectra/instrumental recordings available with the report?		
4.	Was any related current and past investigation reported in the past for said products?		
5.	Was the similar type of results obtained in previous stability interval?		

(continued)

Table 6
(continued)

S. no.	Phase 1 laboratory investigation	Yes/No/NA	Remarks
	Parameters to be checked		
6.	Are the results in increasing/decreasing trend?		
7.	Others, if any _____		
Obvious error identified—Yes ☐ No ☐; if yes—no further investigation required			
Hypothetical testing required—Yes ☐ No ☐			
Obvious error not identified—Hypothetical testing to be done Yes ☐ No ☐ If no—Justification required			
Hypothetical testing—for HPLC and GC analysis			
Reinjection from same vial			
Re-vial original working sample			
Re-dilute sample from original stock sample solution and/or refilter from the original sample(if applicable)			
Prepare new standards			
Use a second instrument			
Analyze blanks and/or placebo preparation			
Sonication of the original sample			
Any other (specify)			
Hypothetical testing - for TLC and non-chromatographic analysis, dissolution, UV assay, and titrimetric include the following as appropriate			
Reevaluate the original working standard solution			
Reevaluate the original working sample solution			
Re-dilute the stock sample solution			
Use a reserve sample that gave expected results			
Remeasurement			
Any other (specify)			
Conclusion of hypothetical testing			
Conclusion			
Results of repeat testing:			
Conclusion of repeat testing			
Conclusion:			
Phase II laboratory investigation			
Allot the analysis to a second chemist. If the result of second analyst is found to be in concordance with that of the first analyst, OOS/OOT is confirmed			

(continued)

Table 6
(continued)

S. no.	Phase 1 laboratory investigation		Yes/No/NA	Remarks
	Parameters to be checked			
Reanalysis with second analyst results:				
If in agreement with the trend repeat analysis performed with the first/third analyst to confirm the result of the second analyst				
Results of repeat analysis with the first/third analyst:				
Summary of OOT/OOS investigation				
Disposition of OOS/OOT:				

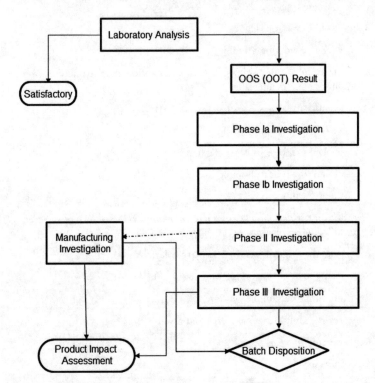

Fig. 3 Flowchart of OOS/OOT investigation

approaches are based on statistics that take the variability of the data into account when setting limit, like regression control chart method, time point method, and slope control chart method.

For degradation products and impurities, it is difficult to identify OOT unless the data reporting routines are changed. The within-batch methods are more difficult to implement than the between-batch methods because of the sparse data within a batch, especially at early time points.

A flowchart of OOS/OOT investigations is presented in Fig. 3. During investigation, root cause analysis tool (fishbone diagram) is

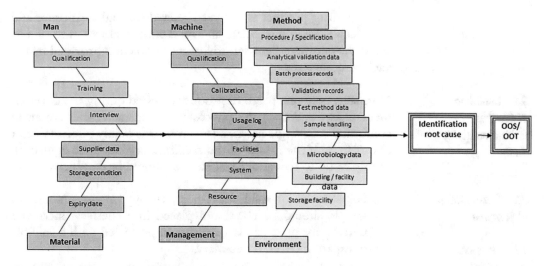

Fig. 4 Root cause analysis flow diagram

used to find out the obvious root cause. The fishbone diagram along with Is/Is not problem-solving tool can be used, as this tool comprises man, machine, method, material, management, environment, and problem statement (*see* Fig. 4).

9 Photostability Testing

The aim for the photostability study is to evaluate the effect of light exposure on the drug product packed in different packs like primary and secondary and also upon open exposure. The intrinsic photostability characteristics of new drug substances and products should also be evaluated to demonstrate that, as appropriate, light exposure does not result in an unacceptable change. Under some circumstances, these studies should be repeated if certain variations and changes are made to the product (e.g., formulation, packaging). The study is protocol driven and the pre-approved protocol should define the testing requirement for the exposed samples. The following sequence is preferred to understand any changes arising during exposure of the samples:

1. Tests on the active substance.
2. Tests on placebo samples.
3. Tests on the exposed product, and if necessary.
4. Tests on the product in the immediate pack, and if necessary.
5. Tests on the product in the marketing pack.

The drug product is analyzed after direct light exposure and upon exposure in immediate and marketing packs so as to understand the nature of light sensitivity and protection provided by the packaging material.

9.1 Selection of Batches for Photostability Study

Normally, only one batch of product is tested during the development phase, and then the photostability characteristics are again confirmed on a single batch, if the product is clearly photostable or photolabile. If the results of the confirmatory study are equivocal, testing of up to two additional batches should be conducted.

9.2 Presentation of Samples

9.2.1 Presentation of Drug Substance

1. For samples of solid substances, an appropriate amount of sample should be taken and placed in a chemical inert and transparent glass or plastic dish and protected with a suitable transparent cover, if necessary.

2. Solid substances should be spread across the container to give a thickness of typically not more than 3 mm.

3. Substances that are liquids should be exposed in chemically inert and transparent containers.

9.2.2 Presentation of Drug Products

1. Where practicable, when testing samples of the product outside of the primary pack, these should be presented in a way similar to the conditions mentioned for the drug substance. The samples should be positioned to provide maximum area of exposure to the light source (e.g., tablets, capsules, etc. should be spread in a single layer).

2. If direct exposure is not practical (e.g., due to oxidation of a product), the sample should be placed in a suitable chemically inert and transparent container (e.g., quartz).

3. If testing of the product in the immediate container or as marketed is needed, the samples should be placed horizontally or transversely with respect to the light source, whichever provides for the most uniform exposure of the samples. Some adjustment of testing conditions may have to be made when testing large-volume containers (e.g., dispensing packs).

4. Liquids should be exposed in the chemically inert and transparent containers. Samples can be exposed side by side with a validated/calibrated photostability system to ensure that the specified light exposure is done.

5. If protected samples (e.g., wrapped in aluminum foil) are used as dark controls to evaluate the contribution of thermally induced change to the total observed change, these should be placed alongside the authentic sample.

Testing should progress until the results demonstrate that the product is adequately protected from exposure to light. For some products, where it has been demonstrated that the immediate pack is completely impenetrable to light, such as aluminum tubes or cans, testing should normally be conducted on directly exposed product. If the temperature control option is not available in the photostability chamber, then analysis of the exposed sample should be performed as mandatory with the protected samples used as dark controls. Immediate (primary) pack is that constituent of the packaging that is in direct contact with the substance or product and includes any appropriate label. Marketing pack is the combination of immediate (primary) pack and other secondary packaging, such as a carton.

9.3 Sample Storage After Exposure

If possible, samples should be subjected to the analysis immediately. If it is not possible, the samples should be stored in a closed container and should be protected from light. These samples should be stored under ambient conditions until subjected to the analysis.

9.4 Drug Substance Analysis

After exposure, study samples should be subjected to the physical/chemical analysis as per the following tests mentioned below or specified recommended tests:

1. Appearance.
2. Assay.
3. Water by KF/loss on drying.
4. Related substances as per the finalized method.

Where solid substance samples are involved, sampling should ensure that a representative portion is used in the individual tests and it should be homogeneous.

9.5 Drug Product Analysis

Normally, the analysis on products should be carried out in a sequential or parallel manner, starting with testing the directly exposed product, and then progressing as necessary to the product in the immediate pack, and then in the marketing pack. The testing should be done for universal (appearance, assay, and degradation products) and selected test parameters among those specified for different types of drug products either in the in-house specification sheet, applicable pharmacopoeia, or those given in regulatory guidelines (also *see* Chapter 2, Table 7).

9.6 Evaluation of Results

If results of sample analysis, whether of drug substance or a product, are not falling into the laid-down acceptance criteria for any parameter, it can be concluded that the sample is unstable to light. Usually, analysis of drug substance or product in primary or secondary pack should give light protection and meet all specifications. The packaging is finalized accordingly. In certain situations, even the drug product may also require employment of

Table 7
Checklist for preaudit stability program evaluation

S. no.	Checkpoints	Availability		
		Yes	No	N/A
1	List of stability chambers	☐	☐	☐
2	List of products in stability chambers	☐	☐	☐
3	URS for all chambers	☐	☐	☐
4	Equipment qualification package for all chambers	☐	☐	☐
5	List of stability chamber-related procedures	☐	☐	☐
6	List of incidents, OOS, and OOT related to stability products (opened)	☐	☐	☐
7	List of analysts involved in stability analysis	☐	☐	☐
8	Analyst qualification and training records for analyst who involves in stability studies	☐	☐	☐
9	Daily temperature monitoring records	☐	☐	☐
10	Calibration/performance verification records for chambers	☐	☐	☐
11	Preventive maintenance procedure for stability chambers	☐	☐	☐

photostabilization approaches like entrapment of drug in cyclodextrins, use of colored coating on tablets, specific colored capsules, and light-protective primary packing (e.g., colored blisters, amber glass containers). This selection of the mode of stabilization depends on the outcome of analytical results of samples exposed sequentially (*see* Subheading 9.2.2).

9.7 Photostability Protocol

A typical photostability protocol should have the following contents:

1. Aim.

2. Batch details indicating batch number, size, source of drug substance with batch number/AR number.

3. Label claim.

4. Packing details indicating primary packaging (e.g., HDPE bottles (100's count)) or unpacked (e.g., tablets placed in petri plate under open exposure): Dark control samples of the above pack type samples should be prepared by sealing them in aluminum foil.

5. Test parameters to be checked (*see* Subheadings 9.4 and 9.5).

6. Storage conditions (e.g., 1.2 million lux h fluorescent light and 200 Watt h/m^2 UV light), testing frequency, number of

samples charged, and number of samples to be withdrawn per frequency [4].

7. Study duration (exposure time) should be based on the calibration data available to achieve the exposure of the product for the mentioned storage condition. Numbers of samples depend upon the method of analysis and number of tests required to be analyzed.

8. Photostability study summary providing all data relating to identification of the study.

9.8 Light Sources

The light sources described below may be used for photostability testing. The applicant should either maintain an appropriate control of temperature to minimize the effect of localized temperature changes or include a dark control in the same environment, unless otherwise justified. For both options 1 and 2, a pharmaceutical manufacturer/applicant may rely on the spectral distribution specification of the light source manufacturer.

9.8.1 Option 1

Any light source that is designed to produce an output similar to the D65/ID65 emission standard such as an artificial daylight fluorescent lamp combining visible and ultraviolet (UV) outputs, xenon, or metal halide lamp: D65 is the internationally recognized standard for outdoor daylight as defined in ISO 10977 (1993). ID65 is the equivalent indoor indirect daylight standard. For a light source emitting significant radiation below 320 nm, an appropriate filter(s) may be fitted to eliminate such radiation.

9.8.2 Option 2

For option 2, the same sample should be exposed to both the cool white fluorescent and near-ultraviolet lamp.

1. A cool white fluorescent lamp designed to produce an output similar to that specified in ISO 10977 (1993).

2. A near-UV fluorescent lamp having a spectral distribution from 320 to 400 nm with a maximum energy emission between 350 and 370 nm: a significant proportion of UV should be in both bands of 320–360 nm and 360–400 nm.

10 Sample Management Through Laboratory Information Management System

Many LIMS packages are designed with features to assist in stability tests and shelf-life studies, and to reduce human errors. In a well-established stability facility, LIMS is integrated with the stability chambers and other instruments/equipment for automatic recording of the events and results. The stability management module usually covers the activities like registration of storage conditions, storage chambers, stability protocols, sample storages, unscheduled withdrawals, certificate of analysis (COA) templates, sample allotments, worksheet headers, sample log-in templates, sample log-ins (auto generation), sample log-ins (on demand), sample log-ins (by tolerance), and test(s) allotments.

10.1 Storage Conditions

This option provides the facility to register and manage each distinctly different storage conditions of temperature and relative humidity, along with details and a unique identity.

10.2 Storage Chambers

LIMS is integrated with the entire stability facility and an option in LIMS provides for registration of each storage chamber, along with its details, as a master data entity and provides real-time status of a chamber without opening it.

10.3 Sample Log-In Template

A stability sample may need to be identified with a specified set of details to be filled in the respective fields at the time of log-in. The required sets of fields may be configured and registered with a uniquely identified sample log-in templates. This option provides the facility to register and manage the identity and details of each sample log-in template as a master data entity.

10.4 Certificate of Analysis Template

A COA needs to be generated for the tests conducted on a stability sample. The template for a COA may vary with the stability sample type and based on the COA type to be used for a with-specification sample or without-specification sample. Thus, there will be only one COA template per COA type per sample type. A template for the COA with header and footer is standardized as the format for its use in all identical situations. To maintain consistency and to avoid error-prone and tedious repetitions, COA templates are registered as a master entity. This option provides the facility to register and manage the identity and details of each stability sample COA template as a master data entity.

10.5 Worksheet Header

A worksheet needs to be created for each test conducted on a stability sample. Based on the individual worksheet, a consolidated worksheet may be prepared for a test plan to execute the sample in the LIMS. A stability worksheet is required to have a header that is commonly used on worksheets, to fill the standard information. To maintain consistency and to avoid error-prone and tedious repetitions, stability worksheet headers may be standardized and registered as a master entry. This option provides the facility to register, and manage the identity and details of each stability worksheet header template as a master data entry.

10.6 Stability Protocol

Stability protocols are the documents that contain the details of a product sample registered for stability study, like storage conditions, test plan, and sampling intervals. As soon as a product is considered for stability test, a protocol is defined for the purpose.

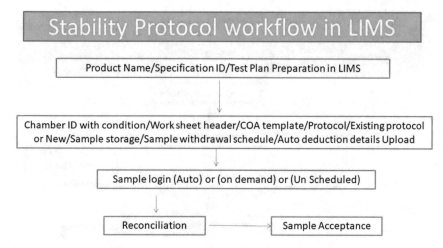

Fig. 5 Stability protocol workflow

This protocol contains full details of the sample (to be registered on the due date/s), including the details of the tests required on it. The protocol will define the schedule with reference to a starting date for the sample "pulls" or "withdrawals" from the storage locations. Stability protocols must be registered with care. Details like the number of samples to be withdrawn at each frequency, the location from, the quantity, whether a withdrawal can be made before the scheduled date (with predefined tolerance), or only if needed (demand) on or after the scheduled date must be carefully recorded. If necessary, an already registered protocol may be modified. This option provides the facility to register and manage each stability protocol, along with its details, as a master data entry. A sample stability protocol workflow is shown in Fig. 5.

10.7   Sample Storage

The samples meant for stability studies are stored at specific shelves and positions in the storage chambers. The details of the stability samples and the storage locations, and the quantity details, may be registered for records. This option provides the facility to register and manage each different stability sample storage location with a unique identity, consisting of a formatted concatenation of protocol ID/storage chamber ID/shelf location.

10.8   Sample Log-In (Auto)

Sample log-in task may be accomplished in any of the three modes: "auto generation" (as scheduled), "tolerance" (earlier than the scheduled date), or "on demand" (only if required for testing, on or after the scheduled date). Sample log-in cannot be done unless the protocol is registered (for which the COA template and worksheet header should also have to be registered).

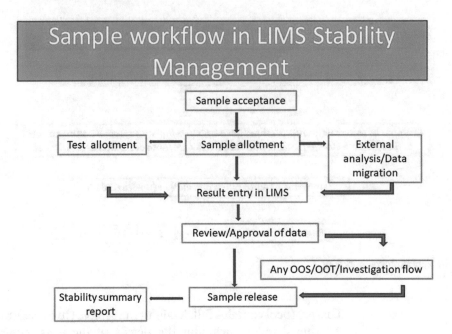

Fig. 6 Stability workflow in LIMS stability management

10.9   Sample Acceptance

Sample acceptance would be useful to track the sample acceptance checklist. After sample withdrawal, the system will show an option to verify the sample and accept for the sample analysis (*see* Fig. 6).

10.10   Sample Allotment

Sample allotment is the process of entrusting the responsibility to an authorized user for various tests to be conducted on a sample. The sample is allotted to a user, who will be the sample incharge. One or more categories of tests on the sample may be allotted to one or more other authorized users, who will become the test category incharges of the concerned test categories. The details of an already registered sample allotment may also be modified, if necessary.

10.11   Test Allotment

Test allotment is the process of entrusting the responsibility of individual test(s) to be conducted on a sample. The test category incharges may allot (delegate) individual test(s) to the other user (s) of a role (level) equal or lower than himself or herself, who will then become the individual test incharge. It may also be possible that the sample incharge may also be a test category incharge as well as a test incharge, and a test category incharge may as well be a test incharge.

10.12   OOT Configuration

OOT configuration master will provide an option to set the OOT limits for the respective tests under the selected test plan. An option to set the OOT limits for the "Initial Pull" and "Previous Pull" by means of % value of the lower limit and upper limit also usually exists.

11   Archival

Good documentation practices are a systematic procedure of preparation, reviewing, approving, issuing, recording, storing, and archival of any documents. All electronic and manual records are documented and archived in a secure manner (e.g., fire/waterproof).

The retention period for stability documents and records must be in compliance with applicable good manufacturing and distribution practices (GMP and GDP).

Access to the archives must be restricted. No information must be lost during the defined retention period. Security administration, access, and control procedures must be specified for electronic systems. Original documentation must be managed in a controlled manner. During the retention period, originals or copies of records must be readily available at the establishment where the activities described in such records occurred. Documents and records that are no longer required, because of the applicable record retention requirements, must be removed from the system and destroyed. Traceability to original hard copy documents or files must be available. Retention periods must be specified in predefined procedures (SOPs) in accordance with regulatory and legal requirements.

12   Audit Handling in Stability Management

Auditing is a critical function within a pharmaceutical company. It provides management with information about how effectively the company controls the quality of their processes and products. The audit process includes reviewing the programs; it ensures that procedures and systems are consistent with contractual and regulatory requirements.

The general definition of an audit is an evaluation of a person, organization, system, process, enterprise, project, or product. Table 7 gives checkpoints (not limited to) with respect to stability program requirements to be evaluated before audit.

13   Conclusion

Implementation of robust stability management systems in a well-established stability facility is the key to the evaluation of stability of the pharmaceutical products. In addition, thorough investigation and analysis of the stability test results enhance the quality and integrity of the stability data facilitating successful regulatory approval of the tested drug products. Integration and implementation of LIMS with module for stability management help in making the system robust, efficient, and reliable.

References

1. US FDA (2003) Guidance for industry part 11, electronic records; electronic signatures—scope and application. https://www.fda.gov/downloads/regulatoryinformation/guidances/ucm125125.pdf. Accessed 29 Sept 2017

2. European Commission (2010) Good manufacturing practice medicinal products for human and veterinary use annex 11: computerised systems. https://ec.europa.eu/health/sites/health/files/files/eudralex/vol-4/annex11_01-2011_en.pdf. Accessed 29 Sept 2017

3. Guidance for industry Q1D bracketing and matrixing designs for stability testing of new drug substances and products (2003) U.S. Department of Health and Human Services, Food and Drug Administration, Center for Drug Evaluation and Research (CDER)

4. US FDA (1996) Guidance for industry Q1B photostability testing of new drug substances and products. https://www.fda.gov/downloads/drugs/guidancecomplianceregulatoryinformation/guidances/ucm073373.pdf. Accessed 29 Sept 2017

Chapter 8

User Requirements and Implementation of a Risk-Based, Compliant Stability Management System

Susan Cleary, Parsa Famili, and Pedro Jorge

Abstract

This chapter evaluates the benefits of a compliant stability system, stability system components, stability user requirements based on inherent risks, new FDA guideline entitled "Data Integrity and Compliance with CGMP", and recommend solutions to various risks. Included in the chapter is a case study that illustrates the success of one company who implemented a complaint stability study management software application.

Key words Compliance, Data integrity, Stability management, Stability study, Risk based, Stability software, LIMS, Software requirements, User requirements, Validation

1 Introduction

The Merriam-Webster dictionary defines risk as the possibility of loss, injury, disease, or even in extreme cases death. In pharmaceutical manufacturing, risk is from a broad range of sources, and technology plays a key part in reducing risks associated with various processes. Data integrity, which is better achieved through automation, is an important component of industry's responsibility to ensure the safety, efficacy, and quality of drugs.

This chapter evaluates the benefits of a compliant stability system, stability system components, stability user requirements based on inherent risks. It also includes discussion on compliance to data integrity, 21CFR Part 11 and good automated manufacturing practice (GAMP) requirements. It recommends implementation of all these through an off-the-shelf (OTS) stability study management software.

Sanjay Bajaj and Saranjit Singh (eds.), *Methods for Stability Testing of Pharmaceuticals*, Methods in Pharmacology and Toxicology,
https://doi.org/10.1007/978-1-4939-7686-7_8, © Springer Science+Business Media, LLC, part of Springer Nature 2018

2 Low-Risk and High-Value Models

Life science corporations have different interpretations of the regulatory aspects of pharmaceutical manufacturing; therefore, the FDA (www.fda.gov) has issued a number of guidances such as "PAT - A Framework for Innovative Pharmaceutical Development, Manufacturing and Quality Assurance" [1]; "Current Good Manufacturing Practice Requirements for Combination Products" [2]; and "Sterile Drug Products Produced by Aseptic Processing - Current Good Manufacturing Practice" [3].

These FDA initiatives are intended to encourage utilization of modern and innovative technologies by various pharmaceutical and biotech companies. Automation plays an important role in managing the stability program, which requires quality units of the manufacturers to not only control the process, but also prove that it is under 'state of control'.

In the past, while risk-related parameters embraced virtually every decision in business, they often remained ambiguous at the senior management level. As regulations change and the governance practices evolve, more senior executives are endeavoring to rectify this, by defining and quantifying risk boundaries. There are three levels of risk parameters, viz., risk capacity, risk tolerance, and risk appetite. They form a co-relational hierarchy.

1. *Risk capacity*: This is defined as the highest level of risk. It establishes the boundaries of risk that a corporation producing drugs, drug substance, excipient, medical device containing drug(s), and the like could conceivably undertake. This limit is often expressed in global regulations, quality standards, safety standards, or financial terms.

   The precise quantification of risk capacity in safety terms is complex. This requires understanding the regulations, manufacturing conditions, intended product use, resources available, corporation infrastructure, and final quality sought.

2. *Risk tolerance*: This reflects the limit of risk set by the regulatory bodies and quality organizations based on sound scientific knowledge that it would not willingly exceed. This outside limit can be expressed in quantifiable terms, such as level of invested capital, quality of product, stability of the product, patient safety, and amount of allocated resources, both human and infrastructure. It may also include other subjective limits such as reputational risk in case of regulatory citations, warning letters, or recalls. Risk tolerance should not be determined in isolation. Risk tolerance should be considered in the context of the quality and stability of the product.

   Senior quality executive discussions about risk tolerance may appear to be theoretical rather than strategic. Defining risk tolerance provides an opportunity for the quality executives and management to reach consensus on the parameters for strategic decision-making. For example, the boundaries might include impurity levels in a given product, based on initial clinical studies. Executives should embrace these parameters, as they provide means to establish standard operating procedures and provide discipline in scoping appropriate strategic plans.

3. *Risk appetite*: Risk appetite is the level of risk that the enterprise willingly accepts in pursuit of its longer-term goals. Risk appetite should always be considered in conjunction with regulatory standards and dynamic to changes in business environment.

How do these three parameters interrelate? One can understand the risk capacity in the framework of defining risk tolerance. The disparity involving risk capacity and risk tolerance signifies the margin of error in risk tolerance, which serves as a measure of safety. Risk tolerance offers an important guideline for sound decision-making. Risk appetite drives activities to achieve the corporation's quality goals.

Effective decision-making in a quality systems environment is based on an informed understanding of risks. Elements of risk should be considered relative to intended use of a product, and in the case of pharmaceuticals, patient safety, while ensuring market availability of critical and important drug products. Management should assign priorities to activities or actions based on an assessment of the risk including both the probability of occurrence, of harm, and of the severity of that harm.

It is important to engage appropriate parties when assessing the risk, which include top management, regulatory, clinical affairs, quality, manufacturing management, and other stakeholders. Implementation of quality risk management includes assessing the risks, selecting and implementing risk management controls commensurate with the level of risk, and evaluating the results of the risk management efforts.

Since risk management is an iterative process, it should be repeated and updated if new information is developed that changes the need for, or nature of risk. In a manufacturing quality systems environment, risk management is used as a tool in the development of product specifications and critical process parameters.

2.1 Identifying Areas of Risk

Each corporation must perform a general SWOT (Strengths, Weaknesses, Opportunities and Threats) analysis to determine areas of risks and improvements.

1. Strengths: What are we good at?
2. Weaknesses: Where are the problem areas?

3. Opportunities: How do we provide better, cost-effective, high-quality products and services?

4. Threats: Regulatory issues, competitive products, quality problems, etc.

Next, the corporation should perform specific risk analysis for various processes in each business units. Tools such as failure modes and effects analysis (FMEA) allow for a systematic, proactive method of evaluating a process to identify risks and where and how a process might fail and to assess the relative impact of different failures, to identify the parts of the process that are most in need of change. One of these areas is the stability program.

2.2 Benefits of a Compliant Stability System

There have been number of FDA citations, both 483s and warning letters given for inadequate stability programs. In recent years, the number of FDA warning letters has increased substantially (*see* Fig. 1).

Most problems identified by the FDA are not technical in nature. An analysis of the FDA's warning letters of past 3 years (2014–2016) shows that one of the top ten citations is related to quality process, including inadequate stability program. Following are some examples of recent warning letters related to stability studies and stability programs.

FDA citation: Failure to have laboratory control records that include complete data derived from all laboratory tests conducted to ensure compliance with established specifications and standards.

The audit trail for high performance liquid chromatography (HPLC) instrument showed multiple integrations conducted on

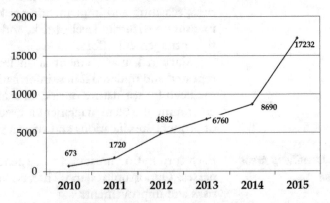

Fig. 1 FDA warning letters (Source: http://www.fda.gov/downloads/ICECI/EnforcementActions/UCM484400.pdf)

the 18-month stability tests for unknown impurity content for (……), without appropriate documentation, justification, and investigation [4]. Data management has been the focus of many of the citations because maintaining the quality and quantity of data generated from stability studies is challenging to manage for most organizations. Following are few examples of such citations.

FDA citation: Failure to follow and document laboratory controls at the time of performance. Our investigator observed inconsistently dated laboratory records. For example, your executed protocol records show that a 24-month time-point stability testing sample of (…… .) entered the laboratory on February 14, 2015. HPLC chromatogram printouts show that the sample was tested on February 12 and 13, 2015, 1 or 2 days before your protocol shows that the samples even entered the lab [4]. FDA citation: The official High Performance Liquid Chromatography (HPLC) impurity data for … .. Tablets batch … .., 3-month stability time-point @ 25 °C/ 60% RH only included the most favorable result obtained from multiple test results without any justification. The data from this batch was submitted to the U.S. FDA as an exhibit batch [5].

3 Recent FDA Guideline for "Data Integrity"

FDA and MHRA have both introduced guidances for data integrity [6, 7], which refer to the completeness, consistency, and accuracy of data. These guidelines are the response to number of observations worldwide (*see* Fig. 2), and provide for use of innovative technologies to capture and store the data in computerized formats.

Data integrity elements include:

1. Audit trail/e-signatures/data validation.

2. All data must be included in cGMP decision-making (including raw data, in-process data), or a proper justification provided.

3. Data changes to be performed by authorized personnel, with justification.

4. Audit trail to be reviewed (not just data) prior to final approval.

5. Control of: blank forms or cells, printing, missed samples.

6. "Testing into compliance" is prohibited.

7. Personnel should be trained in detecting data integrity issues - if issue is found, ensure steps are taken to remedy situation.

FDA expects that companies follow ALCOA when dealing with data, which should be attributable, legible, contemporaneously recorded, original or a true copy, and accurate.

Also, FDA requires that the quality system adequately ensures the accuracy and integrity of data to support the safety,

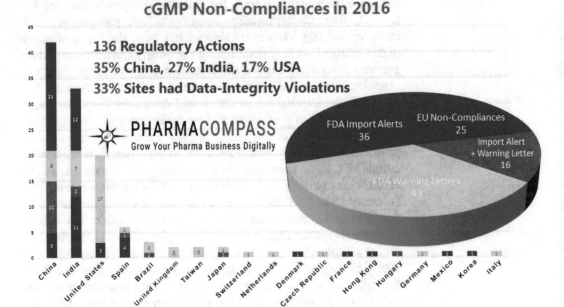

Fig. 2 Non-compliance 2016 (Source: http:/www.pharmacompass.com/radio-compass-blog/2016-a-year-of-data-integrity-issues-and-pharma-non-compliances)

effectiveness, and quality of the drugs being manufactured. On many different occasions the FDA requested that companies provide information to determine the extent of data integrity issues [4].

A comprehensive investigation into the extent of the inaccuracies in data records and reporting is necessary. In the investigation, the following criteria should be included:

1. A detailed investigation protocol and methodology; a summary of all laboratories, manufacturing operations, and quality systems covered by the investigation; and a justification for any part of operations that is excluded.

2. Discussions and third-party interviews with recent and previous staff to identify the reason, nature, scope, and root cause of data inaccuracies.

3. An assessment of the extent of data integrity deficiencies in the facility. Identify omissions, alterations, deletions, record destruction, non-contemporaneous record completion, and other deficiencies.

4. A comprehensive retrospective evaluation of the nature of the data integrity deficiencies.

Additionally, a current risk assessment of the potential effects of the observed failures on the quality of drugs, including analyses of the risks to patients caused by the release of drugs, and risks posed by ongoing operations, should be performed.

Finally, a management strategy that includes the details of corrective action and preventive action plan should be prepared. It should include:

1. A detailed corrective action plan that describes how the reliability and completeness of all the data generated including analytical data, manufacturing records, and all data submitted to the FDA is ensured.

2. A comprehensive root cause investigation of data integrity gaps, including evidence that the extent and depth of the current action plan is proportionate with the findings of the investigation and risk assessment.

3. Whether individuals responsible for data integrity gaps are currently working in positions that can influence cGMP-related decision or drug application data.

4. Interim measures describing the current or future actions to protect patients and ensure the quality of drugs being manufactured, including additional testing, recalls and client notifications, adding lots to your stability programs to assure stability, drug application actions, and enhanced compliance monitoring.

5. Long-term measures describing remediation efforts and enhancements to procedures, processes, methods, controls, systems, management oversight, and human resources (e.g., training, staffing improvements) designed to ensure the integrity of data.

In a paperless automated stability process, all data are quickly and easily acquired in electronic formats and stored in a secure, compliant database. Procedures are stored and accessed electronically, and are executed and documented in full compliance with data integrity guidelines.

The computer system assists in determining the risk areas scenarios, root cause analysis, trending of results, and shelf-life analysis of the product and product lines.

4 Stability User Requirements Based on Inherent Risks

There are several risks associated with a stability program such as:

1. Irregular testing intervals.

2. Inadequate pulling of samples.

3. Inadequate detailing of locations (sample storage and conditions).

4. High volume of data, difficult to track/manage.

5. Lack of effective shelf-life analysis.

6. Missed samples.

7. Notifications on any deviation found are communicated manually.

8. Manual reconciliation of actual vs. planned samples taken/pulled.

9. Regulatory compliance.

10. Costly validation.

11. Low operational efficiency.

In order to build an adequate program, measures should be in place to reduce, alleviate, or completely eliminate the risks.

The stability program should be evaluated to identify the inherent risks. Employee training & accountability plays a critical role in adequacy of the program.

Additionally, the program should inherently enforce best practices ensuring the consistency and accuracy of the scientific approach, methodology, and data.

The stability user requirements should be planned based on the following points in order to address the inherent risks with the stability program. The main components of the stability user requirements are:

1. 21 CFR Part 11 Compliance (Audit trail, time stamp).

2. Communication between cross-functional teams.

3. Metrics & Trending dashboards to measure improvements and effectiveness.

4. Manage system users (roles and responsibilities).

5. Workflow - Sample scheduling (date and time sensitive pulling of samples).

6. Notification and visual cues (email, change of color).

7. Important product information (name, ID, lot number, packaging).

8. Protocol and monograph (defining specifications and limits).

9. Inventory management (ensuring adequate number of samples in specified conditions).

10. Chain of custody (proper sample management and flow in the labs).

11. Using automation such as bar coding (tracking and tracing the samples rapidly and accurately).

12. Workload management (testing, reviewing, and approving the sample test results within the allocated timelines).

13. Management visibility across multiple sites and departments.

14. Out of specification (OOS) and out of trend (OOT) investigations and root cause analysis.

15. Data Integrity.

16. Reporting and dedicated statistical analysis.

The following case study is an example of how a new computerized system assisted a pharmaceutical company to address and remedy a warning letter due to improper stability program.

4.1   Case Study

Following an unannounced audit by the FDA, a warning letter was issued to a pharmaceutical company, which included the following deviations:

1. Failure to establish proper testing programs designed to assess the stability characteristics of drug products.

2. Failure to test stability samples at the scheduled intervals. During the course of the inspection, the investigator documented at least seven lots of product that were subsequently recalled after errors were discovered in the expiration dates.

In response to the warning letter, the company proposed to automate their stability program thus reducing or eliminating the risk of missing post market study commitments, missing sample pull schedules, as well as a variety of other possible risks. Further, with the recently released data integrity regulations, the company clearly needed to improve their data integrity and process efficiency.

The company initiated the process of finding and evaluating software systems specifically designed to meet the need of fully managing their stability program. This case study illustrates the key steps the company followed to accomplish this goal, and also provides details of the features required to both remediate the intrinsic risks in the stability program, including data integrity elements required in the software system, based on which decisions influencing product quality and patient safety were supposed to be made.

4.1.1   Defining the Requirements

The company commenced with the initial evaluation of vendors and quickly realized that a traditional LIMS system would not meet their needs. The typical LIMS systems are designed to manage all generic samples passing through a lab without consideration to the distinct requirements for stability test samples in regard to calculations across time points in tests such as weight/moisture loss, or out-of-trend calculations for samples at the various time points using data from all previous testing from both earlier time points and common product/packaging/storage combinations.

Thus the requirement was for a system that was designed and dedicated to the process of managing stability studies from initiation to completion which not only included the cross study and cross time point calculations, but would also fulfill all regulatory and reporting needs as well as having the statistical analysis for shelf-life estimations.

To define the requirement of the system, the company assembled a team of cross functional personnel including LIMS system users, IT specialists, stability subject matter experts, statistical specialists, and regulatory specialists. This expert team contributed to the user requirements and the end result was a detailed user specification document, which could be used to perform a gap analysis against any vendor system; further this document served them during the execution of the performance qualification (PQ).

4.1.2   Process Workflow

In light of the data integrity and compliance guidance released by FDA in April 2016, and the need to implement the best possible system, the company included the stability workflow details as an integral part of the User Requirement Specification (URS) (*see* Fig. 3). The goal of including the workflow was to provide a clear picture to the vendors as well as having a better understanding of the scope of the system they were defining and a clear path to follow.

4.1.3   21 CFR Part 11: Compliance and Data Integrity

Compliance, security, and data integrity go hand in hand and must be built into the system; these important regulations equate to numerous features. All users have their own system login/password to represent their electronic signature. No user could access or interact with the system with any login, other than its own. Each user would be a member of a permission group, which would allow or disallow access to the features, windows, and reports throughout the system. These permission groups would include every feature in the system without exception.

Audit trails should record all changes to data within the system. They include the time stamp, unique name of the user executing the operation affecting the data, nature of the operation, and modified data (individually the old and new values). Finally, both the reason for the change and, where applicable, a change control number should be captured.

The following are the specific software requirements specified in 21 CFR part 11 [8]:

1. Validation of systems to ensure accuracy, reliability, consistent intended performance, and the ability to discern invalid or altered records.

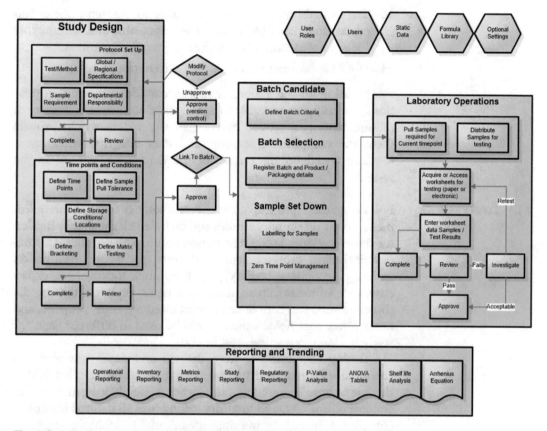

Fig. 3 Stability user requirement specification flowchart

2. The ability to generate accurate and complete copies of records in both human readable and electronic form.

3. Protection of records to enable their accurate and ready retrieval throughout the records retention period.

4. Limiting system access to authorized individuals.

5. Use of secure, computer-generated, time-stamped audit trails.

6. Use of operational system checks to enforce permitted sequencing of steps and events.

7. Use of authority checks to ensure that only authorized personnel can use the system, electronically sign a record, access the operation or computer system input or output device(s), alter a record, or perform the operation at hand.

8. Use of device/system checks to determine the validity of the source of data input or operational instruction.

9. Confirmation that personnel who create, maintain, or use electronic record/electronic signature systems have the education, training, and experience to execute their assigned task.

10. The establishment of, and adherence to, written policies and procedures that hold individuals responsible and accountable for actions executed under their electronic signatures.

11. Use of appropriate controls over system documentation.

By using all the above regulatory considerations and regulations, the company was able to define and document a robust set of requirements that would ensure that the system would provide them the compliance, security, and data integrity, which were required based on the nature of the data being housed in the system.

4.1.4 Stability Study Set

Following their process flow, the company defined the requirements to set up stability studies and included all the details needed for status tracking. Study registration required all product information including product name and code, packaging information (primary, secondary, tertiary), batch number, formulation, expiry date, date of manufacture, drug substances, seals, containers, the source of seals and containers, hazard category, study purpose, and many other data fields which would be used in different ways for study tracking, reporting, and filtering.

Testing requirements were defined and detail was given to ensure all different and unique testing could be handled within the one system. The testing, ranging across weight loss, dissolution, content uniformity, and impurity testing, was all defined for different criteria including multiple specifications, multiple stages of testing, calculated results, multiple results on which calculations would be executed, and the variations in the types of result (s) which would be reported for each different test type.

Some of the other key requirements of this section were: the ability to enter specification for different regions for the same test and the ability to dynamically filter reports specific to those regions.

Also, a formula library tool was included in the requirements that could be used to create mathematical equations, which could then be used to execute validated calculations on the raw data entry within the system, thus eliminating the need for external Excel sheets or manual calculations.

Finally, any type of stability study was to be supported in the system; these include accelerated, intermediate, long-term conditions, forced degradation, photo-stability, as well as transport studies. For each of these types, any number of time points could be defined with hours, days, weeks, or months as the unit of time, and would include pull tolerance settings.

4.1.5 Inventory and Sample Management

Sample storage, sample management, and sample tracking are all key elements for successful stability study management. The stability coordinator considered requirements for the overall inventory requirement, time point sample management, and chain of custody.

The efficiency of the workflow in regard to pulling samples and distributing them as needed to both the chemistry and microbiology labs were also considered.

The current company process was changed to achieve greater efficiency and integrity for sample management. Each sample would be labeled with a unique identification bar-coded label, each with a unique identifier, which could be scanned into the system. These samples were not dedicated to any specific interval, they were placed in boxes, the boxes were labeled to be easily recognized and then placed into environmentally controlled chambers.

At sample pull time, the stability coordinator would be able to enter the chamber and take any number of samples as required, and scan them out of storage using the barcode label affixed on each sample, and link them to a specific time point (interval). Weight loss samples were stored in their own box and the unique sample labels identified them specifically as the weight loss samples.

Pulling samples and all transfers of sample possession, from sample pull to sample discard, at the time point level, should be logged in the system, in a chain of custody feature. This feature should provide the complete history of each and every sample transaction and where samples were divided for different testing the company required reference labels to relate the divided sample to the specific test(s) it was being used for.

The company required all sample transactions to be executed using the scan operation, thus ensuing the correct number of samples was being pulled, and in the case of weight loss samples put back in storage, also that the correct samples were being used, and then finally discarded.

4.1.6 Notifications

Considering how time-dependent stability studies are, and that some of the biggest risks in a stability are missing samples and testing time points, the company clearly defined the automated notifications that would be needed to mitigate the risk of missing any due dates. Some of the email notifications, which were required on a daily basis, were:

1. Samples within pull tolerance.

2. Sample pull required today.

3. Overdue sample pulls.

4. Testing completion due within 5 days.

5. Testing completion due today.

6. And overdue testing.

Each of these emails and others were required to be sent automatically to a defined group of users.

Further to the automated notices, the company also required a series of reports which could be printed from the system on demand and filtered for any given date range. Using these filtered reports, the company would be able to review sample/testing schedules for any given study and for any given time range (day, week, month, quarter).

4.1.7 Laboratory Operations

Operational requirements consisted primarily of workload management that included testing samples, entering results and other method-related data, and reviewing/approving the sample test results all within the allocated timelines. To facilitate this process, the company defined requirements which would support GxP procedures and would include fail safes to minimize or completely remove the possibility of errors.

Some of the key requirements were data visibility across, or limited to multiple sites and multiple departments. Real-time notifications in the form of email, and visual cues based on field specific color change for OOS or OOT result status, as well as for ongoing or completed investigations.

Navigation within the system was also defined, including the ability to scan to any test or sample data using the barcode labels. Also, easy to filter and find views for individual tests, all interval test, tests within a certain department, all tests for a given storage condition, or all testing for all time points in a given study.

4.1.8 Reporting and Statistical Analysis

A robust reporting package must be present in the system. The company divided their reporting requirements into four sections.

Metrics to measure the efficiency of the sample pulls, meeting the testing time frame requirements, review, and approval due date various reports with this information were required to be in the system. *Dashboards* for operational reporting were also required; these included all the current status of the sample pulls, ongoing testing, as well as the review and approval statuses. *Study data reports* for external use were required for the regulatory submission purpose. The fourth was a *Statistical Reporting Package*, which would be dedicated to stability data and provides the calculation of the shelf-life. The statistical package had to include both linear regression and multiple regression, and user required the ability to trend across multiple batches, and other study criteria. The system was required to calculate both the shelf-life and the predicted expiry date for any given batch or study. To achieve this the "p value test" which verifies the poolability of batches and study dataset(s) was needed, as well as the calculation and output of ANOVA tables both before and after pooling on eligible datasets.

Another statistical requirement was the RH-modified Arrhenius equation to quantify drug product stability as a function of temperature and RH. Further statistical requirements included the scatter plot graph but more importantly was the out of trend evaluation based on already entered and approved study data from corresponding batches for the same product and packaging. All tabular and graphical presentations were to be printed to reports.

The critical requirement for the statistical analysis section was that it was required to be built into the system. The company made it clear to all possible vendors, that they were not interested in any system where the data would have to be exported to a third party statistical analysis tool.

Based on current data integrity requirements, exporting the data from the system means the data are no longer housed in a validated and compliant system and the manipulations of data are no longer controlled. Since the point of the system is to adhere to data integrity regulations, exporting it would have defeated the purpose.

4.1.9 Vendor Selection

The company followed a standard process for selecting a vendor by compiling a list of possible vendors, sending out the Request for Proposal (RFP) and then reviewing the responses to create a "Short List" of Vendors.

One of the key criteria on which the vendors were short-listed was that any one which had an extensive configurable system was removed. This decision was made in conjunction with the entire team. The company had experience in the past with systems that required extensive configuration; these projects ended up costing much more than originally budgeted.

Further, this requirement for the system to be OTS also stemmed from a specific time commitment made to the FDA. Extensive configurations not only cost more, but they also take more time to implement, and much more time to test and particularly to validate based on GAMP 5 software categories.

A Gap analysis was performed; the URS created by the project team was used as a tool to evaluate the vendors' systems and ensure that the requirements for compliance, data integrity, and stability process workflow were met.

The final vendor selected met 95% of the defined requirements OTS and the system inherent workflow was specific to the stability process detailed in the URS. Following the vendor postal audit, as per the company procedure for out of the box systems, the stability software program was purchased.

The company also purchased professional consulting services to compliment the resources available in the corporation. The services included:

1. Customization and configuration of about 5% of the system to meet 100% of the URS.

2. Hands on training services.

3. Process mapping of current process to the new process using the software.

4. Validation services including installation qualification (IQ) and operational qualification (OQ).

5. Services for writing new SOPs related to computerized stability program.

6. PQ support.

4.1.10   Implement and Validate

Validation is much more than just testing. Its scope is broader than testing and it has an emphasis both on achieving a validated state and on maintaining the validated state. A "Risk Based Approach" using GAMP was taken by the company to determine how to best focus their validation efforts.

GAMP 5 [9] has classified software under different categories based on its complexity, and also recommends evaluating the reliability based on extended use in the industry, and the likelihood of failure (Table 1). GAMP suggests the identification and evaluation of risks throughout the life cycle of the software. Critical risk areas must be identified and efforts concentrated on the point of risk.

The validation efforts were optimized by focusing on the key and critical functionality and the functionality that was the highest

Table 1
GAMP 5 categories

Category	GAMP 5
1	Infrastructure software – Established or commercially available layered software including operating systems, databases, office software, and the like. – Infrastructure software including virus protection, network management tools, and so forth.
2	Discontinued – Firmware I now treated as software in one of categories 3, 4, or 5
3	Non-configured products – Off-the-shelf products which cannot be changed to match the business processes. – Also, includes configurable products where only the default configuration is used.
4	Configured products – Software applications that are configured to meet user specific business needs. – Biggest and most complex category. – Software can be configured to return different outputs and as a result can require a much higher level of validation than GAMP 5 category 3.
5	Custom applications – Bespoke software is a software that is generally written from scratch to fulfill the business need. – Highest risk of the software categories

risk which was determined using risk analysis and GAMP 5 categorization. Also, the focus was on validation of the computer system for its intended use and testing for the functioning of the complete stability workflow.

The core of the selected system was OTS; the company considered the 95% requiring met portion to be category 3, and the remaining 5% requirement gap, which the vendor customized specifically for the company, was considered category 5.

The lion's share of the validation effort was focused on the following areas: the bespoke 5%, electronic signatures, 21 CFR part 11 requirements, statistical analysis, and shelf-life determination.

The company also took into consideration the maturity of the quality processes of the vendor, taking the opportunity to leverage their experience in the process of validating the system. The vendor provided a complete set of validation documents, including design specification, functional specification, installation guide, user guide, IQ, OQ, and PQ template. Finally, a complete traceability matrix, linking all requirements to testing being executed, was included. The validation approach followed the standard validation V-model (*see* Fig. 4).

The left side of the V represents the specifications—user requirements, functional specifications, hardware and software design, and module specifications. The right side of the V represents the system testing against the specifications. The bottom of the V indicates the code modules.

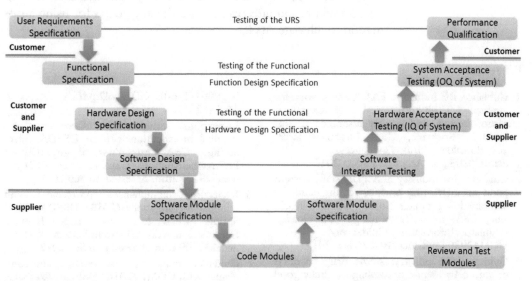

Fig. 4 Validation V-model

5 Conclusion

There is an enormous amount of data required to support the stability of pharmaceutical products. This is amplified when there are several presentations or doses of the same products destined for multiple jurisdictions. There are many things that can go wrong internally that present risks to compliance and potentially safety of the product in the field. Data integrity requirements are extremely important in the industry. As described using the case study, the impacted company was able to define the risks, translate them into proper user requirements, look for a solution and vendor, initiate a project to deliver a final validated solution, and go live with the system to complete the remediation to the warning letter within the agreed time frame. All risks were mitigated and reduced. The system was implemented successfully and met all user requirements, including remediation of past risks, efficiencies for the future, and improved governance of the stability program as a whole. After implementing the Stability Management Software, the company experienced a significant improvement in their laboratory operations throughput; they were able to implement a regular review process of all the system metrics to achieve a continuous improvement approach for stability study management.

Every industry can create better products and services from analyses of available data. Computerized systems assist corporations with this analysis. Management visibility across multiple plants/departments, communication between cross-functional teams, metrics & trending dashboards allowing the measurement of improvements and effectiveness are the key points for using automation to alleviate risks.

References

1. Guidance for industry: PAT-A framework for innovative pharmaceutical development, manufacturing, and quality assurance (2004) USFDA, Rockville, USA. https://www.fda.gov/downloads/drugs/guidances/ucm070305.pdf. Accessed 26 Sep 2017

2. Guidance for industry and FDA staff: current good manufacturing practice requirements for combination products (2017) USFDA, Rockville, USA. https://www.fda.gov/downloads/RegulatoryInformation/Guidances/UCM429304.pdf. Accessed 26 Sep 2017

3. Guidance for industry: sterile drug products produced by aseptic processing—current good manufacturing practice (2003) USFDA, Rockville, USA. https://www.fda.gov/ohrms/dockets/dockets/05d0047/05d-0047-bkg0001-Tab-09-GDL-vol2.pdf. Accessed 26 Sep 2017

4. Inspections, compliance, enforcement, and criminal investigations (2016) USFDA, Silver Spring, USA. http://www.fda.gov/ICECI/EnforcementActions/WarningLetters/2016/ucm529237.htm. Accessed 26 Sep 2017

5. Inspections, compliance, enforcement, and criminal investigations (2015) USFDA, Silver Spring, USA. http://www.fda.gov/ICECI/EnforcementActions/WarningLetters/2016/ucm432709.htm. Accessed 26 Sep 2017

6. Guidance for industry: data integrity and compliance with CGMP (2016) USFDA, Rockville, USA. https://www.fda.gov/downloads/drugs/guidances/ucm495891.pdf. Accessed 26 Sep 2017

7. MHRA GxP data integrity definitions and guidance for industry (2016) MHRA, UK. http://academy.gmp-compliance.org/guidemgr/files/MHRA_GxP_data_integrity_consultation.pdf. Accessed 26 Sep 2017

8. Guidance for industry: part 11, electronic records; electronic signatures-scope and application (2003) USFDA, Rockville, USA. https://www.fda.gov/downloads/regulatoryinformation/guidances/ucm125125.pdf. Accessed 25 May 2017

9. Wyn S GAMP® 5—a risk-based approach to compliant GxP computerized systems (2008). International Society for Pharmaceutical Engineering (ISPE), Enabling innovations. Available via https://www.ispe.org/publications/guidance-documents/gamp-5.

Chapter 9

Stability Considerations in the Life Cycle of Generic Products

Sanjay Bajaj, Srinivasan Rajamani, and Mona Gogia

Abstract

Generic products are the chemical, pharmaceutical, and biological equivalents of the innovator product that is already registered and currently in use in one or more countries. During development, generic products are subjected to a battery of stability tests to guide the choice of excipients, packaging material and processing conditions, and help establish shelf-life, storage conditions, hold time, and transportation environmental control. This chapter discusses key aspects of stability testing through the life cycle of a generic product.

Key words Generic products, Development, Life cycle, Regulatory submission, Stability testing

1 Introduction

Generic products are typically introduced into the market after expiry of the patent filed by the innovator. As a general understanding, the generic product must be equivalent, in terms of quality, efficacy, and safety, to that of the innovator's product already available in the market. It shall be comparable to the innovator's product in terms of dosage form, strength, route of administration, quality, and intended use. A generic product is expected to match even the stability laid down by the innovator.

Conceptually and practically, stability testing for a generic product is no different from that for an innovator's product. However, the objectives, outcome, and implication may vary with the stage of life cycle at which the drug or product is subjected to the stability testing based on market and packaging requirements. Stability requirements for the approval of a generic product are not harmonized globally. Multiple climatic zones [1] correspond to different long-term stability test conditions. Moreover, the requirements of packaging usually differ from country to country. Such incremental country-specific requirements add to the cost of the generic product that is typically launched at one-tenth of the price

Sanjay Bajaj and Saranjit Singh (eds.), *Methods for Stability Testing of Pharmaceuticals*, Methods in Pharmacology and Toxicology, https://doi.org/10.1007/978-1-4939-7686-7_9, © Springer Science+Business Media, LLC, part of Springer Nature 2018

of the innovator's product. Several stability related factors that need due consideration and are of prime importance during various stages of life cycle product development of simple generics are discussed in this chapter. Specific categories of drugs like herbal products (*see* Chap. 14) and biologicals (*see* Chap. 15) have been dealt with separately in this book, while novel drug delivery systems, multi-component generics, aerosols, medical devices, etc., which require special considerations, have been kept out of the scope of this chapter.

Stability studies are carried out in three stages during the life cycle of a generic product, i.e., during product development; for regulatory submission and post-approval to support any changes.

2   Stability Considerations During Developmental Stage of a Generic Product

Most of the times, a generic product is launched initially at a significantly lower price as compared to that of the innovator's product. The price keeps on lowering as more and more generics enter the market. To utilize the window of opportunity available to the first few generics, each manufacturer would make efforts to develop and launch the generic product as early as possible. A significant amount of time is spent on designing a stable generic product, and therefore, potential stability issues need to be addressed early during the development stage. Typically, when a generic product is being developed, the stability profile of the drug substance is well known. Also, the innovator's product is in the market with established storage conditions and shelf-life. A generic development is, therefore, targeted toward a formulation that is comparable with the innovator's product and can be assigned similar storage conditions and shelf-life. Stability of a pharmaceutical product can be best achieved through the principles of Quality-by-Design (QbD). Within the framework of QbD and the Question-based-Review (QbR) implemented by regulatory authorities, the generic manufacturers are able to identify the potential stability issues, and hence design the formulation, manufacturing process, and the container closure system accordingly. Typically, in a pharmaceutical industry, during the generic product development phase, stability studies are carried out initially to support the selection of excipients, packing material, and formulation development. This is then followed by the formal full-scale stability study conducted on registration batches to seek the generic product approval and the same is then extended to the commercial production batches according to the specific regulatory requirements.

Stability-related key considerations during development of a generic drug product are discussed in the following sections.

2.1 Drug Substance Stability Considerations

It is acknowledged that at the time of generic product development, the stability of the drug substance is known. However, there may be differences in quality of the drug substance with respect to the impurity profile and polymorphism due to differences in the route of synthesis, starting materials, solvents, processing conditions, packaging, and storage conditions used by various drug substance manufacturers. An understanding of intrinsic stability of the drug molecules and their degradation pathway enables a formulation scientist to design the pharmaceutical product such that the degradation is minimized. Forced degradation studies on the drug substance provide an insight into the possible degradation mechanisms and facilitate pharmaceutical development, manufacturing, production, and packaging where knowledge of chemical behavior can be used to improve drug product stability. Impurities in the drug products are required to be controlled as per ICH Q3B [2]. Most of the requirements stated in this guidance also apply to the generic products. Specific guidance for the generic products is also available from US FDA [3].

The drug product is expected to have process impurities controlled at the same level as that in the drug substance. It is important to identify the impurities in the drug substance that result from the process and which are formed as a result of degradation. While the process impurities from drug substance may not increase in the drug product, the degradation impurities tend to rise during storage of the formulation.

Different polymorphic forms may have differences in therapeutic efficacy. Generic products are required to establish therapeutic equivalency to that of innovator's product. Therefore, it is essential to establish that polymorphic form of the drug substance does not change over the time. The decision tree in USFDA's Guidance for the Industry ANDAs: Pharmaceutical Solid Polymorphism [4] very clearly explains the approach to be followed for the control of polymorphic forms in the drug substance and the drug product.

In general, a review of the retest period assigned to the drug substance as well as the storage conditions on the package label may give useful insight into the potential instability of a drug substance to be considered during the development of a generic product.

2.2 Excipient Information

A possible source of impurities in a drug product may be the excipients used in the formulation. Instability of the product due to the impurities originating from excipients is studied during product development stage. Although the generic product formulation have a flexibility to use excipients other than what are present in the innovator's product, a generic manufacturer usually prefers to use the same excipients, unless its use is limited by a patent. This is to ensure that the generic product is formulated as close as possible to the innovator's product. Many excipients especially the diluents, disintegrants, and binders are commercially available in different grades. The publicly available innovator product information lists out the name of the excipients but not the grades and quantities. The cost of the specific grade excipient may also be a key consideration for its selection. Further, the innovator may have used customized excipients for the specific application (e.g., ready-to-use coating composition with different pigment and polymer ratio, flavor mixtures). Therefore, during generic development, it is justified to conduct drug-excipient compatibility studies to rule out any drug-excipient or excipient-excipient interaction as that may also affect the stability of the generic product.

2.2.1 Drug-Excipient Compatibility Study

A typical drug-excipient compatibility study design is carried out in the following steps:

1. Equimolar mixtures of the drug substance and chosen excipients (e.g., 1:1 ratio) are intimately mixed, so as to allow good interaction, and are then transferred, preferably into the glass vial.

2. The vial is kept in open and closed condition.

3. The samples are exposed to long-term and accelerated stability test conditions so as to gain knowledge of all possible physical and chemical interactions.

Table 1 gives the details of the study design. If new excipients are used in the generic product, a full characterization is required to be carried out to rule out the contribution of the new excipient in the instability of the generic product.

Table 1
Typical drug-excipient study design

Vial code	Name of drug substance (D)	Name of excipient (Ex)	Ratio (D:Ex)	Initial Closed	25 °C/60% RH, 1 month Open	25 °C/60% RH, 1 month Closed	40 °C/75% RH, 1 month Open	40 °C/75% RH, 1 month Closed
1a	D	Ex-1	1:1	√	–	–	–	–
1b	D	Ex-1	1:1	–	√	–	–	–
1c	D	Ex-1	1:1	–	–	√	–	–
1d	D	Ex-1	1:1	–	–	–	√	–
1e	D	Ex-1	1:1	–	–	–	–	√
2a	D	Ex-2	1:1	√	–	–	–	–
2b	D	Ex-2	1:1	–	√	–	–	–
2c	D	Ex-2	1:1	–	–	√	–	–
2d	D	Ex-2	1:1	–	–	–	√	–
2e	D	Ex-2	1:1	–	–	–	–	√

2.3 Packaging Considerations

Packaging plays a significant role in ensuring stability of a drug product. For a product intended to be marketed globally, stability needs to be demonstrated in each type of packaging. As such, the container-closure system for a generic product is expected to match that of the innovator's product. Various packaging materials are now available for pharmaceutical products; therefore, selection of container-closure system for a generic product is carried out during the early development stages. Since cost of packaging contributes significantly to the overall cost of the generic product, selection of the most cost-effective material that provides protection to the product over the intended shelf-life is critical. However, the selection becomes challenging when the product is expected to be marketed globally. This is because each country has its own dispensing practices and typically, pack type and sizes. Table 2 explains how bracketing may be considered when more than one pack size but same pack type (e.g., High-density polyethylene (HDPE) bottles) is considered for marketing. A guide to selection of packing based on stability considerations is given in Table 3. Critical parameters tested on packaging materials during screening and stability testing are:

1. Release of chemicals from components of packaging materials (extractables and leachables).

2. Release of visible and or subvisible particles.

3. Adsorption or absorption of pharmaceutical components by packaging material.

4. Chemical reaction between pharmaceutical product and packaging material.

5. Degradation of packaging component in contact with pharmaceutical products.

6. Influence of manufacturing process of the container.

7. Water vapor transmission rate (WVTR).

Table 2
Bracketing for HDPE bottle pack—various counts

Strength	30 mg			60 mg			90 mg		
Pack size	30's count	50's count	100's count	30's count	50's count	100's count	30's count	50's count	100's count
Batch 1	T	–	T	–	–	–	T	–	T
Batch 2	T	–	T	–	–	–	T	–	T
Batch 3	T	–	T	–	–	–	T	–	T

Note: *T* - Sample tested

Table 3
Guide to selection of suitable packing

Material of construction/type	Critical properties	Area of use
Polymer/blister pack		
PVC (Polyvinyl Chloride) 200/250/350	Low barrier/simple unit pack/aesthetic	Stable products
PVC/PVdC (Polyvinylidine Chloride) (250/40)	Low barrier better than PVC	Product not very sensitive to moisture and gases
PVC/PVdC (250/60)/(250/90)/(250/120)	Good barrier	Moderate to highly sensitive products
PVC/PE/PVdC (250/25/60)/(250/25/90)/(300/30/90)	Good barrier	Highly sensitive products
PVC/Aclar (10–100 μm)	Excellent barrier	Extremely moisture sensitive products
OPA (Oriented Polyamide)/Alu foil/PVC	Excellent barrier	Extremely moisture sensitive products
OPA/Alu foil/PVC with desiccant	Excellent barrier	Extremely moisture sensitive products
Aluminum foil with HSL (Heat Seal Laquer)	Excellent barrier	Lidding foil for blister packing
Aluminum foil (hard tempered with special coating	Excellent barrier	Lidding foil for blister packing
Aluminum foil/poly 30–40 microns soft tampered	Excellent barrier	Strip packing of very sensitive products
Aluminum foil/VMCH (Vinyl chloride vinyl acetate copolymer resin) 30–40 microns soft tampered	Excellent barrier	Strip packing of very sensitive products
Container-closure system		
HDPE (High-density polyethylene) container	Good barrier to moisture, gas, and light	All kind of products from solid oral and dry syrup
PET (Polyethylene terephthalate)/PP (Polypropene) (Amber)	Moderate barrier	Light sensitive products
Glass bottles	High barrier	Highly sensitive products
Glass vials (USP I and USP II)	High barrier	Injectable products
Glass vials (USP III)	High barrier	Dry syrup, suspension, and powder for injection
PFS (Prefilled syringes) (glass/PE)	Moderate to high	Unit dose injectables

(continued)

Table 3
(continued)

Material of construction/type	Critical properties	Area of use
Rubber stopper	Chemical resistant, low permeability, low water/solvent	Injectable products
Desiccant silica gel bags Activated carbon Molecular sieves	Desiccant will effectively alleviate moisture and odor problems	Moisture sensitive products Product releasing odor/gas Highly moisture sensitive products

Additionally, testing of package integrity is an important point of consideration as failure in an otherwise impervious container-closure system may occur due to the failure in the seal integrity at the interface. Disruption of the integrity of pack may affect the drug product stability due to ingress of moisture, oxygen, or even microbial contamination. Some examples of typical integrity testing involve the tests on different packaging like bubble test for blister/strip pack and liquid bottles/cap; pressure decay test for vials, ampoules, blisters, pouches, and intravenous bags; and vacuum decay test for vials and ampoules.

2.4 Manufacturing Considerations

Information gained from the early developmental stability studies can provide an insight into specific and controlled environmental conditions to be maintained during routine manufacturing process. Few examples of manufacturing considerations important for ensuring a stable product are given in Table 4. Further, to ensure that the quality is maintained throughout the shelf-life, the maximum permissible hold time for the intermediate products at each manufacturing stage is determined under manufacturing conditions applicable for the commercial batches. Such a protocol-bound study may be carried out during development on pilot scale batches or during process validation studies. A typical program implemented by generic manufacturers to determine the hold time of intermediate products at each manufacturing stage is given in Table 5.

2.5 Determining Stability of Reference Product

Generic products are formulated to be interchangeable with the innovator's product. Stability evaluation of the innovator's product may provide a pathway to the qualification of impurities in the generic product. US FDA guidance on "ANDAs: Impurities in Drug Products" [5] allows the ANDA applicants to use the information generated on the reference listed drug (RLD) to provide a rationale for establishing the acceptance criteria for impurities.

Table 4
Manufacturing considerations based on product type

Type of product	Manufacturing conditions
Photosensitive products	Conditioned lighting in manufacturing area
Moisture-sensitive products	Low humidity conditions in manufacturing area
	Silica gel bags are used in bulk holding containers for the intermediate stage products
	Solvent coating in place of aqueous-based coating
	Use of moisture-free compressed air
Oxygen-sensitive products	Processing time to be limited
	Inert gas flushing
	Oxygen busters are used in the bulk hold containers for the intermediate stage products

During generic product development, it is useful to determine the impurity content of three batches of RLD with different residual shelf-life and also to carry out a short-term stability on at least two batches in comparison to the generic product using same validated analytical methods. This enables the formulation scientist to predict the potential degradation and set limits for the generic product accordingly.

2.6 Stress Testing as a Tool to Evaluate Degradation Mechanisms and Establishment of Stability-Indicating Analytical Methods

During method development, analytical scientists carry out stress testing or forced degradation testing of drug substance and drug product to understand the degradation mechanism and evaluate the stability-indicating nature of the analytical method. Such studies can also serve as a useful tool for the formulation scientist to predict the possibility of degradation during long-term storage. Results from an appropriately designed stress testing program can be used not only to select excipients and packaging material but also to support the transit conditions and determine the possible impact of temperature excursions during shipment. Stress studies are usually carried out on unpackaged generic product. There are no official guidances available on how the stress testing program should be carried out; however, typical stress conditions and duration of exposure for various dosage forms are listed in Tables 6, 7, and 8.

2.7 Polymorphic Change in Generic Products

Polymorphs are known to have different chemical and physical properties that can have a direct impact on the quality/performance of drug products such as stability, dissolution, and

Table 5
A typical hold time study program

Product type and process	Hold time study intermediate stage	Time points	Suggested tests
Uncoated tablets (Direct compression/ Dry granulation)	Blend before lubrication	0, 7, 15, 30 d	Description, water content, assay, related substance, microbiological enumeration test
	Lubricated blend	0, 7, 15, 30 d	Description, water content, assay, related substance, microbiological enumeration test.
	Uncoated tablets	0, 7, 15, 30, 60, 90 d	Description, water content, assay, related substance, resistance to crushing, dissolution, microbiological enumeration test.
Coated tablets (Wet granulation)	Dry mix blend	0, 7 d	Description, water content, assay, related substance, microbiological enumeration test
	Binder solution	0, 12, 24, 36, 48, 72 h	Description, viscosity, microbiological enumeration test
	Wet granules	0, 12, 24, 36, 48, 72 h	Description, water content, microbiological enumeration test
	Blend before lubrication	0, 7, 15, 30 d	Description, water content, assay, related substance, microbiological enumeration test
	Lubricated blend	0, 7, 15, 30 d	Description, water content, assay, related substance, microbiological enumeration test
	Uncoated tablets	0, 7, 15, 30, 60, 90 d	Description, water content, assay, related substance, resistance to crushing, dissolution, microbiological enumeration test.
	Coating solution	0, 12, 24, 36, 48, 72 h	Description, viscosity, microbiological enumeration test
	Coated tablets	0, 15, 30, 60, 90 d	Description, water content, assay, related substance, resistance to crushing, dissolution, microbiological enumeration test
Liquids (Syrups, Oral Solutions, Suspensions and Linctus)	Un-filtered solution	0, 1, 2, 5, 7 d	Description, pH value, weight per mL, assay, related substance, viscosity and microbiological enumeration test
	Filtered solution	0, 1, 2, 5, 7 d	Description, pH value, weight per mL, assay, related substance, viscosity, microbiological enumeration test
Suspensions (Powders for oral suspension, if the processed by simple blending and filling)	Blend powder	0, 7, 15, 30 d	Description and water content assay, related substance, microbiological enumeration test.

Note: 0-initial time point; water content may also be presented as loss on drying (LOD), as is applicable for the sample

Table 6
Typical stress conditions during pre-formulation studies [6]

Stress factor	Conditions	Concentration of Drug[a]	Time
Heat	60 °C	1:1 with diluent[b], solid state	1–10 d
Humidity	75% Relative humidity or greater	1:1 with diluent[b], solid state	1–10 d
Acid	0.1 N Hydrochloric acid	2:1 in 0.1 N Hydrochloric acid	1–10 d
Base	0.1 N Sodium hydroxide	2:1 in 0.1 N Sodium hydroxide	1–10 d
Oxidation	3% Hydrogen peroxide	1:1 in 3% hydrogen peroxide	1–10 d
Photolysis	Metal halide, Mercury, Xenon, or Ultraviolet-B fluorescent lamp	1:1 with diluent[b]	1–10 d
Metal ions (optional)	0.05 M Fe^{2+} or Cu^{2+}	1:1 with solution of metal ions	1–10 d

Note: [a]When testing degradability of drug substance in combination, the drug substance should be in the same ratio as in the fixed dose combination
[b]In each case, the diluent is either an excipient or all excipients in the formulation in the same ratios as in the formulation. Other ratios of diluent may also be appropriate, e.g., the approximate ratio in which the drug and excipients will be used in the formulation

Table 7
Typical stress testing storage condition for solid oral dosage forms [7]

Storage conditions	Duration of the study[a]
40 °C/75% RH	3 months
50-60 °C, ambient RH	3 months
Photostability	According to ICH Q1B

Note: [a]Time period should be reduced according to degradation, either 3 months or 5–15% level of degradation, whatever comes first

bioavailability. A change in polymorphic form may occur in response to changes in environmental conditions, processing, or over time. Conversion is also possible during drug product manufacturing unit operations (e.g., milling/micronization, wet granulation, heating, compression, and spray-drying). The drug substance in a generic product should essentially be "same" as that of the reference drug product and "sameness" can be demonstrated in terms of identity. The generic product must demonstrate that it meets the standards for identity, stability, and is

Table 8
Typical stress testing conditions for drug substance in solution forms [7]

Storage conditions	Duration of the study[a]
At about pH 2, room temperature	2 weeks
At about pH 7, room temperature	2 weeks
At about pH 10–12, room temperature	2 weeks
Hydrogen peroxide, 0.1–2% at neutral pH, room temperature	24 h

Note: (1) Stress testing of drug substance in solution form at elevated temperature may be of interest on case to case basis, e.g., to predict the stability during autoclaving of solution form
(2) Stress testing in solution should be conducted on dissolved samples; additives may be used to enhance the solubility
(3) Suspensions are not recommended because degradation might be influenced by the presence of particles, and sensitive products liable to degradation can be protected if suspension formulation is used
[a]Time period should be reduced according to degradation, either the above storage condition or 5–15% level of degradation, whichever comes first

bioequivalent to the reference product, but may not be required to have the same physical form (particle size, shape, or polymorphic form) as the drug substance in the reference product. One polymorph may convert to another during manufacturing and storage, particularly, when a metastable form is used. The possibility of multiple polymorphs of drug substance being formed, the properties of individual polymorphs, and the desired polymorph for the generic product and its stability should be investigated and understood during early development stages. The decision trees in US FDA's guidance for industry "ANDAs: Pharmaceutical Solid Polymorphism" [4] can then be applied to the information gained to determine if a specification is required to confirm the nature of the polymorph present in both bulk substance and product. When concerns regarding polymorph do exist, regulatory authorities expect that generic producers determine that there is no change in the polymorphic form as a result of manufacturing process and upon long-term storage.

2.8   Designing Stability Specifications

Stability specifications of a generic product must be inclusive of testing all attributes that are indicative of quality, safety, and efficacy and are susceptible to change during storage. The physical, chemical, and microbiological attributes to be monitored on stability for various dosage forms are listed in Table 7 of Chap. 2. The testing frequency is mentioned in ICH Q1A(R2) [8]. While all critical tests have to be tested at all intervals, it is acceptable to conduct some of them at the end of proposed shelf-life or at less frequent intervals to show compliance. Release test results, development batches stability results as well as expected analytical and manufacturing variables should be considered when setting up stability limits.

3 Stability Studies for Regulatory Submission

A standard stability package for the generic product is required to be included in the marketing authorization application (MAA). Stability must be demonstrated for all packaging configurations intended to be placed in the market. Usually, bracketing is applied for various pack sizes of the same pack type in order to reduce the number of samples being tested. Although ICH Q1D [9] allows bracketing and matrixing design approach to different strengths also, it is recommended to generate the entire stability data set for a generic product intended to be marketed globally. As a general requirement, the accelerated and long-term stability data are required to be submitted for three primary batches that are manufactured using two or more batches of drug substance. Two of the three batches of drug product must be of pilot scale or larger and the third could be smaller. Most generic manufacturers conduct stability studies on three batches of drug product since there are many countries where smaller than pilot scale batches for stability studies are not considered.

While the accelerated stability conditions are common across various zones, the long-term stability conditions are based on the zonal classification of countries where the products are intended to be marketed. The entire world has been divided into four climatic zones [1] and the conditions selected for long-term stability should conform to the respective zone in which the product is intended to be marketed. The stability studies of generic product intended to be marketed in countries falling in more than two zones could be designed such that samples and analysis can be kept to a minimum. The stability data to be included in the MAA is essentially 6 months of accelerated data and 6 months of long-term data. The latter, however, differs from country to country and up to 24 months long-term data may be required for some nations. Most of the countries allow extrapolation of limited long-term stability data to determine the shelf-life of the drug product, as outlined in ICH Q1E [10].

Due to dispensing practices in the USA, FDA has mandated stability testing of split tablets as review criteria for approval of an abbreviated new drug application (ANDA) for a scored generic product. As per the guidance for industry entitled "Tablet Scoring: Nomenclature, Labeling, and Data for Evaluation" [11], split tablets are required to demonstrate adequate stability for a period of 3 months at long-term conditions of $25\,°C \pm 2\,°C/60\%\,RH \pm 5\%$ RH. In most countries, breakability of scored tablets as per pharmacopoeia is required to be demonstrated at the end of shelf-life.

In addition to the standard accelerated and long-term stability studies, the test results of the following are also required to be included in the MAA for the approval of a generic product, as applicable.

3.1 In-Use Stability

In-use stability is required for products that are packed in containers with multiple doses or are to be reconstituted before administration [12]. There is no official guidance on how to conduct such a study. However, the study design should simulate the actual use and storage of the product. The length of the study should cover the time period over which the product is intended to be used and the number of doses in the pack. Thus, pharmacy packs of solid oral products may have an in-use period of 9 months whereas the eye and ear drops may have an in-use period of 30 days. Reconstituted oral suspension/solution may have an in-use period of 14 days, whereas reconstituted injection may have an in-use period of few hours.

The objective of in-use stability is to demonstrate that the physical and chemical properties of the product remain unaffected with repeated opening and closing of the container. Sterility cannot be assured once the integrity of the pack has been breached. Microbiological testing as a part of in-use study is, therefore, limited to determine the change in microbial burden after the container has been opened and this is highly dependent on the environmental conditions in which the opened container is stored.

At least two pilot scale batches of the drug product must be subjected to in-use stability testing. One of the two batches should preferably be near the end of projected shelf-life. At the predetermined time intervals, the product is tested using same validated methods as used for initial testing. All physical and chemical parameters indicative of stability of the product are tested and must comply with the shelf-life specifications. Generic products may have their own established in-use period that is justified by data and the number of doses in the pack.

3.2 Photostability

Understanding how light affects the drug product is useful to establish the type of packaging as well as storage conditions during usage of the product. As per ICH Q1B [13], a typical photostability program is designed with an approach to determine whether or not the exposed unpacked drug product, drug product in immediate primary pack, and drug product in the final marketed pack are photolabile. A preliminary photostability testing must be carried out during development and the confirmatory testing is required to be carried out on one pilot scale batch. Depending on the extent of change, special labeling or packaging is recommended to mitigate the risk associated with exposure of the product to light.

3.3 Stability Data Package

A standard stability data package for a generic product may be as follows:

1. 6 months accelerated stability data.
2. 6 months long-term stability data at conditions specified for the zone.

3. 12 months intermediate stability data if the product does not comply with pre-set specifications at accelerated conditions.

4. In-use stability data if the product is intended to be marketed in multidose containers or if the product is to be reconstituted before use.

5. Photostability data.

6. 3 months long-term stability data for split tablets.

4   Post Approval Stability

4.1   Annual Stability Testing Program

The stability studies do not actually stop once the drug product is approved but it is an ongoing process, which continues till the last batch of the approved product remains in the market. Thus, all drug products on the market must be monitored in a continuous program in order to demonstrate stability and quality over their entire market life. The objective of annual stability studies is to identify the minor changes in manufacture of drug product that may have an adverse effect on the quality of the product. The understanding behind these studies is to ensure that the products maintain their quality attributes while being subjected to the actual environmental conditions that might be different from the conditions when the batches for stability data package were manufactured. Annual stability studies are carried out on one batch each year (if commercial batch has been manufactured) only at long-term stability conditions as included in the stability data package for the approval of the product. Very often, matrixing and bracketing approach are applied to the annual stability program to keep the testing of stability samples to a minimum. Outcome of such annual studies are included in the annual product quality review (APQR).

4.2   Stability Testing Upon Post Approval Changes

After the product has been approved, there may be many changes in the drug product (e.g., change in drug substance source, manufacturing site, composition, process, primary packaging material, batch size). From a regulatory perspective, these changes may be annual reportable or a notification for change or may require prior approval of regulatory authorities before implementation. Some of these changes may be significant and require a substantial amount of stability data while others are minor and may only require a stability commitment. Guidance documents are available from various regulatory authorities US FDA [3], EMA [13], etc. that help manufacturers in designing stability studies for changes post approval of the product.

4.3   Supportive Stability Studies

Transportation of generic products should preferably be carried out under temperature conditions as finalized for the storage of the product unless it has been demonstrated that quality of the product is unaffected by minor excursions in temperature for a predefined time period. There are presently no official guidelines for testing pharmaceutical products in order to define suitable transport conditions. Although exposure to low temperature conditions are known not to effect solid oral dosage forms, liquids and semisolids may have an untoward effect when exposed to low or freezing temperature conditions. Studies must be carried out to predict the stability of the product throughout the conditions of shipment route and seasonal variations in the environmental conditions must also be considered. Exposure to high temperature as well as low/-freezing temperature conditions must be evaluated (*see* Chap. 12). For highly sensitive products, such studies should be carried out both during development stage and on batches for which the standard regulatory stability data package was generated.

4.3.1   Temperature Excursions During Transit

Pharmaceutical manufacturers face increasing regulatory pressure to provide data to support claims that product quality is unaffected by transient excursions in temperature and humidity extremes encountered during storage, distribution, and end use outside of storage conditions stated on the label. Alternative is to use expensive packaging and stringent shipping control measures.

Specific protocols have been proposed to study temperature and humidity excursions.

Two types of studies are in vogue:

1. Single excursion studies.
2. Repetitive cycling studies between two conditions.

In either case, one leg may be a control condition, or both legs may be extremes.

Packages intended for transport of goods are required to fulfill the primary function of physical protection to the contents. The packages are transported normally by road, sea, and air, and also inland water ways, either by one or a combination of these modes. The nature of the hazards that are confronted during transport varies widely depending on the distribution system, handling methods, and skills of staff employed.

The purpose of the study is to provide the documented evidence that transportation has no impact on the quality of the drug product.

5   Evaluation of Stability Data

The objective of the stability studies conducted as a part of submission package for product approval is to assign a shelf-life and storage condition to the product. This can be done with a critical evaluation of complete set of stability data obtained at various conditions. It is important to compare the stability results across batches and with the development batches to identify any results that do not follow the expected trend. Further, it is important that any investigation for out-of-specification (OOS) stability results is conclusive enough to determine the root cause of such results. While concluding the investigation, it should be clear whether the OOS results were actually related to the instability of the product or were probably due to analytical errors or improper batch manufacturing. While a true stability failure may need a redevelopment of the product, an improperly investigated OOS may conclude instability of an otherwise stable product.

ICH Q1E [3] provides a decision tree for stability data evaluation to estimate the shelf-life of a drug product intended to be stored at and below room temperature. If accelerated stability data shows significant changes, intermediate condition data and/or long-term stability data are considered for estimation of shelf-life. Significant change is described in ICH Q1A(R2) [1].

When 6 months accelerated data show no significant change and long-term data show no variability, extrapolation of data to assign the shelf-life beyond the period covered by long-term data is allowed. Such a shelf-life granted on the basis of extrapolation is verified by the actual long-term data for the time point corresponding to the end of the extrapolated shelf-life. As a part of stability commitment, long-term stability studies of the batches included in the stability package for product approval have to be continued till the end of proposed shelf-life.

If significant change occurs during accelerated stability, long-term data needs to be used for analysis and intermediate data for a period of 12 months and long-term data are required for the approval of the product. Extrapolation of data to assign the shelf-life beyond the period covered by long-term data is allowed and this is verified by the actual long-term data for the time point corresponding to the end of the extrapolated shelf-life. If intermediate data also shows significant changes, then shelf-life is granted based on the time period for which long-term stability data are available. No extrapolation of the stability data are allowed for determination of shelf-life in such situations.

For products intended to be stored in a freezer or below $-20\ ^{\circ}C$, the above-stated extrapolation is not applicable and the shelf-life is estimated based on the long-term data. Appropriate storage statements are included on the label based on the intended storage conditions and the outcome of photostability and in-use stability results. OOS results of batches under the annual stability program are very critical as these batches are in the market. Where safety and efficacy of the batch is affected, a recall is warranted. As a part of post approval commitment, any OOS results of batches under the annual stability program have to be reported to the regulatory authorities.

6   Stability-Related Information for Healthcare Professionals

Including information generated from stability studies in product information, e.g., package leaflet and summary of product characteristics, may be very useful for a healthcare professional. There have been instances when the color of solution for injection changes over time without affecting the quality of the product. A statement regarding the same in package leaflet would address the concerns when the color change is noted by a healthcare professional. Such a change, needs thorough investigation.

7   Conclusion

The development of a generic product, which is a therapeutic equivalent to that of the innovator's, requires testing for stability throughout the life cycle. Even for a generic product, elaborate stability-linked preformulation studies are essential to determine the quality attributes that are anticipated to affect the stability performance of the product subsequent to marketing. The prototype formulations are subjected to a variety of stability testing protocols, which are outlined in this chapter. The generic pharmaceutical industry must take responsibility that the products manufactured by it maintain their quality till used by the patients. It has to be clearly understood that stability testing is key to drug quality and hence is indispensable and must be implemented as per best practices that have been established by regulatory over the years.

References

1. WHO (1996) Technical report series, Guidelines for stability testing of pharmaceutical products containing well established drug substances in conventional dosage forms, 863. http://apps.who.int/medicinedocs/pdf/s5516e/s5516e.pdf. Accessed on 24 Sep 2017
2. ICH (2006) Impurities in new drug products Q3B(R2), Geneva. https://www.ich.org/fileadmin/Public_Web_Site/ICH_Products/Guidelines/Quality/Q3B_R2/Step4/Q3B_R2_Guideline.pdf. Accessed on 24 Sep 2017
3. US Department of Health and Human Services, FDA (1998 draft) Stability testing of drug substances and drug products, Rockville. https://www.fda.gov/ohrms/dockets/98fr/980362gd.pdf. Accessed on 24 Sep 2017
4. US Department of Health and Human Services, FDA (2007) ANDAs: pharmaceutical solid polymorphism, Rockville. https://www.fda.gov/downloads/Drugs/Guidances/UCM072866.pdf. Accessed on 24 Sep 2017
5. US Department of Health and Human Services, FDA (2010) ANDAs: impurities in drug products, Rockville. https://www.fda.gov/downloads/drugs/guidancecomplianceregulatoryinformation/guidances/ucm072861.pdf. Accessed on 29 Sep 2017
6. WHO (2005) Technical report series, No. 929, Annex 5, Guidelines for registration of fixed-dose combination medicinal products, Appendix 3, Pharmaceutical development (or preformulation) studies. http://apps.who.int/iris/bitstream/10665/43157/1/WHO_TRS_929_eng.pdf. Accessed on 29 Sep 2017

7. Klick S et al. (2005) Towards a generic approach for stress testing of drug substance and drug products. Pharm Tech 48–66. http://alfresco.ubm-us.net/alfresco_images/pharma/2014/08/22/5cd50f8c-cc0e-425a-b94b-66091196f691/article-146294.pdf. Accessed on 29 Sep 2017

8. ICH (2003) Stability testing of new drug substances and products Q1A(R2), Geneva. http://academy.gmp-compliance.org/guidemgr/files/Q1A(R2)STEP4.PDF. Accessed on 24 Sep 2017

9. ICH (2002) Bracketing and matrixing designs for stability testing of new drug substances and products Q1D, Geneva. http://www.ich.org/fileadmin/Public_Web_Site/ICH_Products/Guidelines/Quality/Q1D/Step4/Q1D_Guideline.pdf. Accessed on 24 Sep 2017

10. US Department of Health and Human Services, FDA (2004) Guidance for industry, Q1E evaluation of stability data, Rockville. https://www.fda.gov/downloads/drugs/guidancecomplianceregulatoryinformation/guidances/ucm073380.pdf. Accessed on 29 Sep 2017

11. US Department of Health and Human Services, FDA (2013) Guidance for industry, Tablet Scoring: nomenclature, labeling, and data for evaluation, Silver Spring. https://www.fda.gov/downloads/drugs/guidances/ucm269921.pdf. Accessed on 29 Sep 2017

12. WHO (2009) Technical report series, Stability testing of active pharmaceutical ingredients and finished pharmaceutical products, No. 953. http://apps.who.int/medicinedocs/documents/s19133en/s19133en.pdf. Accessed on 29 Sep 2017

13. ICH (1996) Photostability testing of new drug substances and products Q1B, Geneva. https://www.ich.org/fileadmin/Public_Web_Site/ICH_Products/Guidelines/Quality/Q1B/Step4/Q1B_Guideline.pdf. Accessed on 24 Sep 2017

Chapter 10

Predictive Stability Testing Utilizing Accelerated Stability Assessment Program (ASAP) Studies

Helen Williams

Abstract

Predictive stability studies allow the long-term stability characteristics of a drug substance or drug product to be characterized from extrapolation of results from a short-term stressed stability study. These studies are typically one month in duration and focus on chemical degradation. This chapter focuses on accelerated stability assessment program (ASAP) studies as one method of predicting stability. The main phases of performing an ASAP study are described including designing the protocol, setting down the studies, storing and analyzing the samples followed by reviewing and modeling the data and performing predictions. The applications of predictive stability studies are also discussed including in regulatory submissions.

Key words Predictive, Stability, ASAP, Accelerated, Packaging, Arrhenius, Solid-state kinetics

1 Introduction

The stability testing of pharmaceutical products during both the development and commercial phases places a significant burden on the industry, in terms of cost, resource, and time. Predictive stability methods utilize shorter stability studies under accelerated or stressed conditions, and are designed such that extrapolation of the degradation kinetics can be performed back to ambient storage conditions [1–5]. In this manner, the stability characteristics of a drug substance or drug product can be investigated in a short study of typically one-month duration. From a predictive stability study, not only can suitable long-term storage conditions be determined but also appropriate packaging selected [3, 4, 6] and the retest period or shelf-life predicted.

The most commonly used predictive stability study type is the Accelerated Stability Assessment Program (ASAP) study [3–5, 7], which focuses on chemical degradation monitored either by the formation of a degradation product or by the loss of the drug substance. These studies are based on standard Arrhenius kinetics for solutions or liquids and on a modified Arrhenius equation for

Sanjay Bajaj and Saranjit Singh (eds.), *Methods for Stability Testing of Pharmaceuticals*, Methods in Pharmacology and Toxicology, https://doi.org/10.1007/978-1-4939-7686-7_10, © Springer Science+Business Media, LLC, part of Springer Nature 2018

solids [2], to also take into account the effect of humidity on the rate of reaction as shown below.

Arrhenius equation - for solution/liquid kinetics

$$\ln(k) = \ln(A) - \frac{Ea}{RT} \tag{1}$$

Modified Arrhenius equation - for solid state kinetics

$$\ln(k) = \ln(A) - \frac{Ea}{RT} + B(RH) \tag{2}$$

where k = reaction rate

$\ln(A)$ = collision frequency

Ea = activation energy (kcal/mol)

R = gas constant (kcal/(K·mol))

T = temperature (K)

B = humidity factor

RH = relative humidity (%)

Predictive stability and ASAP studies have a wide range of applications throughout the development and commercial lifetime of a material [7]. These include formulation screening, setting initial retest periods and shelf-lives early in development, control strategy support, specification setting and justification, investigating batch-to-batch variability [8], investigating the effect of drug substance particle engineering on drug product stability [9], and supporting pack changes. ASAP studies are also particularly useful to assess the impact of any change during the development of a drug substance or a drug product on the chemical stability characteristics (e.g., if a minor drug substance route change or formulation change is made, an ASAP study can be performed to investigate the impact of this change on the chemical stability). If the ASAP study demonstrates equivalence with the existing drug substance or drug product, then no further stability testing on the new drug substance or drug product may be required at that time. ASAP studies are also useful for handling excursions during development. Predictions can be performed from the ASAP study data to help define a suitable excursion statement for a drug product. Similarly, if an excursion has occurred, then the ASAP data and predictions can be used to justify the suitability of the batch.

The aim of an ASAP study is to chemically degrade the sample to the relevant specification limit (in terms of potency or degradation product level) at a range of stressed stability conditions, where both temperature and humidity are varied independently of each other. This allows the time taken to reach the specification (or the reaction rate to specification) to be determined under each condition tested. For solving the relevant Arrhenius equation, the collision frequency ($\ln(A)$), the activation energy (Ea in kcal/mol) and the humidity factor (B), where relevant, for the specific reaction need to be determined. These values can then be used to predict the reaction rate to the specification limit at any given condition and so as to determine a suitable long-term storage condition and retest period/shelf-life for the sample [3–5]. It is important that the samples are degraded to the same extent (typically the relevant specification limit) at each storage condition, such that the degradation kinetics remain similar across the study, a concept called isoconversion [2–4]. This aims to overcome the complexity of heterogeneous solid-state kinetics and then allows extrapolation to the long-term storage condition.

ASAP studies can be used to investigate the chemical stability of a range of pharmaceutical materials including drug substances, raw materials, intermediates, tablets, capsules, granules, solutions, lyophiles, and other formulations [7]. ASAP studies conducted to date in the pharmaceutical industry have typically been applied to small molecules, but they can also be applied to larger biomolecules [7, 10] particularly when chemical degradation may be the shelf-life limiting attribute. Alternative models of predictive stability may also be considered, which have been discussed by Clancy et al. [11]. The authors have highlighted the applicability of other models and the use of water vapor pressure, instead of relative humidity when modeling certain hydrolysis reactions, given that hydrolysis could occur with water vapor in the atmosphere rather than liquid water adsorbed on a solid.

As with any stability study, the data generated from an ASAP study reflects the quality of the analytical methods used. It is important that the methods are designed to be stability-indicating. Specifically, for related organic impurity methods by liquid chromatography (LC), the degradation products should be suitably separated from the main component. Therefore, it is proposed that some forced degradation studies are performed, and the degraded samples are used to aid method development, in advance to an ASAP study. In silico tools can also be used to predict likely degradation products from a chemical structure, so as to aid in the design of a forced degradation study or method development. Examples of in silico tools include Zeneth, a rule-based system [12], and bond dissociation energy calculations [13]. For a chiral molecule, the potential formation of any enantiomers should also be considered, and if necessary, chiral analysis is included in the ASAP protocol.

One important prerequisite of an ASAP study is that the entity of interest does not change physical form during the study. Any form change could result in a change in the degradation kinetics and so invalidate any extrapolations to the long-term storage condition. Therefore, for designing the ASAP study protocol, it is important to assess any critical temperatures or humidities beyond which the sample or a component of the sample may change its form, and the protocol is adjusted accordingly.

Packaging predictions can be performed, the relative humidity inside a pack during the shelf-life of a product [6]. These predictions depend on the moisture vapour transmission rate (MVTR) of the packaging used, the ability of the sample to pick up moisture, the packaging conditions, and the external storage conditions. If both an ASAP study and packaging predictions have been performed for a specific product, it is further possible to predict the extent of degradation in different packaging configurations, without actually performing stability testing in the different pack types. From these predictions, a suitable packaging format and configuration can be selected. For example, the effect of changing the tablet count in a bottle can be determined, along with the effect of increasing the level of desiccant on the degradation of a sample susceptible to humidity. Predictions of the humidity in a pack can also be performed during the in-use scenario [14, 15]. These predictions take into account the opening and closing of a bottle, for example, and removing a number of tablets on each occasion.

One limitation of ASAP studies is that they tend to be focused on chemical degradation and this may not be the shelf-life limiting attribute for a specific formulation. Other stability-indicating attributes should also be considered and investigated where necessary, when setting a predicted shelf-life, for example, physical stability for a drug substance, dissolution for an oral solid dosage form [16] or for a solution formulation precipitation, change in pH or microbial growth. Results from a survey of the International Consortium for Innovation and Quality in Pharmaceutical Development (IQ) [17] member companies in 2016 suggested that across the industry in general ASAP predictions were based on assay or impurities but some companies also reported modeling physical stability such as disintegration, dissolution, hardness, and form changes [7]. Clancy et al. reported using predictive stability studies to model both hydrate formation and solvate loss [11].

While ASAP studies are currently not covered by International Council for Harmonisation (ICH) guidelines or guidance from specific regulatory authorities, the applications of ASAP studies are increasing within regulatory submissions. Freed et al. published the regulatory experiences from Pfizer of using predictive stability in submissions [18]. They reported submitting ASAP data to support an initial shelf-life of not more than 12 months for numerous drug products, without submitting standard stability data, in early clinical submissions in a range of markets. The survey of the IQ member companies performed in 2016 [7] ascertained that of the 19 companies surveyed 16 were using predictive stability studies. Ten of the companies surveyed reported using standard ASAP studies, with other companies using in-house predictive stability tools. Ten companies also reported using predictive stability data in regulatory filings, mostly in clinical submissions but also in some marketing submissions and to support post approval changes. Across the survey responses, it was evident that submissions involving predictive stability data have been approved in at least 23 countries.

2   Materials

2.1   Salt Solutions

Saturated salt solutions can be used to maintain certain humidity levels at different temperatures [19]. They should be prepared at least 24 h before use with an excess of solid to maintain saturation. The use of hot water to prepare the salt solutions may aid in achieving saturation. It is important to be aware that the solubility of some salts increases significantly as temperature is increased, so a salt solution that is saturated at room temperature may not still be saturated at higher temperatures used in the ASAP studies. Enough salt must be used to maintain excess solid salt and, therefore, saturation at the chosen storage temperature. Humidity capsules can also be purchased to achieve specific humidity at specific temperatures.

3   Methods

3.1   Designing an ASAP Protocol

1. Existing knowledge of the stability of the sample is useful when designing an ASAP protocol. The specific conditions and time points should be designed to degrade the sample to the specification limit and not too far beyond. Time points that bracket specification with one at least half way to specification and another not more than 150% of specification are ideal.

2. At least four conditions are required in an ASAP study but ideally at least five or six should be used.

3. Replicate samples are required to determine an accurate measurement for the initial time point, but also to determine the error in the study. Typically, a single analysis is performed for most time points, but at one intermediate condition and time point, multiple replicates are required such that a relative standard deviation (RSD) can be determined. This value can then be applied to the data from the whole study, to reduce the number of samples for testing.

4. It is also important to consider the aim of an ASAP study when designing the protocol. A typical protocol for a study to rank the stability of a number of solid oral dosage form prototypes is shown in Table 1 and a typical protocol to set a shelf-life of the same formulation type given in Table 2. For the ranking study,

Table 1
Typical protocol for a formulation prototypes ranking study

Temperature (°C)	Humidity (% RH)	Time point (weeks)
NA	NA	Initial (duplicate)
50	75	2, 4, S
60	11	2, 4, S
60	50	2 (triplicate), 4, S
70	30	1, 2, S
70	75	1, 2, S

Note: S - spare

Table 2
Typical protocol for a shelf-life determination study

Temperature (°C)	Humidity (% RH)	Time point (weeks)
NA	NA	Initial (triplicate), X, C
50	30	2, 4, S
50	75	2, 4, S
60	11	2, 4, S
60	50	2 (fivefold repeat), 4, S
70	30	1, 2, S, X, C
70	75	1, 2, S, X, C

Note: S - spare, X - solid state sample, C - chiral sample (if relevant)

a minimum of five conditions are suggested with at least duplicate analysis of the initial samples and triplicate analysis of an intermediate condition and time point. For a shelf-life setting study that could potentially be used in a regulatory submission, at least six conditions are suggested with triplicate analysis of the initial and a fivefold repeat of an intermediate sample.

5. Temperature and humidity should be varied independently in an ASAP study as demonstrated in Figs. 1 and 2 for the protocols shown in Tables 1 and 2, otherwise the independent effects of each variable cannot be determined (*see* **Note 1**).

6. If existing knowledge of the stability of the sample is limited as is often the case in early development, an initial scouting study or a flexible type protocol, with a number of spare samples at each condition, as shown in Table 3, can be used (*see* **Note 2**).

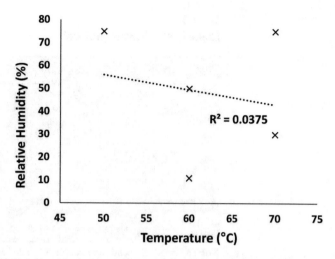

Fig. 1 Relationship between temperature and humidity for ASAP protocol in Table 1

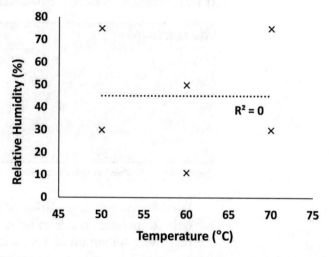

Fig. 2 Relationship between temperature and humidity for ASAP protocol in Table 2

7. One important criterion of an ASAP study as described in Sect. 1, is that the sample does not change physical form during the study. Therefore, it is key to understand the boundaries in terms of both temperature and humidity for a particular sample (*see* **Note 3**). For ASAP studies of formulations, these boundaries apply to the excipients as well as the active ingredients, as a change in the form of an excipient could also change the kinetics of the degradation of the active ingredient (*see* **Note 4**).

8. ASAP protocols for solution formulations are typically much simpler than for solids as there is generally no impact of

Table 3
Example of a flexible protocol

Temperature (°C)	Humidity (% RH)	Time point (weeks)
NA	NA	Initial (triplicate), X, C
50	30	2, S x 2
50	75	2, S x 2
60	11	2, S x 2
60	50	2 (fivefold repeat), S x 2
70	30	1, 2, S, X, C
70	75	1, 2, S, X, C

Note: S - spare, X - solid state sample, C - chiral sample (if relevant)

Table 4
Typical protocol for a solution formulation

Temperature (°C)	Time point (weeks)
NA	Initial (triplicate)
40	2, 4, S
50	2, 4, S
60	1, 2, S
70	1, 2, S, C

Note: S - spare, C - chiral sample (if relevant)

humidity on the degradation of the majority of solutions, so only temperature needs to be varied, as shown in Table 4. In this case, a minimum of three conditions are required.

9. For all protocols, irrespective of the sample type, it can be useful if a spare sample is included at each condition. The spare can be pulled if there is an issue with the analysis of samples at a particular time point and a repeat is required or pulled at a later time point, if further degradation is required in order to reach close to or bracket the specification limit.

10. When designing the protocol for an ASAP study, attention should be given as to what analysis should be performed, the methods used, and at which time points and conditions. For a typical drug substance or oral solid dosage form, impurities analysis by LC is most common. As discussed in Sect. 1 the method should be stability-indicating, as for any stability study.

11. At the last time point at the harshest conditions, solid state and chiral analysis should be considered when relevant, to confirm

that no change in the form or chirality has occurred during the study. If conversion to the enantiomer is thought to be the main degradation mechanism, then chiral analysis should be performed at all the conditions and time points.

12. Description analysis should also be considered when studies might be used to support a shelf-life claim in a regulatory submission. For different formulation types, other analysis methods may be more relevant (*see* **Note 5**).

13. When designing the protocol, the amount of sample needed for each time point should be calculated, based on the amount required for each analysis. For a formulation prototype ranking study, the amount of sample may be limited and the analysis may need to be performed using only one or two formulations at each time point for each condition.

3.2 Setting Down an ASAP Study

1. A representative batch or batches should be chosen for the ASAP study. It should be noted that the previous history of the sample, in terms of exposure to humidity, may be important (*see* **Note 6**).

2. ASAP samples can be stored in ovens using saturated salt solutions to control the humidity, in stability chambers that control both temperature and humidity, or using automated robotic storage systems (*see* **Note 7**).

3. Irrespective of the mode of storage, it is vital that the exact temperature and humidity that the samples are exposed to is measured, particularly for shelf-life prediction studies to support regulatory submissions (*see* **Note 8**).

4. It is critical that all the degradation that occurs during an ASAP study is caused by the effect of either temperature or humidity. If a sample is sensitive to photodegradation, it is important to protect from light on storage under the ASAP conditions.

5. The error in the analysis of ASAP study samples, and so in the resulting prediction, should be minimized wherever possible. As such, it is ideal to minimize the number of LC runs required. This can be achieved by staggering the set down of the study such that all time points pull on the same day (Fig. 3), and typically can be analyzed in one LC run including the initial samples. The initial samples, and samples for time points before they are set down, can be stored in the fridge or freezer, as relevant until required. If running a flexible ASAP protocol, as shown in Table 3, the samples cannot be tested in one LC run, plans should be followed where the number of runs ideally are still minimized.

3.3 Analyzing the ASAP Samples

1. Area percent analysis is typically sufficient for impurities analysis for an ASAP study. For a shelf-life determination study, which

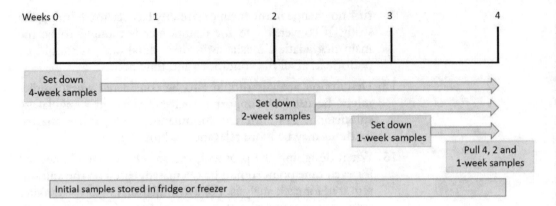

Fig. 3 Schematic of a staggered set down

could be used in a regulatory filing, it may be relevant to demonstrate mass balance via the use of external standards, by performing both assay and impurities analysis and applying knowledge of any relevant response factors. In the early phases of development, this may well not be possible as the relevant standards may not be available and response factors may not also be known. In such cases, area percent results may be sufficient.

2. It is also important to randomize the order of the samples throughout the LC run; this includes the replicate initial and intermediate samples, to avoid systematic errors affecting the subsequent predictions.

3.4 Reviewing the ASAP Data

1. When the analysis is completed, the data should be reviewed before any modeling is started.

2. For impurities analysis, the main degradation product that is likely to be shelf-life limiting needs to be determined from the data and not assumed from prior knowledge.

3. If multiple degradation products are formed, it may be necessary to model them all individually to determine which one is going to limit the shelf-life under certain long-term conditions.

4. The total level of degradation products should also be considered. In the case where multiple degradation products are formed at low levels, it may actually be the total level that fails specification before any individual impurity.

5. When the main degradation product(s) has been determined, the data should be reviewed to confirm whether at each condition the samples have degraded at least half way to specification and not too far past specification, as discussed previously.

6. Conditions where no degradation has occurred may need to be excluded from the model (*see* **Notes 9** and **10**). Time points

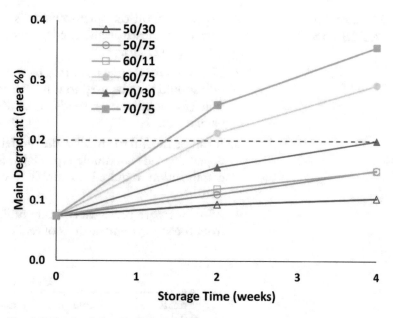

Fig. 4 Example of visualization of ASAP data

where degradation has exceeded 150% specification may also need to be excluded (*see* **Note 11**). Visualization of the data, such as that shown in Fig. 4, is always recommended.

7. When the conditions and time points to be used in the ASAP model have been identified, the mean value for the initial samples should be calculated from the multiple repeats and the RSD calculated for both the initials and intermediate condition/time point replicates. The higher of the RSD values should then be applied to the data across the whole study.

8. The degradation kinetics used to fit the data then needs to be decided. In the majority of cases a linear fit will be sufficient (*see* **Note 12**). The use of other fits should be justified scientifically (*see* **Note 13**).

9. Irrespective of the fit used, data at all conditions should be fitted using the same kinetics. If the extreme condition does not seem to fit the same kinetics as the rest of the conditions, this may be evidence that this condition is too harsh for the particular sample and not relevant to long-term storage conditions. As such it should be removed from the model. The removal of intermediate conditions from the model is much harder to justify scientifically.

10. When the data at each condition have been fitted the time taken to reach the specification limit and the degradation rate to specification under each condition can be determined.

3.5 Modeling the ASAP Data

1. Commercial off-the-shelf software is available to model ASAP data. Some pharmaceutical companies have developed custom software [11, 20].

2. The resultant degradation rate to specification at each condition should then be used to solve the relevant Arrhenius equation (for solutions or solids) and determine the Arrhenius parameters.

3. It can be helpful to visualize the model, either in 2D or in 3D, depending on the sample type (Figs. 5 and 6). The extent of extrapolation required to ambient conditions can also be visualized.

4. ASAP software packages typically utilizes the error calculated from the storage and analysis of replicate samples to determine

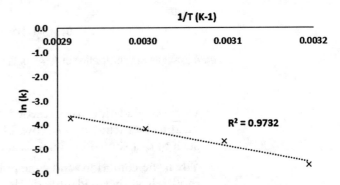

Fig. 5 Example of visualization of ASAP model for solution samples

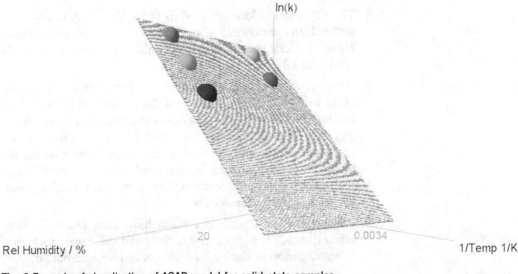

Fig. 6 Example of visualization of ASAP model for solid-state samples

the error in the time to reach specification at each condition. This error in turn then propagates through to the resultant error in the Arrhenius parameters and so gives confidence limits on the predicted degradation under long-term conditions.

5. The model generated is then critically evaluated. The Arrhenius constants determined should be within the expected range (*see* **Note 14**). Each condition should fit the model within the error determined. This can be determined from the R squared term (which should ideally be greater than 0.9) and the residuals. At this point, it may become obvious that one condition is an outlier in the model. Again, if this is the harshest condition, it can potentially be removed from the model. If it is an intermediate condition, it is harder to scientifically justify omitting it from the model (*see* **Note 15**). Leave-one-out cross-validation can also be performed to determine the Q squared term (which should ideally be greater than 0.8) and investigate the robustness of the model.

6. If the model generated is shown to be a reliable model, predictions can then be performed at the relevant long-term storage conditions. These predictions can then be used to rank formulation prototypes or predict retest periods or shelf-lives (*see* **Note 16**). A typical ASAP prediction versus a specification limit of 0.2% for the main degradation product is shown in Fig. 7. This example prediction can be seen to support a shelf-life of 12 months within the upper 95% confidence limit.

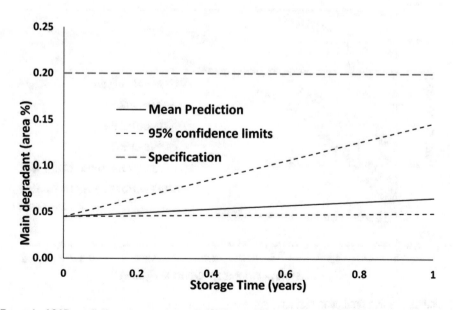

Fig. 7 Example ASAP predictions to support a shelf-life

7. In some cases, the degradation kinetics may not follow the assumptions of the modified Arrhenius equation and different models may need to be used (*see* **Note 17**).

3.6 Packaging Predictions

1. To predict a shelf-life in a packed product the MVTR of the pack should be determined either experimentally or via calculations. Standard test methods are available for polymer sheets or films (ASTM E96) and for pharmaceutical bottles and blisters (ASTM D7709).

2. The ability of the drug substance or product to pick up moisture at different humidities also needs to be determined, using dynamic vapour sorption (DVS) instrument.

3. Commercially available off-the-shelf software or pharmaceutical company's custom-built software [14] can then be used to determine the humidity in the pack over the time based on a number of variables. These include tablet count, size, and amount of desiccant for a bottle pack configuration.

4. Using the Arrhenius parameters from the ASAP study, the humidity in the pack can be converted to degradation level in the pack over the time on storage. By this method, different pack types and configurations can be compared, as shown in Fig. 8, without even performing any stability testing of the packed product.

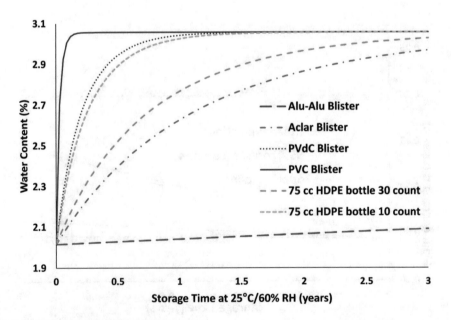

Fig. 8 Typical packaging prediction results

4 Notes

1. A hexagonal protocol design is one such option, such that there is no correlation between temperature and humidity [11].

2. An initial scouting study can be performed to determine the conditions and time points that are necessary to degrade the sample to specification. This is ideal but can significantly increase the amount of resource required. Instead of running a scouting study, the ASAP study itself can be designed in a flexible way such, that samples are tested at all conditions at an intermediate time point, for example, 2 weeks. Results from this testing can determine whether additional time points are required in order to degrade to specification, or alternatively if the degradation levels exceed specification, extra samples may be set down for a shorter period.

3. Examples of form changes to consider include conversion of amorphous material to crystalline, conversion of one crystalline polymorphic form to another, hydration or dehydration, melting, glass transition, deliquescence, and even sublimation. It is advisable to check the solid-state form of the ASAP samples stored under the harshest conditions at the last time point and compare to the initial sample, to ensure that no change has taken place. Typically, samples from the highest temperature and humidity conditions are analyzed, but also the lowest humidity at high temperature should be considered, as this condition may instigate a form change, for example, dehydration of a hydrate. Therefore, prior knowledge of the solid-state properties of the material can prove beneficial.

4. Solvates can prove challenging to design a suitable protocol for, as low humidity conditions could potentially pull off the solvate and under high humidity the solvate molecules could be replaced by water molecules. Amorphous solids also offer a challenge, as the conditions need to be chosen to ensure that the solid remains below the glass transition temperature. It should be noted that the glass transition temperature varies with humidity, consequently, the temperature range may be limited at high humidity. Similar limitations apply to studies of lyophile formulations. For suspensions, it is important that the solubility of the drug substance does not change under the stressed conditions. Gelatin capsules offer a specific challenge in that they are sensitive to both high and low humidity (becoming soft and brittle, respectively) and high temperatures. Therefore, ASAP studies for gelatin capsules use less harsh conditions than standard protocols, while also avoiding low humidity and typically require longer time points to achieve degradation to the specification limit. A standard

ASAP study protocol can be considered for the capsule contents.

5. For solution formulations, color change can be used to monitor degradation. In addition, it may be necessary to confirm that there has been no change in pH during the study or that no precipitation has occurred. If precipitation of the active ingredient is observed at an ASAP condition, data from that condition should not be used in the ASAP model, as some of the active ingredient might have undergone a change in physical state and the degradation kinetics may have also been affected.

6. For solid-state samples, the previous history of the sample may affect the degradation kinetics, particularly if the sample has been exposed to high humidity previously and then subsequently dried at low humidity [21].

7. Saturated salt solutions (as described in Sect. 2) are available that control at a range of humidities across a range of temperatures [19]. The relevant salt solution can be placed along with the required samples in sealed jars or desiccators and stored in an oven. In this way, conditions with different humidity can be stored in one oven and, in general, only three or four ovens are required to run multiple ASAP studies at the same time. If stability chambers are used, then typically six are needed, one for each condition, and if multiple studies are run simultaneously using different conditions, even more would be required. Automated robotic systems offer an efficient way to perform ASAP studies, particularly if the system also automates the sample preparation and analysis, but they require significant upfront investment. It should be noted that solid dosage forms can take 1–2 d to equilibrate with humidity. Therefore, solid dosage form samples for ASAP studies should be exposed to humidity for at least 24 h at ambient temperature before being set down at the higher temperatures, as per the ASAP study protocol. This is particularly important for coated tablets and capsules.

8. Accurate measurement of the temperature and humidity, which the samples are exposed to, will increases the accuracy of the ASAP model. This can be achieved by using temperature and humidity sensors. Many ovens and stability chambers automatically record temperature and humidity, where appropriate, but it is important that they maintain uniform conditions across the oven. Probes that measure both temperature and humidity can also be used and placed in jars or desiccators with the samples and salt solutions. Special ASAP stability pods are also available (http://www.amebisltd.com/small-scale-stability-testing?id=108) that continuously monitor both temperature and humidity and wirelessly transmit the data, so that the

temperature and humidity can be monitored remotely as the study progresses.

9. If conditions are to be removed from the model, it is important that enough conditions remain to generate it. Since three parameters need to be determined to solve the modified Arrhenius equation, four or five conditions are required as a minimum to result in one or two degrees of freedom [3]. In addition, humidity and temperature still need to be varied independently across the remaining conditions. For example, if very little degradation is seen under the low humidity conditions and these are subsequently removed from the model, the remaining conditions will all be at higher humidity, so the effect of humidity on the degradation can no longer be determined. In this case, it may be better to leave the low humidity conditions in the model, despite the low level of degradation observed. The limit of this scenario is when no degradation is observed in an ASAP study. While this may appear to be an ideal situation, in that it demonstrates that the sample being tested is very stable, it makes extrapolating a shelf-life harder as no model can be generated. This issue was addressed in the IQ survey [7] and three companies responded, indicating that in this situation they tend to default in assigning a retest period or shelf-life of at least 12 months.

10. When significant degradation cannot be achieved under each condition, extrapolation is required to determine the time when the degradation level will reach its specification. This extrapolation introduces additional errors into the ASAP model. Clancy et al. suggest that fitting kinetic models to the data obtained, rather than purely determining the time taken to reach specification (the isoconversion approach), may result in less error [11]. They also suggest that the need to design a protocol in order to degrade to specification, results in the use of relatively harsh conditions. This in turn then increases the extrapolation required from the rate measured at the harsh conditions to the predicted rate under ambient storage conditions, again increasing the error in the predictions.

11. If the level of degradation in an ASAP study has exceeded the specification limit, the kinetics of degradation may change. Therefore, it is important to stay below approximately 150% of the specification limit. This will minimize errors when generating the ASAP model and extrapolating to ambient conditions.

12. Standard kinetic models can be used to model the ASAP data at each condition including zero, first, and second order kinetics. If only a limited number of time points are used in an ASAP

study, typically a zero order (linear model) will be fit for purpose. First and second order kinetics can often be approximated with a linear fit to typical pharmaceutical specification limits due to the low values of typical pharmaceutical impurity limits ($<0.2\%$ to $<0.5\%$). For solid-state samples, the degradation kinetics are likely to be complex and heterogeneous. However, since specification limits are typically low for pharmaceutical products and it is only the degradation kinetics to the specification limit that are being modeled, the complex solid-state kinetics can be modeled by much simpler models. Typically, a linear zero order fit will suffice for a large percentage of ASAP studies.

13. Diffusion, Avromi-Erofeyev or other models can also be used where relevant and scientifically justified. These models however typically need more time points to achieve a satisfactory fit. For an autoxidation mechanism that is autocatalytic or when a reaction rate is governed by inhibitor loss, the Avromi-Erofeyev fit may be appropriate. When mobility is rate limiting or for a degradation product formed via degradation of a synthetic impurity present at a finite amount, the diffusion fit type may be valid.

14. The activation energy determined should typically be within the range of 15–40 kcal/mol and the B term can vary from 0 to 0.1 [3]. Occasionally a negative B term may be determined, i.e., the reaction rate slows as humidity is increased. If the B term is negative, but effectively zero within the error determined, then there is effectively no impact of humidity on the degradation. If the B term is negative across the error range, then a full scientific understanding and justification is necessary before any predictions can be made. Secondary degradation may be one possible explanation when the rate of degradation of the primary degradation product to the secondary degradation product increases at high humidity. A negative B term may also be evidence of a solid-state form change at high humidity (e.g., amorphous material converting to crystalline) affecting the rate of reaction, so no predictions can be made in this case.

15. Certain outliers can legitimately be removed from a model, for example, when at the most extreme condition the degradation kinetics seem to have changed and are no longer the same as the less harsh conditions. It is much harder to justify removing any other condition that may be an outlier from a model. Different statistical approaches can be applied to demonstrate that a condition is an outlier, but the scientific reason for excluding the condition is not always obvious. In this case, no predictions can be made from the model.

16. When a retest period or shelf-life is determined via an ASAP study, it is suggested that the retest period or shelf-life claim should be valid within the 95% confidence limits of the ASAP predictions. Typically, ASAP predictions are performed at 25 °C/60% RH and 30 °C/75% RH to cover storage in the majority of global territories. It should be noted that these predictions assume that the product is exposed to the humidity stated. In fact, the majority of packaging options offer some protection from humidity, so the ASAP predictions in this case may overpredict the level of degradation. This will be particularly significant when a product is stored with a desiccant. In this case, the ASAP predictions can be performed at a relative humidity more relevant to the product, determined by packaging predictions.

17. When water is a reactant in a degradation mechanism, the exponential relationship with humidity, which is assumed in the modified Arrhenius equation, may not hold true and water may need to be considered more as a typical reactant in the kinetics [11]. It should be noted that the drug substance is also obviously a reactant in the degradation kinetics, but because the level of degradation to specification is typically very low, there is effectively no change in the drug substance concentration during the reaction, so it becomes part of the constants in the equation [11]. Clancy et al. also discussed the applicability of water vapor pressure instead of relative humidity, particularly when modeling certain hydrolysis reactions, given that hydrolysis can occur with water vapor in the atmosphere rather than liquid water adsorbed on a solid.

Acknowledgements

The author would like to thank Faye Turner, Dr. Steve Cosgrove, Anna Powell, and Dr. Jonathan Bright from AstraZeneca for their contributions.

References

1. Waterman K, Adami R (2005) Accelerated aging: prediction of chemical stability of pharmaceuticals. Int J Pharm 293:101–125

2. Waterman K, Carella A, Gumkowski M et al (2007) Improved protocol and data analysis for accelerated shelf-life estimation of solid dosage forms. Pharm Res 24(4):780–790

3. Waterman K, Colgan S (2008) A science-based approach to setting expiry dating for solid drug products. Regulatory Rapporteur 5(7):9–14

4. Waterman K (2011) The application of Accelerated Stability Assessment Program (ASAP) to Quality by Design (QbD) for drug product stability. AAPS PharmSciTech 12(3):932–937

5. Waterman K, Swanson J, Lippold B (2014) A scientific and statistical analysis of accelerated aging for pharmaceuticals. Part 1: accuracy of fitting methods. J Pharm Sci:1–7. https://doi.org/10.1002/jps.24075

6. Waterman K, Macdonald B (2010) Package selection for moisture protection for solid oral drug products. J Pharm Sci 99(11):4437–4452

7. Williams H, Stephens D, McMahon M et al (2017) Risk-based predictive stability—an industry perspective. Pharm Tech 41(3):52–57

8. Colgan S, Watson T, Whipple R et al (2012) The application of science- and risk-based concepts to drug substance stability strategies. J Pharm Innov 7:205–213

9. Kougoulos E, Smales I, Verrier H (2011) Towards integrated drug substance and drug product design for an active pharmaceutical ingredient using particle engineering. AAPS PharmSciTech 12(1):287–294

10. Oliva A, Fariña J, Llabrés M (2012) An improved methodology for data analysis in accelerated stability studies of peptide drugs: practical considerations. Talanta 94:158–166

11. Clancy D, Hodnett N, Orr R et al (2016) Kinetic model development for accelerated stability studies. AAPS PharmSciTech online. https://doi.org/10.1208/s12249-016-0565-4

12. Kleinman M, Baertschi S, Alsante K (2014) In silico prediction of pharmaceutical degradation pathways: a benchmarking study. Mol Pharm 11:4179–4188

13. Andersson T, Broo A, Evertsson E (2014) Prediction of drug candidates' sensitivity toward autoxidation: computation estimation of C-H dissociation energies of carbon-centered radicals. J Pharm Sci 103(1):1949–1955

14. Remmelgas J, Simonutti A-L, Ronkvist Å (2013) A mechanistic model for the prediction of in-use moisture uptake by packaged dosage forms. Int J Pharm 441:316–322

15. Waterman K, Chen L, Waterman P et al (2016) Modeling of in-use stability for tablets and powder in bottles. Drug Dev Ind Pharm 42:1571–1578. https://doi.org/10.3109/03639045.2016.1153648

16. Li H, Nadig D, Kuzmission A et al (2016) Predictions of the changes in drug dissolution from an immediate-release tablet containing two active pharmaceutical ingredients using an accelerated stability assessment program. AAPS Open 2:7. https://doi.org/10.1186/s41120-016-0010-5

17. International Consortium for Innovation and Quality in Pharmaceutical Development. http://iqconsortium.org

18. Freed A, Clement E, Timpano R (2014) Regulatory responses to the use of various lean stability strategies in early drug development. Regulatory Rapporteur 11(7/8):5–8

19. Greenspan L (1977) Humidity fixed points of binary saturated aqueous solutions. J Res Natl Bur Stand A Phys Chem 81A(1):89–96

20. Fu M, Perlman M, Lu Q, Varga C (2015) Pharmaceutical solid-state kinetic stability investigation by using moisture-modified Arrhenius equation and JMP statistical software. J Pharm Biomed Anal 107:370–377

21. Waterman K, Gerst P, Macdonald B (2012) Relative humidity hysteresis in solid-state chemical reactivity: a pharmaceutical case study. J Pharm Sci 101(2):610–615

Chapter 11

Statistical Methods and Approaches to Avoid Stability Failures of Drug Product During Shelf-Life

B. V. Suresh Kumar, Priyank Kulshrestha, and Sandeep Shiromani

Abstract

Generation of stability data is an important part of a drug product's life cycle. Various statistical approaches can be used to identify patterns and predict the behavior of the drug products. The ICH guidance Q1E for industry provides nonbinding recommendations on evaluation of the stability data. This chapter compliments those guidelines and describes specific statistical methods to assess the long-term stability data. The primary objective of this chapter is to demonstrate statistical approaches to predict the likelihood of drug product failure during its shelf-life. The key methodologies discussed are estimation of release limits using stability data, predicting batch failure rate and assessment of process performance statistics like CpK and PpK. The chapter describes the regression modeling techniques, application of empirical cumulative distribution function, and estimation of defects per million opportunity using process performance indices. To avoid erroneous statistical estimations, the diagnostic techniques to verify the validity of statistical methods used are also discussed. The ultimate application of the outcomes of these statistical approaches is to support sound business decisions. Failure of drug products during their shelf-life can lead to market recalls, which not only affects the profitability of a company but also impacts its reputation and credibility. These statistical approaches help in backing the decisions on prioritization of process improvement projects and tightening the batch release strategies.

Key words Long-term stability data, Regression, Fixed and mixed effects models, Release limits, Batch rejection rate, Empirical cumulative distribution function, Process performance indices, Diagnostic tests for statistical methods

---

1 Introduction

The whole purpose of a stability study is to ensure that a drug product does not lose its critical quality attributes (CQA) during the course of its shelf-life. Typically, stability studies are performed at the storage conditions as per the climatic zone of marketing location. The stability studies are conducted under long-term and accelerated test conditions [1]. The storage conditions for accelerated stability studies are harsher as compared to the long-term studies. Observation of significant change over the time at accelerated storage condition for any of the CQA triggers the analysis of

Sanjay Bajaj and Saranjit Singh (eds.), *Methods for Stability Testing of Pharmaceuticals*, Methods in Pharmacology and Toxicology, https://doi.org/10.1007/978-1-4939-7686-7_11, © Springer Science+Business Media, LLC, part of Springer Nature 2018

the stability data generated for long-term storage condition. The statistical assessment of the data generated for long-term storage condition is crucial in preventing the drug product failure during its shelf-life. ICH guideline Q1E provides recommendation on statistical approaches to evaluate the stability data and recommendations on statistically establishing the drug product shelf-life [2]. However, the practical aspects of these statistical approaches are not covered in the ICH guideline Q1E. This chapter will cover the application of statistical approaches and methods that can be used to identify the patterns in the stability data and predict the probability of drug product failures.

According to the ICH guideline Q1E, it is recommended that the stability data for each quantitative CQA be assessed separately [2]. Typically, regression models are developed with linear or nonlinear functions for statistical assessment of the stability data. The appropriateness of these regression models is demonstrated by the extent of information they reveal about the change over the time, overall variability, and error component. A regression model can be improved by allowing random effects in the model and by reducing the models with only significant factors. Such models are also known as mixed effects models. These statistical approaches eventually help in managing the manufacturing risks by estimating release limits and predicting batch rejection rate. Release limits are actually the limits on the registered specifications based on the change over the time modeled from the long-term stability data and the variability components [3]. These release limits assure that the CQA of the drug product remain within the specifications until the end of the shelf-life. The percentage of the batches, which breach the release limits actually have higher chances of having certain CQA going out-of-specifications (OOS) during the shelf-life of the drug product. Therefore, such batches are recommended to be rejected from releasing into the market. Percentage of failing batches out of the total manufactured batches is known as the actual batch rejection rate. The estimate of release limit from the stability data can be used to calculate the predicted rate of rejection for the whole population based on the validity of the normality assumptions. Higher predicted batch rejection rate indicates that there is a need to bring in some change in the process or correct the shelf-life of the drug product so that stability failures can be avoided. This chapter will also briefly touch upon the concepts of statistical assessment of process performance against these release limits [4]. If the process performance indices (e.g., CpK and PpK values) are below the industry standard of less than 1.33 for a particular CQA, it means that the process is not statistically stable and a process improvement initiative should be taken so that batch failure rates can be minimized.

The statistical analysis used in the subsequent sections of this chapter can be performed using standard software like Minitab,

SAS-JMP, and R. The scope of this chapter does not include performing the statistics part but to make reader understand how these statistical indices can be inferred for better process understanding.

2 Stability Studies and Design

Stability data required for statistical analysis can be planned and acquired according to various stability designs available in literature [5]. These designs can be basic or specialized, based on the reduced amount of effort for data collection or resolution, etc. Each data collection plan has some pros and cons [6]. Therefore, it is for the management to decide which stability design to follow. ICH guideline Q1E lists down various approaches that can be used for acquiring stability data. In this chapter, no specialized design for acquiring stability data is used, rather traditionally or commonly used full factorial design has been followed.

3 Regression Models

ICH guideline Q1E suggests that at least three batches should be tested for stability [2]. This is foremost step in estimating release limit, expiry or shelf-life of the drug product. This section lists down few statistical approaches used for analysis of stability data and same approach can be used for samples put on stablity from manufacturing batches.

3.1 Poolability of Batches

Poolability is a statistical test that enables data-driven decision by statistician to decide whether the batches under study belong to same population or not. To establish poolability, analysis of covariance (ANCOVA) is used, where time is considered covariates to test for difference in slopes and intercepts [7, 8]. This method can be used to evaluate scenarios where batches from two different hypothesized populations are tested statistically. Poolability can be established for below cases for same drug products:

1. Stability data obtained for two different packagings.
2. Stability data for two climatic zones.
3. Stability data obtained for two different dosage strengths.

Poolability of the batches is established before performing any statistical analysis. Poolability can be checked for either equality of slopes or intercepts. Consider assay of a drug product, which decreases with time. This can be modeled by linear regression given by Eq. 1 [8]:

$$y_{ij} = \alpha_0 + \alpha_i + (\beta_0 + \beta_i)t_{ij} + \varepsilon_{ij} \tag{1}$$

where y_{ij} = response of ith batch at sampling time t_{ij}
α_0 = common intercept of all batches
α_i = deviation of individual intercept of ith batch from α_0
β_0 = common slope for all batches
β_i = deviation of individual slope of ith batch from β_0
t_{ij} = sampling time (months)
ε_{ij} = error factor, such that $\varepsilon \sim N(0, \sigma)$

Test of hypotheses for equality of slopes and intercepts gives an idea about the homogeneity among the decreasing lines in case of assay of the drug and increasing lines in case of the degradation product. Pooling test for slope is established among the batches followed by intercept test. Test hypotheses for equality of slopes are of the following two types:

| Null hypothesis | $H_{0\beta}: \beta_i = 0$ |
| Alternative hypothesis | $H_{a\beta}: \beta_i \neq 0$ |

Once alternative hypothesis is rejected, this means that all the batches tested have common slope. In the next step, we test hypotheses for equality of intercepts, which are again of the two types:

| Null hypothesis | $H_{0\alpha}: \alpha_i = 0$ |
| Alternative hypothesis | $H_{a\alpha}: \alpha_i \neq 0$ |

Depending on the acceptance of null hypothesis in test for slope, we can determine whether the batch can be pooled or not for statistical analysis. If the null hypothesis is accepted in test for slope and null hypothesis is rejected in test for intercept, still data can be combined for estimating common slope. If both tests are rejected, data are not poolable and separate analysis should be done. In such a case ICH guideline Q1E suggests assigning the shelf-life based on worst batch.

Therefore, four different scenarios can occur when establishing poolability of batches:

1. $H_{0\beta}: \beta_i = 0$ and $H_{0\alpha}: \alpha_i = 0$ Data are poolable.
2. $H_{0\beta}: \beta_i = 0$ and $H_{a\alpha}: \alpha_i \neq 0$ Data are poolable to estimate common slope.
3. $H_{0\beta}: \beta_i \neq 0$ and $H_{0\alpha}: \alpha_i \neq 0$ Data are not poolable.
4. $H_{0\beta}: \beta_i \neq 0$ and $H_{0\alpha}: \alpha i = 0$ Data are not poolable.

While evaluating the batches for poolability, significance level (p-value) considered is 0.25 [9]. This value seems to be high, but is chosen because, we should be confident enough due to low number of batches used for stability test.

Consider data in Table 1 acquired during stability testing of a drug AA which is to be marketed for two different climatic zones 25 °C/60% RH and 30 °C/75% RH.

Case 1: Common Slopes and Common Intercepts: If the poolability hypothesis is not rejected, it is considered that all batches are from the same population of batches. In such a case, the model reduces to the form in Eq. 2.

Table 1
Stability data for climatic zones 25 °C/60% RH and 30 °C/75% RH

Batch	Months (T)	Storage temp	CQA1	CQA2	CQA3	CQA4
A	0	25 °C/60% RH	99.8	99	0.2	12
A	12	25 °C/60% RH	98.7	98	0.3	14
A	24	25 °C/60% RH	97.2	97	0.3	15
A	35	25 °C/60% RH	95.5	97	0.5	15
B	0	25 °C/60% RH	98.8	102	0.3	15
B	12	25 °C/60% RH	102.8	100	0.3	14
B	24	25 °C/60% RH	102.5	99	0.3	12
B	33	25 °C/60% RH	99.2	97	0.2	14
C	0	25 °C/60% RH	98.8	99	0.2	16
C	12	25 °C/60% RH	98	95	0.2	13
C	24	25 °C/60% RH	99.3	98	0.3	13
C	36	25 °C/60% RH	98.2	103	0.4	14
D	0	30 °C/75% RH	98.1	104	0.4	11
D	12	30 °C/75% RH	98.6	98	0.4	13
D	24	30 °C/75% RH	98.4	101	0.8	14
D	35	30 °C/75% RH	98.7	97	1.2	15
E	0	30 °C/75% RH	97.6	104	0.3	12
E	12	30 °C/75% RH	99.1	96	0.5	14
E	24	30 °C/75% RH	100.4	100	0.6	14
E	36	30 °C/75% RH	98.2	95	0.3	12
F	0	30 °C/75% RH	102.3	103	0.4	13
F	12	30 °C/75% RH	99.6	97	0.4	14
F	24	30 °C/75% RH	97.7	100	0.5	11
F	35	30 °C/75% RH	99.7	99	0.8	15

$$y_{ij} = \alpha_0 + \beta_0 t_{ij} + \varepsilon_{ij} \qquad (2)$$

Under these conditions, pooled stability data from the batches provide a better least square estimation of slope and intercept. Therefore, the above model is sufficient to explain shelf-life of the drug product.

The model output for CQA1 of the drug where poolability is established between storage conditions 25 °C/60% RH and 30 °C/75% RH has been presented in Table 2.

Case 2: Common Slopes but Different Intercepts: Consider CQA4 for the drug product as in Table 1, where variation in slopes is not significant and variation of intercept is significant. In such a case, the model is reduced to the form as in Eq. 3.

$$y_{ij} = \alpha_i + \beta_0 t_{ij} + \varepsilon_{ij} \qquad (3)$$

Similar to Case 1, pooled data from stability batch provide better least square estimation. The model output for dissolution of the drug where poolability is established between storage conditions 25 °C/60% RH and 30 °C/75% RH has been presented in Table 3.

Case 3: Different Slopes and Different Intercepts: If the poolability hypothesis is rejected, it is considered that all batches are not from same population. In such a case, the model is reduced to the form as in Eq. 4.

$$y_{ij} = \alpha_i + \beta_i t_{ij} + \varepsilon_{ij} \qquad (4)$$

Table 2
Effect test

Source	Nparm	DF	Sum of squares	F ratio	Prob > F
Storage condition	1	1	0.0049753	0.0016	0.9680
Time (M)	1	1	3.0476811	1.0084	0.3273
Storage condition × time (M)	1	1	0.6638738	0.2197	0.6444

Note: P-value of the F-test (0.6444) for $H_{0\beta}$: $\beta i = 0$ is greater than 0.25. The p-value of the F-test (0.9680) of $H_{0\alpha}$: $\alpha i = 0$ is greater than 0.25

Table 3
Effect test

Source	Nparm	DF	Sum of squares	F ratio	Prob > F
Storage condition	1	1	3.4053533	1.9754	0.1752
Time (M)	1	1	1.6920211	0.9815	0.3337
Storage condition × time (M)	1	1	2.3503159	1.3634	0.2567

Note: P-value of the F-test (0.2567) for $H_{0\beta}$: $\beta i = 0$ is greater than 0.25. The p-value of the F-test (0.1752) of $H_{0\alpha}$: $\alpha i = 0$ is smaller than 0.25

Table 4
Effect test

Source	Nparm	DF	Sum of squares	F ratio	Prob > F
Storage condition	1	1	0.39640283	14.5196	0.0011
Time (M)	1	1	0.24750395	9.0657	0.0069
Storage condition × time (M)	1	1	0.06165610	2.2584	0.1485

Note: P-value of the F-test (0.1485) for $H_{0\beta}$: $\beta i = 0$ is smaller than 0.25. The p-value of the F-test (0.0011) of $H_{0\alpha}$: $\alpha i = 0$ is smaller than 0.25

Table 5
Effect tests

Source	Nparm	DF	Sum of squares	F ratio	Prob > F
Storage condition	1	1	4.303045	0.7509	0.3965
Time (M)	1	1	27.168560	4.7410	0.0416
Storage condition × Time (M)	1	1	15.233698	2.6583	0.1187

Note: P-value of the F-test (0.1187) for $H_{0\beta}$: $\beta i = 0$ is smaller than 0.25. The p-value of the F-test (0.3965) of $H_{0\alpha}$: $\alpha i = 0$ is greater than 0.25

The model output for CQA3 of the drug where poolability is established between storage conditions 25 °C/60% RH and 30 °C/75% RH has been presented in Table 4. In this case, worst batch expiry approach is used.

Case 4: Common Intercepts Different Slopes: Similar to case 3, poolability hypothesis is rejected here. It is considered that all batches are not from same population. In such a case, the model is reduced to the form as in Eq. 5.

$$y_{ij} = \alpha_0 + \beta_i t_{ij} + \varepsilon_{ij} \tag{5}$$

The model output for CQA2 of the drug where poolability is established between storage conditions of 25 °C/60% RH and 30 °C/75% RH has been presented in Table 5. For Cases 2 and 3, which have batch-to-batch variability, statistical methods like fixed batch approach or random batch approach can be used.

3.2 Fixed Batch Approach

Fixed batch approach is a linear regression which uses least square estimation for fitting a regression line [10]. Equation 6 is the model equation for fixed batch approach.

$$y_{kl} = \alpha_k + \beta_k t_{kl} + \varepsilon_{kl} \tag{6}$$

where y_{kl} = response of kth batch at time t_{kl}
t_{kl} = sampling time of kth batch
β_k = slope of kth batch

$\alpha_k =$ intercept of kth batch

$\varepsilon_{kl} =$ error factor, such that $\varepsilon \sim N(0, \sigma)$

Considering attributes like assay, which are expected to decrease with time, release limits are calculated using the expression in Eq. 7 [11]. Similar approach can be used to find upper release limits (URL) for attributes like degradation product(s), which increases with time.

$$LRL = LSL - B \times T_{SL} + t_{1-a, k} \times \sqrt{S_T^2 + \frac{S^2}{n}} \text{ for } B < 0 \qquad (7)$$

where LRL = lower release limit
LSL = lower specification limit
$B =$ average slope for fall in assay
$T_{SL} =$ shelf-life
$S_T =$ standard error of average slope $\times$ shelf-life
$S =$ assay standard deviation
$t_{1-a, k} =$ one-sided $(1-a)\%$ critical t value with k degrees of freedom
$n =$ number of replicate assays used for lot release

Above equation is valid, but it does not take into account variability at time. Therefore, an alternative approach is proposed as Eq. 8 to account for this variability [3].

$$LRL = LSL + bT + (z_\alpha + z_{0.05})\sqrt{\sigma_\beta^2 T^2 + \sigma_e^2 \left(\frac{1}{n_T} + \frac{1}{n_0}\right)} \qquad (8)$$

where $n_0 =$ number of samples drawn at time zero
$n_T =$ number of samples drawn at end of study
$b =$ average slope for decresing line
$T =$ shelf-life
$z_{0.05} =$ 95% lower confidence interval for mean potency at time T
$z_\alpha =$ allowable failure rate (%)

3.3 Random Batches Approach

Major advantage of using random model over fixed batch is that the inference deduced from fixed model can be applied for current batch under study and not for the future batches. Main aim of stability study is to predict shelf-life of future batches, therefore, random model seems to be appropriate for this type of predictions. A mixed model with time as fixed components and batch and time by batch interaction treated as a random component is described below. Therefore, Eq. 1 is modified to take care of random coefficients [11, 12].

$$y_{ij} = X'_{ij}\beta_i + \varepsilon_{ij} \qquad (9)$$

where $y_{ij} =$ response of ith batch at jth time point
$X'_{ij} =$ px1 vector of nonrandom covariates

β_i = px1 vector of parameters
ε_{ij} = random error in estimating y_{ij}

An alternative approach mixed effect model [13] uses algorithm to obtain maximum likelihood estimate of regression coefficients.

$$y_{ij} = \mu + \alpha_i + (b + \beta_i)T_{ij} + \varepsilon_{ij} \tag{10}$$

where y_{ij} = response of ith batch at jth time point
μ = mean batch assay at time zero
α_i = random batch effect at time zero, $\alpha_i \sim N(0, \sigma^2_\alpha)$
b = average assay change rate per time unit
β_i = random batch effect on slope, $\beta_i \sim N(0, \sigma^2_\beta)$
T_{ij} = sampling time (months)
ε_{ij} = total random error, $\varepsilon_{ij} \sim N(0, \sigma^2_\varepsilon)$

3.4 Bayesian Statistics

Bayesian statistics based release limit calculation relies on simulation of future lots. To evaluate release limit, we need samples means for posterior distribution of future lots and release test for posterior distribution. Therefore, the model equations considered are given in Eqs. 11 and 12 [14, 15].

$$K_t = \alpha_{0f} + t_{SL}.\beta_{if} \tag{11}$$

$$\Upsilon_{fr} \sim N\left(\alpha_{0f}, \left(\frac{\sigma^2_\varepsilon}{n_r}\right)\right) \tag{12}$$

Where Υ_{fr} = posterior predictive distribution of future release test results.
α_{0f} = Intercept of future batch
β_{if} = Slope of future batch
K_t = Samples from posterior distribution of future batch meanst
t_{SL} = time at end of shelf-life
σ^2_ε = variance in error
n_r = number of stability test values

Equation 11 can be used to form posterior distribution samples of future lots means K_t at end of shelf-life t_{SL}, using parmeters obtained by Markov chain Monte Carlo draw. Equation 12 describes samples of posterior predictive distribution of future release test obtained by simulation from normal distribution N. Using this method a correlation can be established between future batch mean potencies at shelf-life and future release test.

4   Statistical Methods and Approaches for the Assessment of Stability Data and Prediction of Drug Product Failure

4.1   Statistical Assessment of the Long-Term Stability Data

According to the ICH guidelines Q1E, it is recommended that the statistical assessment of the long-term stability data should be performed separately for each CQA. The assessment should be triggered only when there is a significant change over the time observed during the first 3 months of accelerated stability study. Assuming that the accelerated stability data for drug product A show significant change over the time for CQA1, statistical assessment of the long-term stability data to estimate the release limits is done as given in the following steps.

a. Organization of stability data.

b. Development of regression model.

c. Estimation of release limits.

4.1.1   Organization of Stability Data

Before any statistical assessment is performed, it is necessary that the data are organized in a structured way. As a first step, the generated stability data are organized as shown in Table 6, which is the easiest way in which the stability data can be organized in a tabular form. A table heading can have information like the drug product name and the storage condition. The very first row in Table 6 represents the specifications of the respective critical quality attributes CQA1 and CQA2. Please note that CQA1 and CQA2 are mentioned only for example purpose, the specification ranges mentioned are also only to explain the concept and may differ for diffent products and their respective quantitative CQAs. A stability data table should contain data available for all the quantitative stability-indicating attributes. In the given example, the stability data are captured for 60 months for both CQA1 and CQA2. Any OOS observations, missing time points and data points with different testing methods should always be appropriately labeled and explained in the "Key" at the end of the stability data table. The statistical assessment explained in the subsequent sections is based on the assumption that all the stability data generated represents the current manufacturing process for the drug product A and uses the same testing monograph for the analysis of all the CQAs at all the time points. In practice it may happen that the testing methods change; in such cases, data generated from different testing methods should not be pooled or statistically assessed for poolability.

4.1.2   Development of Regression Model

Throughout this section, we shall be referring to Table 6 for stability data of CQA1. It should be noted that "Batch" column is a nominal variable (non-numeric) and "Time" (months) and "CQA1" values are continuous numeric variables. "Batch" and "Time" are independent effect variables. CQA1 is a dependent "response" variable. To model the effect of "Batch" and "Time"

Table 6
Stability data for drug product A at storage condition 25 °C/60% RH

Specifications			
		98.0–102.0%	NMT 0.50
Batch	Time (months)	CQA1	CQA2
B0001	0	100.19	0.047
B0001	12	100.03	0.083
B0001	24	100.06	0.071
B0001	36	99.70	0.103
B0001	48	99.88	0.115
B0001	60	99.10	0.103
B0002	0	100.03	0.088
B0002	12	100.81	0.131
B0002	24	100.00	0.190
B0002	36	100.36	0.153
B0002	48	99.62	0.120
B0002	60	99.55	0.162
B0003	0	100.21	0.077
B0003	12	100.02	0.031
B0003	24	100.11	NT
B0003	36	100.02	0.082
B0003	48	99.98	0.075
B0003	60	99.81	0.151

Note: NT - not tested

on dependent variable "CQA1", regression method will be used. A regression model can be fitted with "Batch", "Time", and the interaction of "Batch" and "Time" as the model effects and CQA1 values as response variable. Such regression models are known as fixed effects models. Figure 1 shows the scatter of all three batches, a regression line modeled using least square method and 95% confidence interval of the regression fit. Table 7 summarizes the statistics of the fit of the overall regression model for all the three batches. It should be noted that this regression model explains almost 59% (coefficient of determination (r^2) = 0.586) of the variability present in the CQA1 data. The adjusted coefficient of determination (r^2_{adj}) and root mean square error (RMSE) of this model are 0.414258 and 0.273247, respectively.

Next, we need to analyze the significance of each of the model effects, i.e., "Batch", "Time", and "Batch - Time interaction" (Batch × Time) on the overall regression fit. The probability

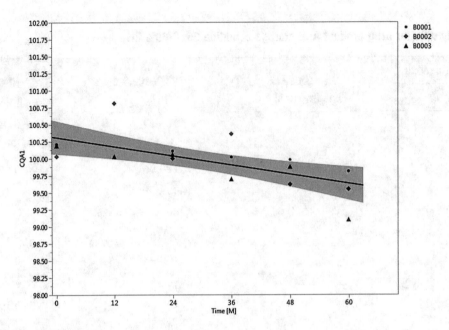

Fig. 1 Regression fit plot

Table 7
Summary of fit for fixed effects model

r^2	0.586535
r^2_{adj}	0.414258
RMSE	0.273247
Mean of response	99.97111
Observations (or sum Weights)	18

Table 8
Effects tests

Source	Nparm	DF	Sum of squares	F ratio	Prob > F
Batch	2	2	0.19181111	1.2845	0.3123
Time	1	1	0.94403048	12.6437	0.0040
Batch × time	2	2	0.13516667	0.9052	0.4304

(p-values) value of F-statistics in Table 8 shows the p-value of each of the model effect. The p-value for "Time" is less than 0.05. Assuming that the acceptance for type I error is 5%, "Time" has significant effect in the fitted regression model. The same can be visually inferred from the downward slope of fitted regression line in Fig. 1. The p-value of "Batch" effect is greater than 0.05. This means that the variation in CQA1 values due to "Batch" effect is not statistically significant. The p-value of "Batch–Time interaction" is also greater than 0.05, this indicates that the difference in the individual slopes of each batch is also not statistically significant. This corresponds to "Case I" mentioned in Sect. 3.1 where poolability of slopes and interactions was explained. However, this does not discount the contribution of "Batch" and "Batch–Time interaction" to the random variability in the CQA1 data.

To capture the random variability due to "Batch" and "Batch–Time" interaction, a mixed effect model should be analyzed. This model will have only one fixed effect, i.e., "Time" because as can be noticed in Table 8, this is the only statistically significant effect. Along with this fixed effect the regression model will also have "Batch" and "Batch–Time interaction" as random effects (hence known as mixed effect model, which includes both fixed and random effects in the regression model).

Table 9 summarizes the statistics of the fit for the mixed effects model. To understand the significance of developing a mixed effects model, Table 8 is compared with Table 9. It is to be noted that the error in the model is still unaffected (RMSE = 0.273247) as compared to the fixed effect model. The r^2_{adj} is improved ($r^2_{adj} = 0.422803$) when compared to the fixed effect model ($r^2_{adj} = 0.414258$). This is because the statistical model is now able to explain the variability in the data better than the fixed effects model.

To get the estimate of random effects of "Batch" and "Batch - Time interaction" in the regression model variability, the REML variance components of the mixed effects are analyzed as shown in Table 10. It is to be noted that the variance component of "Batch - Time interaction" is negative. Any variance component that is smaller than zero does not contribute to the overall variability explained by the model. This means that the "Batch - Time interaction" term is not contributing to explain the variability in the CQA1 data. To further simplify the regression model, a new

Table 9
Summary of fit for mixed (random effects) model

r^2	0.456756
r^2_{adj}	0.422803
RMSE	0.273247
Mean of response	99.97111
Observations (or sum Weights)	18

Table 10
REML variance components estimates

Random effect	Variance ratio	Variance component	Std error	95% Lower	95% Upper	% of total
Batch	0.0474155	0.0035402	0.0167722	−0.029333	0.0364131	4.527
Batch × time	−3.763e-5	−2.81e-6	2.942e-5	-6.047e-5	5.4853e-5	0.000
Residual		0.0746641	0.0304815	0.0383932	0.2034543	95.473
Total		0.0782044	0.030012	0.0415829	0.1978923	100.000

Table 11
Summary of fit for reduced mixed model

r^2	0.471955
r^2_{adj}	0.438952
RMSE	0.27139
Mean of response	99.97111
Observations (or sum Weights)	18

Table 12
Parameter estimates from reduced mixed model

Term	Estimate	Std Error	DFDen	t ratio	Prob > |t|
Intercept	100.30635	0.118728	10.09	844.84	<.0001
Time	−0.011175	0.003121	14	−3.58	0.0030

reduced mixed model will be fitted. This model will have fixed effect "Time" and the random effect of only "Batch". The summary of fit of the reduced mixed effects model can be seen in Table 11.

It should be noted that the error (RMSE = 0.27139) in the reduced mixed model is now lesser as compared to the mixed effects model (*see* Table 9). The r^2_{adj} due to this change in the regression model has also got improved ($r^2_{adj} = 0.438952$) when compared to the mixed effects model ($r^2_{adj} = 0.422803$). It can be observed that at this stage, there is improvement in the regression model by having the effects that explain more variability in the CQA1 data and is simpler than the fixed effects model. Table 12 shows the parameter estimates from the reduced mixed model.

Estimates of intercept and slope from this table can be used to derive the prediction expression as following:

Prediction Expression

CQA1 (at time t) = 100.3063493 + (−0.0111746) × Time (t) + 0.296 \hfill (13)

The first term of prediction expression is the intercept estimate derived from the reduced mixed model. Coefficient of the second term Time (t) represents the estimate of slope obtaind from the reduced mixed model. Third term is the error component in the model. Note that the negative slope in the prediction expression signifies the decreasing pattern. For CQAs like assay, the negative slope is scientifically sound as an unstable drug substance tends to degrade over the time. The value of model error component is estimated by calculating the standard error from mixed model at the end of shelf-life for thisdrug product. In this case, the standard error at 60 months is 0.296.

4.1.3   Estimation of Release Limits

These estimates of slope and variability will now be used to introduce the concept of release limit. A release limit is that value which, if the CQA1 crosses at the time of release, chances that it will fail to meet its registered specification during its shelf-life will be very high. It should be noted here that CQA1 is assumed to exhibit decreasing characteristic and is not expected to increase over the time. This implies that the release limit for CQA1 should be calculated only against the lower registered release specification. Table 13 summarizes the regression model characteristics and calculation of release limit for CQA1.

An interesting way to visualize the application of release limit is to populate the prediction expression, given above, with intercept as 98.97%, slope as 0.011175, time as 60 months, and random variability (ε) at 60 months as 0.296, finally arriving at a value close to 98.0 (98.97−0.6705−0.296). In other words, if CQA1 starts at 98.97 (at release time point, i.e., $t = 0$), then with the change over the time within 60 months and random variability in the nature of the analytical method, it will actually fall as low as 98.0 at the end of its shelf-life. Therefore, if a batch is released with CQA1 value of less than 98.97, then within 60 months of shelf-life it will fail to meet the registered specification of 98.0. To prevent such drug product failure, it is advisable to perform the statistical assessment of the long-term stability data and set the release limit of CQA1 to "not less than 98.97%" so that the drug product remains within the specification during its shelf-life.

It is to be noted that CQA1 is an example of decreasing characteristic, but the same statistical approach can be used for attributes like CQA2 in Table 6, where the change over the time can be positive. In such cases, an upper release limit is set. The

Table 13
Release limits calculations

CQA1			
Expected variability (%)	0.296 (standard error at 60 months)		
Slope (% per month)	−0.011175		
Shelf-life	60 months		
Expected change over the time during the shelf-life (%)	$0.011175 \times 60 = 0.6705\%$		
Upper release specification (URS) (%)	Not more than 102.0		
Lower release specification (LRS) (%)	Not less than 98.0		
Upper release limit (%)	Not applicable		
	LRS Expected change over the time	Expected variability	=
Lower release limit (%)	98.0 + 0.6705	+ 0.296	= Not less than 98.97

upper limit in such case will be a value, above which, if the drug product is released, it will fail to meet the upper specification of not more than 0.50 by the end of 60 months. In case when it is not possible from the process improvement point of view to consistently release the batches within the release limits, it is recommended that the shelf-life of the drug product should be shortened accordingly.

The above example was to demonstrate the statistical approaches to prevent the drug product failure. But it is not necessary to have significant change over the time or even sufficient stability data all the time to perform such analysis. ICH guideline Q1E also provides recommendation for cases as given below.

Case 1: No Significant Change Over the Time Observed but High Estimate of Variability Observed

As per the ICH guideline Q1E, if the change over the time for a CQA is not significant and the registered release specifications are not set based on analytical method and process variability, then the release limit can be calculated with RMSE of the fixed model as measure of variability. The upper release specification should be subtracted with the RMSE to estimate upper release limit, the lower release specifications should be added with RMSE to estimate the upper release limit. If the registered release specifications are set taking analytical method and process variability into the account, then estimation of release limits is not required.

Case 2: Insufficient Data Available to Perform Any Statistical Analysis

The data are considered to be statistically insufficient when there are less than three time points available for a batch, as the degrees of freedom are not enough to fit a line (at least three data points are required for fitting a line). Similarly, if the data are available for less than three batches, the reliability of the statistical model is low. The estimates of slope and intercept from such model will not be appropriate to represent the statistical trend. As more and more batches are added to the statistical model, the power of the model improves and the estimates of slopes and intercepts are more precise. In case when the data are insufficient to perform statistical assessment of slope and variability, the intermediate precision of the method is used to calculate the release limits. Intermediate precision of the method is a measure of repeatability and reproducibility considering man-to-man, machine-to-machine, and man-to-machine variations into account. Release limits must be re-evaluated in such cases with statistical methods as more and more data become available with time.

4.2 Statistical Assessment of Predicted Batch Rejection Rate

Once the value of release limit is estimated for a CQA using the statistical assessment of the stability data, it is important to know how the manufacturing batches are behaving at the release time point. In this second statistical approach, we will demonstrate how the manufacturing data for batches at release time point (i.e., $t = 0$) can be used to statistically predict the batch rejection rate. The statistical assessment for predicting the batch rejection rate is done in the following three steps:

1. Summarizing the batch release data using the histogram.
2. Development of empirical cumulative distribution function.
3. Prediction of batch rejection rate.

4.2.1 Summary of Batch Release Data

In this example, the release data for CQA1 for 40 batches, all representing the same manufacturing process has been collected. The histogram of the release data are plotted as shown in Fig. 2. The reference lines for lower and upper registered specifications are added at 98.0 and 102.0. A reference line corresponding to the lower release limit of 98.97, as estimated in the section above, is also added in the histogram.

It can be easily visualized from the histogram and reference lines that all the batches are within the registered specification limits. However, there are three observations which are within lower registered specification limit but outside the release limit of 98.97. Therefore, the calculated actual batch rejection rate from this sample data will be 7.5% (3/40).

4.2.2 Development of Empirical Cumulative Distribution Function

The actual batch rejection rate may be an overestimation of rejection rate since we cannot generalize this sample data for the whole population of manufacturing data. Assuming that the data are normally distributed, an empirical cumulative distribution function

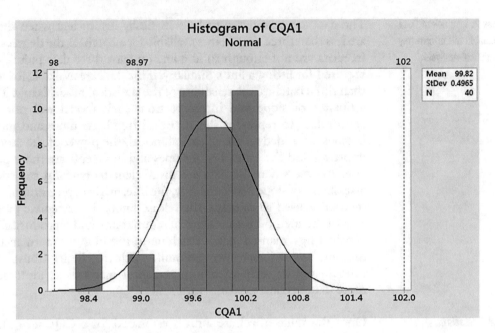

Fig. 2 Histogram of manufacturing batch release data

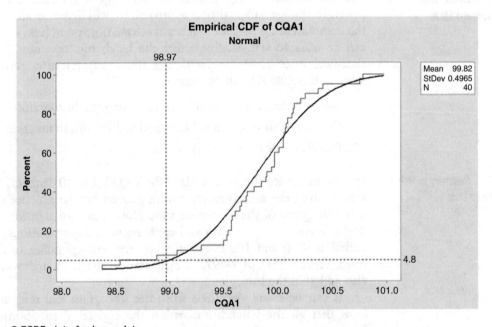

Fig. 3 ECDF plot of release data

(ECDF) plot can be generated for the release data (*see* Sect. 5.3 for details). Figure 3 shows the ECDF plotted using the release data of 40 batch sample and generalized for the whole population. The horizontal reference line at 4.8% on the plot indicates the percentage of population that is expected to fail in meeting the release limit of not more than 98.97% (vertical reference line).

4.2.3   Prediction of Batch Rejection Rate

This percentage area is actually the percentage of batches which are predicted to fail when released at the CQA1 value of less than 98.97 (vertical reference line). In this example, the predicted batch rejection rate, i.e., percentage area on the left of the vertical reference line is approximately 4.8% (contrary to the actual batch rejection rate of 7.5% calculated from the sample of 40 batches in Sect. 4.2.1). In essence, we have used statistical approach of generating an ECDF from a sample data of 40 batches to generalize the whole population and have predicted the frequency of batches which will fail to achieve the release limit. ECDF is an important statistical approach to predict, for a given process, what could be the rate of failure or rejection. This approach is used by manufacturing process owners to decide the need of process improvement initiatives to prevent compromise on the stability failures.

4.3   Statistical Assessment of Process Performance

Both the above mentioned approaches (statistical assessment of the release limits in Sect. 4.1.3 and prediction of batch rejection rate in Sect. 4.2.3) take us closer to predict when a drug product may fail to meet its specifications. It should be noted that whenever a drug product fails at the time of release, predominantly the root cause lies in the manufacturing process or the analytical method. This third approach will briefly touch upon how to statistically assess the process performance. Apparently, a process having better performance statistics will have lesser probability of batch failures at release. Statistical assessment of process performance will be explained in the following steps:

(a) Definition of process performance indices.

(b) Assessment of process performance using the registered specification limits.

(c) Assessment of process performance using the release limits derived from stability data.

4.3.1   Definition of Process Performance Indices

Process performance statistics tells about how well a process meets a set of specifications. CpK and PpK are the two statistical indicators, which describes the process performance. CpK measures how close a process is running to its specification, relative to the natural variability of the process. PpK verifies that the process is capable to meet the specifications. To demonstrate the application of process performance statistics, the release data for the same critical quality attribute "CQA1" that was referred in Sect. 4.2 will be used. CpK and PpK statistics can be calculated as the following equation:

$$\text{CpK}/\text{PpK} = \text{minimum } (|\mu - \text{LSL}, \text{USL} - \mu|)/3\sigma \qquad (14)$$

where μ is the mean of the data, LSL is lower specification limit, USL is upper specification limit, and σ is the standard deviation of

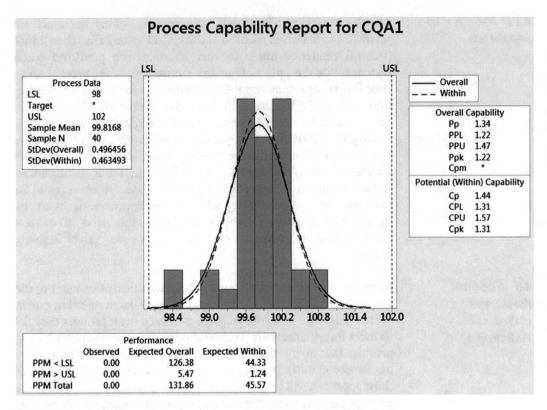

Fig. 4 Process capability report using upper and lower registered specifications

the data. The difference between CpK and PpK lies in the usage of σ. CpK uses variation within the subgroups, whereas PpK uses the overall variation of all the measurements taken.

4.3.2 Assessment of Process Performance Using the Registered Specification Limits

Figure 4 shows the process capability report with the estimate of performance indices. It is to be noted that the PpK value is 1.22 and CpK is 1.31 and the overall standard deviation is 0.496 whereas the subgroup standard deviation is 0.463. Although there is no set benchmark for a good or a bad PpK and CpK value, generally in pharma industry a process with PpK and CpK of 1.33 is considered acceptable and above 2.0 as excellent.

The process performance statistics CpK and PpK indices also have a relationship with the defects per million opportunities (DPMO) and hence with the quality σ level. In between different industries, CpK and PpK are debatable to be used as an indicator of quality. In pharmaceuticals industry, PpK is more acceptable as it considers the long-term variability rather than batch-to-batch variability. A process with PpK value of 2.00 is considered as representing 6σ (6 Sigma) quality, which means approximately 3.4 DPMO. It can be observed from Fig. 4 that the PpK of 1.22 represent the expected overall performance of approximately

132 DPMO. This gives a heads up to the manufacturing process owner to decide whether these many defects are acceptable from quality as well as process economics perspective.

4.3.3 Assessment of Process Performance Using the Release Limits

If the same process performance indices with lower release limit, calculated in Sect. 4.1, are estimated instead of the lower specification limit, the CpK and PpK values change drastically. The CpK and PpK indices have dropped down to 0.61 and 0.57, respectively (*see* Fig. 5). Note that the overall expected process performance is now estimated as approximately 44,047 DPMO. This indicates that in true sense, even though acceptable number of batches may meet the lower specification limits, but with release limits the defects rate may increase drastically. That is where the process owner needs to flag the need of improving the process capability and process stability. In larger organizations, these statistical indices play a key role in prioritizing R&D efforts for process improvement projects so that the chances of batch failures at the time of release and during the shelf-life can be minimized.

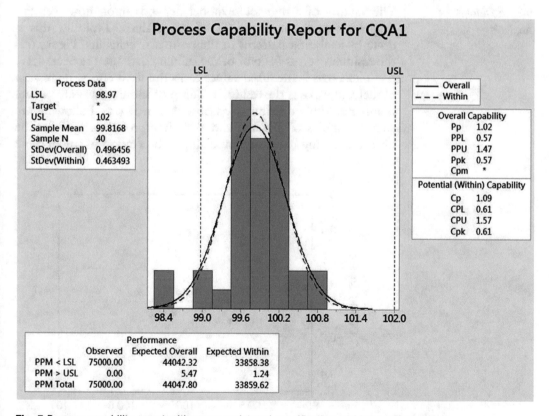

Fig. 5 Process capability report with upper registered specification and lower release limit

5   Diagnostic Tests for Statistical Methods

For statistical methods discussed in this chapter, the following four diagnostic tests are applicable.

5.1   Goodness-of-Fit Statistics

A regression model should always be examined for its key goodness-of-fit statistics. In Sect. 4.1, r^2_{adj} statistics has been consistently used to compare the goodness-of-fit of fixed model with mixed effects model and with reduced mixed effects model. When there is only one independent variable (X) in a statistical model that explains the variability in Y variable, then r^2 and r^2_{adj} are practically interchangeable. As more and more independent variables (Xs) (i.e., effects—fixed as well as mixed) are added to the regression model, the r^2 increases irrespective of how well they are correlated to the Y variable. However, r^2_{adj} provides an adjustment to r^2 such that the independent variable that has a correlation to Y increases the r^2_{adj}. Any variable that does not have a strong correlation will make r^2_{adj} to decrease. Therefore, in the given example we are monitoring the r^2_{adj} to analyze the goodness of fit of the model.

5.2   Residuals Analysis

The validity of a regression model depends upon how well the model meets the assumptions of the analysis. Typically, this is done by analyzing patterns in the residuals versus fits. Figure 6 is the residuals versus fits plot of the stability data used in Sect. 4.1.

The x-axis is the fitted values form the fixed effects regression model and y-axis is the residuals. This plot should always have data points randomly distributed as observed in Fig. 6. Following are some examples of patterns and their interpretations that can be observed during regression modeling. Observation of any of these

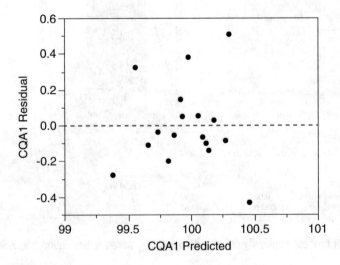

Fig. 6 Residuals versus fits plot

Table 14
Patterns in residuals versus fits plot

Pattern	Interpretation
Fanning or uneven spreading of residuals across fitted values	Variance is not constant over the measurement range
Curvilinear	A missing higher order term in the model
A point far away from zero along y-axis	Outlier
A point far away from the other point along x-axis	Influential point

patterns indicates the violation of assumptions of regression modeling (Table 14).

In case outliers or influential points are observed similar to the last two patterns mentioned in Table 13, an investigation should be performed to identify the root cause. It can be because of wrong data entry or measurement error. Such data entries should be replaced with the correct values, if not, then should be excluded from the statistical assessment. Note that in long-term stability data sometimes OOS observations are flagged as outliers. Caution must be taken while handling such data points. If the root cause of an OOS observation is identified, expected and accepted, then such data points should be excluded from the statistical assessment. If the root cause is not identified for an OOS observation and there is no analytical basis to exclude such data points, then these values should be included in the statistical assessment.

5.3 Normal Probability Plot

Normal probability plot is used to validate the assumption that the data are normally distributed. To examine the validity of a regression model, the residuals should be checked for their normal distribution. Figure 7 displays how a typical probability plot of normally distributed residuals may look like. The residuals should appear to follow the straight line. The data points at the tail sometimes may appear away from the line but should be within the bounds of the specified confidence interval. Data points that are away from the line as well as outside the specified confidence interval, do not follow the normal distribution. Note that along with the visual pattern, the p-value displayed in Fig. 7 (for Anderson-darling (AD) statistics for normal distribution) is greater than 0.05 (usually the chosen alpha). For a distribution plot (in this case normal distribution), AD statistics p-value greater than 0.05 indicates that the data follows the same distribution (in this case normal

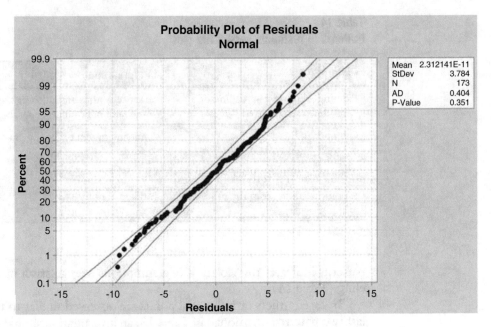

Fig. 7 Typical probability plot of residuals following normal distribution

distribution). *P*-value less than 0.05 would have indicated that the data does not follow the given distribution.

Figure 8 shows the normal probability plot of the residuals from the regression model developed in Sect. 4.1. Although, the residuals do not appear to follow the line consistently, but all the points are within the 95% confidence interval and the *p*-value for AD statistics for normal distribution is greater than 0.05. Therefore, we can assume that the residuals are normally distributed and the model does not violate the regression model assumption.

The normal probability plot also has application in the statistical approach to predict the batch rejection rate as discussed in Sect. 4.2. The validity of ECDF relies on the distribution of the data because the cumulative distribution function gives the cumulative probability of the whole population associated with a distribution. The area under the probability density function up to a specified value can be calculated using the ECDF. For predicting the batch rejection rate in Sect. 4.2, the ECDF was generated with the assumption that the data are normally distributed. Let us examine the normality assumption for the batch release data used in Sect. 4.2. Figure 9 displays the normal probability plot of the batch release data for CQA1. Note that the *p*-value for normal distribution is less than 0.05, which means the batch release data does not follow the normal distribution. Therefore, using the ECDF plot generated with normality assumption will not be a statistically sound decision. In such cases, there are two approaches which are

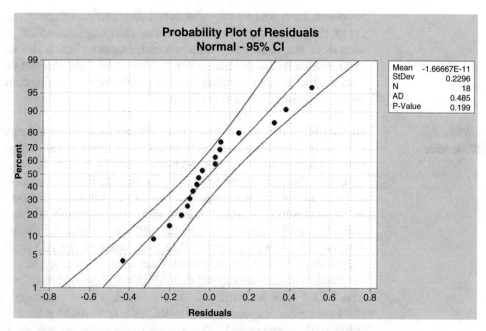

Fig. 8 Normal probability plot of residuals from fixed model developed in Sect. 4.1.2

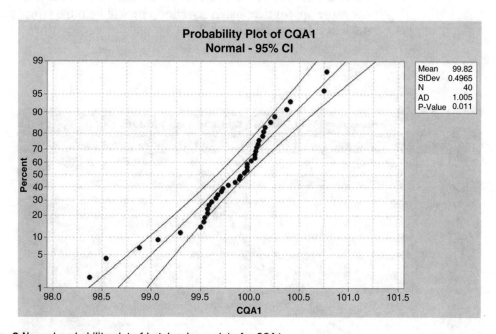

Fig. 9 Normal probability plot of batch release data for CQA1

followed, first, we identify what is the distribution of the data, and create the ECDF based on the identified distribution. Second, if the data does not follow any standard distribution, then it should be modified such that the transformed values follow the normal distribution. In the next section, we will briefly introduce the concept and application of data transformation.

5.4 Data Transformation

In simple words transformation is the application of a function (e.g., logarithmic, square, square root) or their combination to the original data. The transformation function can be selected such that the transformed data fits the normal distribution. In the example in Fig. 10, it has been identified that the Johnson transformation converts the batch release data into normally distributed data. Figure 11 shows the normal probability plot of the transformed data. It is to be noted that the p-value of the AD statistics for normal distribution is greater than 0.05. Therefore, it can be assumed that the transformed data fits into the normal distribution. The ECDF plot with the transformed data is then generated and the area under the curve on the left of transformed release limit value is then calculated. The transformed value of release limit 98.97 is equal to -1.41841. Further, the area under the ECDF curve on the left of -1.418 is approximately 6.0% and, therefore, the more appropriate batch rejection rate will be 6.0% rather than 4.8% as calculated in Sect. 4.2.

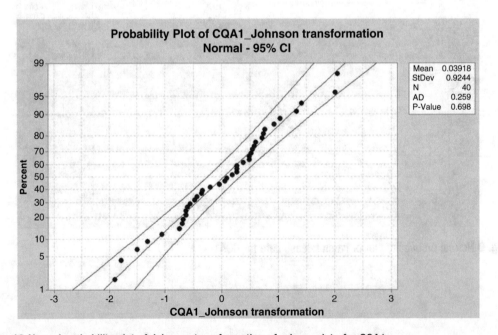

Fig. 10 Normal probability plot of Johnson transformation of release data for CQA1

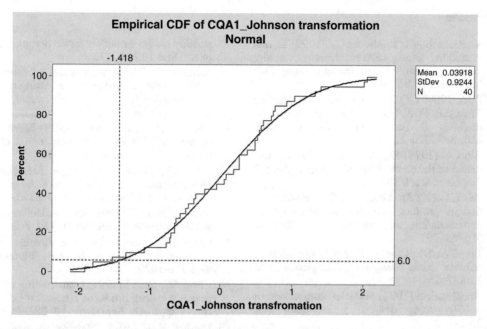

Fig. 11 ECDF plot of Johnson transformation of release data for CQA1

6   Discussion

The drug product failure during its shelf-life is one of the major concerns in pharmaceutical industry. It not only costs millions when a product recall happens but also affects the credibility and reputation in the eyes of patients. Pharmaceutical industry is putting a lot of efforts in conducting stability studies to understand the behavior of the drug products over the time. This chapter starts with the introduction of ICH guideline for assessing the stability data and how those can be extended to avoid stability failures. The chapter discussed briefly about developing the regression models and verifying the validity of assumptions behind the regression statistics. The chapter also demonstrated various statistical approaches to assess the stability data and estimate the statistical indices, which can predict the batch failure rate and provided information about process performance. The statistical methods discussed in this chapter are important part of board room discussions in today's pharmaceuticals industry. These statistics help the business drivers and manufacturing process owners to prioritize the process improvement initiatives and produce stable drug products.

References

1. Kommanaboyina B, Rhodes CT (1999) Trends in stability testing with emphasis on stability during distribution and storage. Drug Dev Ind Pharm 25:857–868

2. FDA (2005) Q1E—Evaluation for stability data Q1E. FDA, US - Published in the Federal Register, 8 June 2004, Vol. 69, No. 110, p. 32010–11

3. Wei GC (1998) Simple methods for determination of the release limits for drug products. J Biopharm Stat 8:103–114

4. Yu LX (2008) Pharmaceutical quality by design: product and process development, understanding, and control. Pharm Res 25 (4):781–791

5. Tsae-Yun DL, Chen CW (2007) Overview of stability study designs. J Biopharm Stat 13:337–354

6. Nordbrock E (1992) Statistical comparison of stability study designs. J Biopharm Stat 2:91–113

7. Ahn H, Chen JJ, Tsae-Yun DL (1997) A two way analysis of covariance model for classification of stability data. Biom J 39:559–576

8. Tsong Y, Chen W, Chen WC (2003) ANCOVA approach for shelf-life analysis of stability study of multiple factor design. J Biopharm Stat 13:375–393

9. Bancroft TA (1964) Analysis and inference for incompletely specified models involving the use of preliminary test(s) of significance. Biometrics 20:427–442

10. Chen JJ, Hwan J, Tsong Y (1995) Estimation of the shelf-life of drugs with mixed effect models. J Biopharm Stat 5:131–140

11. Allen PV, Dukes GR, Gerger ME (1991) Determination of release limits: a general methodology. Pharm Res 9:1210–1213

12. Shao J, Chow SC (1994) Statistical inference in stability analysis. Biometrics 50:753–763

13. Chow SC, Shao J (1991) Estimating drug shelf-life with random batches. Biometrics 47:1071–1079

14. Chow SC, Shao J (1991) Constructing release tragets for drug products: a bayesian decision theory approach. Appl statist 40: 381–390

15. Burdick R K (2017) Stability. In Statistical Applications for Chemistry, Manufacturing and Controls (CMC) in the Pharmaceutical Industry. Springer, Heidelberg, P 269

Chapter 12

Estimation of Stability Based on Monitoring of Shipment and Storage

Manuel Zahn

Abstract

The chemical degradation of drug substances and drug products can be estimated by using the result of standard stability studies, and calculating the degradation rate. This method is also applicable to assess the impact of short-term temperature excursions during shipment in support of the decision whether to destroy a batch or continue to distribute.

Key words Storage, Shipment, Regulatory requirements, Good distribution practice (GDP), Statistical analysis, Arrhenius, Arrhenius plot, Mean kinetic temperature (MKT), Temperature excursion

1 Regulations for Storage and Shipment

Pharmaceutical development aims at delivering products that do not show any change of assay over the time, even if stored or transported at extreme conditions. These stable products contain drugs that shall ideally not interact with excipients and are resistant to temperature, humidity, or light. In the real world, however, most of the substances degrade over the time, in particular at higher temperature and humidity. The most challenging part for pharmaceuticals is shipment from a temperature-controlled environment to a warehouse, pharmacy, or patient. During this shipment period, the product could be damaged due to inappropriate handling (e.g., during storage outside specified conditions by nonqualified courier service providers). Transportation could be delayed or deviate from specified routes, and boxes may be unloaded, stored outside, and reloaded again.

In order to mitigate the risk of unnecessary degradation of the active substances, regulators in the EU [1, 2], Ireland [3], the USA [4, 5], and Canada [6], as well as the WHO [7, 8] have implemented laws and regulations that force the pharmaceutical industry and the courier service providers to monitor or even control the

Sanjay Bajaj and Saranjit Singh (eds.), *Methods for Stability Testing of Pharmaceuticals*, Methods in Pharmacology and Toxicology, https://doi.org/10.1007/978-1-4939-7686-7_12, © Springer Science+Business Media, LLC, part of Springer Nature 2018

temperature in the direct environment of the product during storage and shipment.

All of these guidelines require that

1. "warehousing operations … ensure appropriate storage conditions are maintained" (Reference [2], Chap. 5.5), and that

2. "the required storage conditions for medicinal products (be) maintained during transportation within the defined limits as described by the manufacturers or on the outer packaging" [2].

This can be achieved by continuous monitoring or controlling the temperature and in some cases the humidity inside the warehouse or cool room, refrigerator or freezer as well as during shipment. The conditions are to be measured and recorded in defined short-term intervals, normally 5–10 min, using calibrated and qualified sensors and data loggers.

Good distribution practice (GDP) guidelines contain also the following requirement:

"If a deviation such as temperature excursion … has occurred during transportation, this should be reported to the distributor and recipient of the affected medicinal products. A procedure should also be in place for investigating and handling temperature excursions" (Reference [2], Chap. 9.2).

The distributor is normally consulting the manufacturer of the medicinal product for advice concerning the consequences of temperature excursions during shipment and storage as only the manufacturer is in a position to run calculations based on results of stability studies. In case of products intended to be used in clinical trials, the distributor is normally obliged to report excursions to the sponsor based on a quality agreement between the sponsor and the courier service provider. In the EU, it is up to the qualified person (QP) to decide whether a shipment is affected by temperature excursions and has to be destroyed or can still be used by the patient. This decision requires the definition of a threshold that can be justified by sound scientific arguments.

In the following sections, it is described, how stability data of drug substances and drug products can be evaluated by statistical analysis in support of estimating the shelf-life in situation of temperature excursions. Also, the estimation of the remaining shelf-life after temperature excursions during shipment and storage is explained.

2   Impact of Temperature

Drug substances are unstable over the time; some of them degrade very slowly, e.g., small chemical molecules, others faster, e.g., biotechnologically derived macromolecules. In this chapter, the impact of temperature on small chemical substances is evaluated. All other aspects like the impact of humidity or light on the degradation are neglected here. In general, stability studies are performed by measuring assay and amount of degradation products at pre-defined time points on samples stored at constant temperature (± 2 °C) and relative humidity ($\pm 5\%$) (*see* Fig. 1, Table 1). In order to achieve independent observations, the same samples are assessed at each of the time points, i.e., taken from the same batch, packed in the same container closure system, and stored in the same stability chamber. The increasing amount of degradation product A found at time

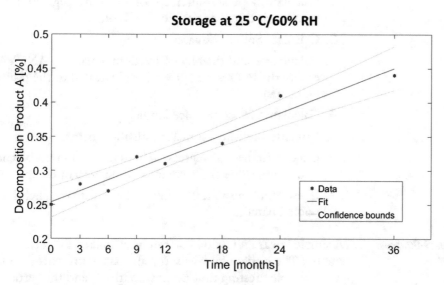

Fig. 1 Increase of degradation product A in a medicinal product stored at 25 °C/60% RH for 36 months (linear regression line, 95% confidence interval)

Table 1
Amount (y) of degradation product A (%) found at 8 time points (x) (months) after storage of a medicinal product at 25 °C/60% relative humidity (RH)

x	y
0	0.25
3	0.28
6	0.27
9	0.32
12	0.31
18	0.34
24	0.41
36	0.44

points 0, 3, 6, 9, 12, 18, 24, and 36 months are used to calculate the linear regression line (*see* **Note 1**). To estimate the shelf-life, the 95% confidence interval of the linear regression line has to be known, which requires some understanding of statistical analysis.

3 Statistical Analysis of Stability Data

3.1 Road Map

A complete statistical analysis of the stability data generated may follow a stepwise approach like this:

1. Calculate slope and intercept of individual regression lines for each batch tested as described in **Note 1**.
2. Calculate Sum of Squares.
3. Calculate F and degrees of freedom; create an ANOVA table; ensure the test results (y) are linearly related to the testing time points (x).
4. Calculate 95% confidence limits.
5. Estimate shelf-lives for each individual batch.
6. Check whether the regression lines from different batches have a common slope and a common time-zero intercept.
7. If yes, combine all test results and calculate the shelf-life of the pooled batches.

3.2 Least-Squares Estimation

A simple linear regression line can be estimated from two variables, x and y. The horizontal x-axis, the abscissa, represents the independent variable "testing time point (months)", and the vertical y-axis, the ordinate, presents the dependent outcome "assay" or "amount of degradation product (%)". A straight line is drawn that best fits between the y-values found (*see* Fig. 2). This line is called the "least-squares" line, as it offers the smallest squares drawn between the values found and the line (*see* Fig. 3). The large areas squares (left) represent the squared vertical distances between the data points and the line, called the "residuals" with respect to the average or mean value ($\bar{y}$), and the areas of the small squares (right) represent the squared residuals with respect to the linear regression.

If the amount of deviations above and below the line were equal, the sum of the residuals should equal zero. Thus, the best fit is the line that results in the smallest value for the sum of the squared unexplained deviations, called "Error Sum of Squares (SS_{Error})". To calculate SS_{Error}, first the sum of the total variation between the values found (y), divided by the number of observations (n), and each observed value (y), called the "Total Sum of Squares (SS_{Total})", have to be known. SS_{Total} can then be derived by Eq. 1:

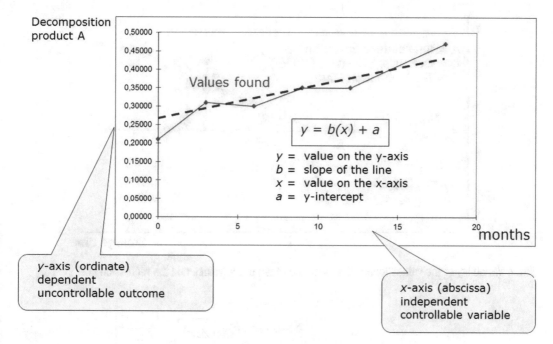

Fig. 2 Linear regression line drawn based on values found

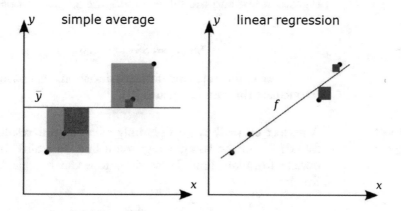

Fig. 3 Size of squared residuals ("errors") for an average line compared to a linear regression line. Source: http:/en.wikipedia.org/wiki/Coefficient_of_determination

$$SS_{Total} = \sum y^2 - \frac{(\sum y)^2}{n} \tag{1}$$

In order to calculate the variability explained by the regression line of the deviations between the mean and the line, called the "Model Sum of Squares (SS_{Model})", the slope of the line is required, which can be calculated as described in **Note 1**. Then SS_{Model} can be calculated by using Eq. 2:

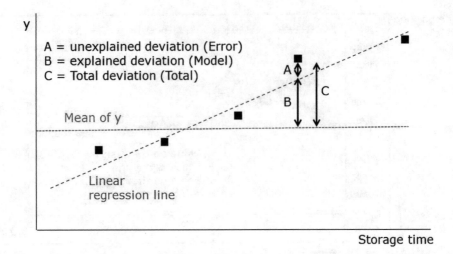

A = unexplained deviation (Error)
B = explained deviation (Model)
C = Total deviation (Total)

Fig. 4 Variability of the values found (y) around the mean of the values and the regression line

$$SS_{Model} = b^2 \cdot \left[\sum x^2 - \frac{(\sum x)^2}{n} \right] \qquad (2)$$

Finally, the remaining unexplained deviation between the regression line and the values found, the SS_{Error}, can be calculated by using Eq. 3:

$$SS_{Error} = SS_{Total} - SS_{Model} \qquad (3)$$

Figure 4 illustrates the different deviations that have been used to calculate the sum of squares [9].

3.3 Coefficient of Determination

A perfect estimate is possible only when all test results (y values found) lie on the straight regression line. In reality, the y-values deviate from the line. These deviations can be calculated using Eq. 4:

$$r^2 = \frac{SS_{Model}}{SS_{Total}} \times 100\% \qquad (4)$$

The coefficient of determination (r^2) represents that proportion of variance in the y-values that is accounted for by variance in the x-values. It measures the exactness of fit of the regression equation to the observed values (y). The better the linear regression fits the data in comparison to the mean, the closer the value of r^2 is to 100% [9].

In addition to r^2, the "adjusted coefficient of determination (r^2_{adj})" is often presented in statistical calculation, adjusted for the number of predictor variables in the model according to Eq. 5:

$$r_{\text{adj}}^2 = 1 - \left(\frac{n-1}{n-p}\right)\frac{SS_{\text{Error}}}{SS_{\text{Total}}} \tag{5}$$

p = number of regression coefficients (including the intercept) (in simple linear regression: $p = 2$)

3.4 ANOVA Table

The final decision on the acceptability of the linear regression model is a result of an Analysis of Variance (ANOVA) that determines whether the values are best represented by a straight line. For this outcome, the statistical hypothesis H_0 that the x- and y-values are not linearly related has to be rejected. ANOVA is a collection of statistical models used to analyze the differences among group means and their associated procedures (such as "variation" among and between groups), developed by the "father" of scientific statistics Sir Ronald A. Fisher (*see* Fig. 5).

In honor of R. A. Fisher, the statistical test showing a particular distribution under the null hypothesis has been named *F-test*, used for comparing the factors of the total deviation by using Eq. 6:

$$F = \frac{MS_{\text{Model}}}{MS_{\text{Error}}} \tag{6}$$

MS = mean square.

The amount of variability explained by the regression line (*Model*) is placed in the numerator of this Eq. 6, and the variability of the unexplained residual (*Error*) is the denominator. The numerator degrees of freedom is df = $2-1 = 1$ for the regression line, since the regression line is based on two parameters (slope and intercept), and the degrees of freedom are the number of parameters minus one. The denominator degrees of freedom is df = $n-2$ [9].

If the amount of explained deviations (*Model*) increases, the F-value will increase, and it becomes more likely that the result will be a rejection of the null hypothesis H_0, which is assuming that x and y are not linearly related.

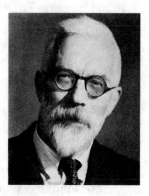

Fig. 5 R. A. Fisher (1890–1962). Source: https:/en.wikipedia.org/wiki/Ronald_Fisher

Table 2
ANOVA table

Source of variation	df	SS	MS	F
Linear regression (model)	1	SS_{Model}	$MS_{Model} = SS_{Model}/1$	MS_{Model}/MS_{Error}
Residual (error)	$n-2$	SS_{Error}	$MS_{Error} = SS_{Error}/n-2$	
Total	$n-1$	SS_{Total}		

Note: SS = Sum of squares
MS = Mean squares

It is generally accepted to use an error rate of $\alpha = 0.05$, which means a probability of <5% is regarded as an "unlikely event". If the calculated F-value is higher than the F-value $F_{1,n-2}(1-\alpha)$, the null hypothesis can be rejected in favor of the alternative hypothesis H_1, which is assuming that x and y are linearly related, and the result is "statistically significant" (see Eq. 7).

$$\text{Reject } H_0 \text{ if } \quad F > F_{1,n-2}(1 - \alpha) \tag{7}$$

In this equation, n equals the number of data points. The critical F-values for $F_{1,n-2}(0.95)$ can be found in statistical textbooks or in computer software programs. A general ANOVA table is presented in Table 2.

3.5 Confidence Intervals

As stated in the ICH Stability Guideline Q1E [10], the purpose of statistical analysis of primary stability batches "is to establish, with a high degree of confidence, a retest period or shelf-life during which a quantitative attribute will remain within acceptance criteria for all future batches manufactured, packaged, and stored under similar circumstances". This "high degree of confidence" is generally accepted as 95%. A 95% confidence ($\alpha = 0.05$) means a 2.5% chance of being wrong to each side of the distribution ($\alpha/2 = 0.025$). With n number of y-values, and $n-2$ degrees of freedom, the corresponding t-values for the Student's t-distribution can be found by using Eq. 8:

$$t_{n-2}\left(1 - \frac{\alpha}{2}\right) \tag{8}$$

For a 95% confidence, the t-values at 0.975 are relevant (see Eq. 9):

$$1 - \frac{\alpha}{2} = 0.975 \tag{9}$$

The $t_{0.975}$-values are presented in Table 3.

For infinite degrees of freedom (df $= \infty$), the resulting t-value is $t_{0.975} = 1.9602$.

Table 3
Student's *t*-distribution for 95% confidence ($\alpha/2 = 0.025$)

Degrees of freedom	$t_{.975}$
1	12.706
2	4.3027
3	3.1824
4	2.7765
5	2.5706
6	2.4469
20	2.0860
∞	1.9602

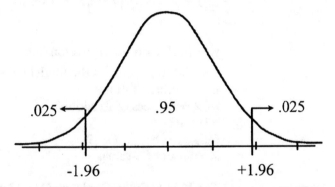

Fig. 6 Distribution with 95% confidence (0.95), i.e., 2.5% error ($\alpha/2 = 0.025$) at each side, and infinite degrees of freedom (df $= \infty$), $t_{0.975} = 1.9602$

An illustration of a symmetrical distribution of values (mean value $= 0$) with 95% confidence is presented in Fig. 6.

The shape of the Student's *t*-distribution is symmetrical and adequate in particular for small sample sizes. When the sample size gets smaller, the range becomes wider. The "Student's t-distribution" has been developed by William Sealy Gosset (*see* Fig. 7).

He was not allowed by his employer to publish results of his scientific research, so he used the pseudonym "Student" in his publication "The Probable Error of a Mean" in Biometrika 6(1), 1–25 (1908). Gosset's concept is, therefore, called "Student's *t*-distribution", and has been applied by R. A. Fisher to the regression analysis.

For any value on the *x*-axis it is possible to estimate a corresponding value on the *y*-axis using the equation $y = b(x) + a$. A confidence interval [9] for the expected *y*-value can be calculated using Eq. 10:

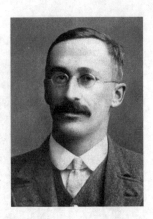

Fig. 7 William Gosset (1876–1937). Source: https:/en.wikipedia.org/wiki/William_Sealy_Gosset

$$y = y_c \pm t_{n-2}\left(1 - \frac{\alpha}{2}\right) \cdot \sqrt{MS_{Error}} \cdot \sqrt{\frac{1}{n} + \frac{(x_i - \bar{X})^2}{\sum x^2 - \frac{(\sum x)^2}{n}}} \quad (10)$$

y_c = y-value on the regression line
t = 95th-percentile of the Student's t-distribution
n = number of values
$n-2$ = degrees of freedom
$\alpha = 0.05$
$MS_{Error} = SS_{Error}/n-2$
$\bar{X}$ = mean of x-values

3.6 Estimation of Shelf-Life

The ICH Stability Guideline Q1E [10] describes the procedure to estimate a retest period or shelf-life as follows:

"An appropriate approach to retest period or shelf-life estimation is to analyze a quantitative attribute (e.g., assay, degradation products) by determining the earliest time at which the 95% confidence limit for the mean intersects the proposed acceptance criterion".

Taking the example of a medicinal product stored at 25 °C/60% RH for 36 months presented above, and assuming a specified acceptance criterion of not more than 0.45% for degradation product A, the upper 95% confidence limit intersects the 0.45%-value at about 32 months, which would, in consequence, set the shelf-life at 24 months (*see* Fig. 8).

Although the 36-month value found (0.44%, *see* Table 1) is not out-of-specification (OOS), the shelf-life has to be estimated in a more conservative approach using the 95% confidence limit.

3.7 Pooling of Batches

The amount of data can be increased by combining batches produced according to the same manufacturing procedure and packed in the same packaging material. Combining batches is called "pooling", and is very helpful as the confidence intervals become smaller

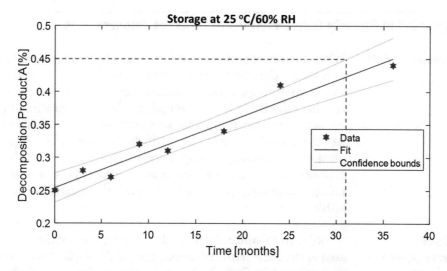

Fig. 8 Estimation of shelf-life assuming a specified acceptance criterion for degradation product A at 0.45% (− − −) in a medicinal product stored at 25 °C/60% for 36 months (linear regression line, 95% confidence interval)

when the sample size increases, as described above. As a consequence, smaller confidence intervals result in longer shelf-lives.

The test procedure for poolability of batches is described in ICH Q1E, Section B2.2 [10].

3.8 Limitations of Statistics

Whenever a statistical evaluation of stability data is conducted, its limitation has to be taken into consideration, i.e.,

1. Manufacturing process must be robust in order to avoid different slopes and intercepts of the regression lines calculated for different batches of the same product.

2. The number of batches is low; normally there are just two or three batches of the same product in the same strength packed in identical packaging material available for stability studies.

3. Only quantitative (chemical) attributes, e.g., assay and amount of degradation products, are amenable to statistical analysis.

4. Linear degradation is assumed, which is not always reflecting reality, in particular when the degradation takes place more pronounced in the first days or weeks after production.

In the ICH Stability Guideline Q1A(R2), Sect. 2.2.9 Evaluation [11], the following statement can be found:

"Where the data show so little degradation and so little variability that it is apparent from looking at the data that the requested shelf-life will be granted, it is normally unnecessary to go through the formal statistical analysis; providing a justification for the omission should be sufficient".

4 Evaluation of Stability Data Generated at Different Temperatures

4.1 Degradation Rate
When the retest period or shelf-life should be estimated based on short-term data or when the remaining shelf-life should be estimated after temperature excursions during shipment and storage, another calculation is recommended using a combination of stability data generated at different temperatures. It is possible to calculate the degradation rate (k), at which the amount of a degradation product is increasing during storage. This rate is increasing in an exponential manner with increasing temperatures, and is higher, i.e., the degradation is faster, when the chemical substance is less stable.

4.2 Slopes of Different Linear Regression Lines
In order to calculate the degradation rate, the stability data generated at the long-term condition, e.g., at 25 °C/60% RH, are taken as presented in Sect. 2. Based on the y-values found, the linear regression line and its slope are calculated as described in **Note 1**.

The slope of the linear regression line of the product stored at the defined condition, e.g., 25 °C, is equal to the degradation rate k_{25} (%/month) at this temperature, and can be calculated as described in **Note 2**.

Storage at 30 °C/75% RH

When stored at higher temperatures, e.g., at 30 °C, the degradation of the drug is faster (*see* Table 4 and Fig. 9).

Again, the regression line and the slope of this line are calculated for the product stored at 30 °C/75% RH. The slope is equal to the degradation rate k_{30} (%/month).

Table 4
Amount (y) of degradation product A (%) found at 8 time points (x) (months) after storage of a medicinal product at 30 °C/75% RH

x	y
0	0.25
3	0.31
6	0.33
9	0.37
12	0.38
18	0.48
24	0.52
36	0.64

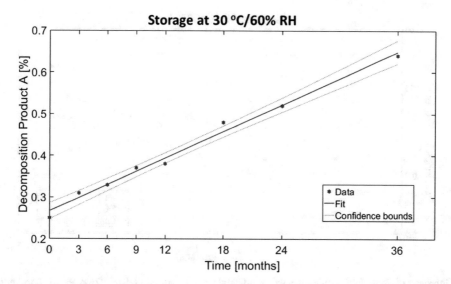

Fig. 9 Increase of degradation product A in a medicinal product stored at 30 °C/75% for 36 months (linear regression line, 95% confidence interval)

Table 5
Amount (y) of degradation product A (%) found at 3 time points (x) (months) after storage of a medicinal product at 40 °C/75% RH for 6 months

x	y
0	0.25
3	0.36
6	0.46

Storage at 40 °C/75% RH

Stored at the accelerated condition 40 °C/75% RH, the product degrades even faster (*see* Table 5 and Fig. 10).

The slope is equal to the degradation rate k_{40} (%/month).

A combination of the stability data from all three storage conditions visualizes the faster degradation at higher temperatures (*see* Fig. 11).

4.3 The Arrhenius Equation

The degradation increases in an exponential manner with increasing temperatures. This has been described by the Swedish chemist Svante Arrhenius[1] (*see* Fig. 12) in 1889 for the first time (Eq. 11).

---

[1] Svante Arrhenius was awarded the Nobel Prize in Chemistry 1903 "in recognition of the extraordinary services he has rendered to the advancement of chemistry by his electrolytic theory of dissociation". Source: http://www.nobel.se/chemistry/laureates/1903/arrhenius-bio.html

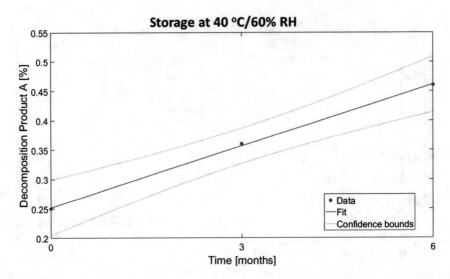

Fig. 10 Increase of degradation product A in a medicinal product stored at 40 °C/75% RH for 6 months (linear regression line, 95% confidence interval)

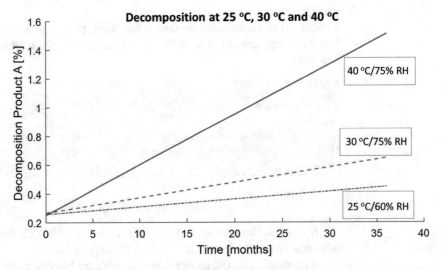

Fig. 11 Increase of degradation product A in a medicinal product stored at 25 °C/60% RH, 30 °C/75% RH, and 40 °C/75% RH (linear regression lines, extrapolated at 40 °C)

$$k = A \; e^{-\frac{E_a}{R \times T}} \tag{11}$$

k = Loss rate constant = chemical reaction rate
A = Pre-exponential factor = Arrhenius factor
E_a = Activation energy (kJ/mol)
R = Universal gas constant = 8.3144 (J/K mol)
T = Temperature (K)

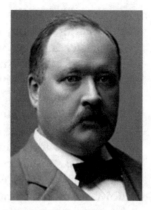

Fig. 12 Svante Arrhenius (1859–1927). Source: http:/www.nobel.se/chemistry/laureates/1903/arrhenius-bio.html

4.4   The Arrhenius Plot

Starting point is a list of the different slopes of the linear regression lines found at different temperatures, e.g., k_{25}, k_{30}, and k_{40}, and the temperatures used to store the stability samples (*see* Table 9).

If the natural logarithm of the degradation rates $\ln(k_{temp})$ is plotted versus the temperature $1/T\,(^{\circ}\mathrm{K}^{-1})$, the so-called "Arrhenius plot" is derived. The degradation of the medicinal product at three different temperatures presented above is used to calculate the Arrhenius plot (*see* **Note 2**).

The logarithmic expression of the Arrhenius equation is (Eq. 12)

$$\ln(k) = \frac{-E_a}{R}\left(\frac{1}{T}\right) + \ln(A) \tag{12}$$

When Eq. 12 is compared to a standard equation describing a linear regression line (Eq. 13), it becomes obvious that $-E_a/R$ is equal to the slope and $\ln(A)$ is equal to the intercept of the regression line.

$$y = b(x) + a \tag{13}$$

$y = \ln(k)$

$b = \text{Slope} = -E_a/R$

$x = 1/T$

$a = \text{Intercept} = \ln(A)$

Based on the slope of the Arrhenius plot, the activation energy E_a can be calculated as follows (Eq. 14):

$$E_a = -b \cdot R \tag{14}$$

$E_a = \text{Activation energy (kJ/mol)}$

$b = \text{Slope of Arrhenius plot}$

$R = \text{Universal gas constant} = 8.3144 \times 10^{-3}\ (\text{kJ/K mol})$

A stable chemical substance requires a higher energy to initiate a chemical reaction, i.e., degradation, compared to a less stable substance. In other words, the higher the activation energy, the more stable the substance is.

The activation energy E_a is also called the "heat of activation" ΔH or ΔE, and the USP [5] recommends to take the value 83.144 (kJ/mol) "unless more accurate information is available from experimental studies". This value has been derived from the overall mean values found in the literature between 1950 and 1980 for 132 active substances [12] used in medicines. Applying this mean value, the result is easy to use, namely $E_a/R = 10,000$. It is, however, more accurate to calculate the activation energy by creating the Arrhenius plot and using the slope of the resulting line, as described in **Note 2**.

Finally, the pre-exponential factor A, also called the "Arrhenius factor", can be calculated (Eq. 15):

$$\ln(A) = y\text{-Intercept of the Arrhenius plot} \qquad (15)$$

As a result, all elements within the Arrhenius equation are known, and the equation can be applied to chemical reactions, i.e., degradation processes, at any temperature.

4.5 Estimation of Shelf-Life Based on Short-Term Data

With the complete knowledge of all elements of the Arrhenius equation, the chemical degradation of a drug in a medicinal product due to the impact of temperature can be estimated, and the shelf-life can be predicted based on short-term stability data.

The first-order reaction of a degradation process can be described as follows (Eq. 16):

$$\frac{dC}{dt} = -k_1 C \qquad (16)$$

which integrates to (Eq. 17)

$$C = C_0 e^{-k_1 t} \qquad (17)$$

C = Content of substance
C_0 = Initial content at time point $t = 0$
k_1 = Degradation rate constant of first-order reaction
t = Time

Stable products degrade very slowly over a long period of time, normally several years. For this kind of products, a zero-order reaction can be assumed, expressed as follows (Eq. 18):

$$C = C_0 - k \cdot t \tag{18}$$

C = Content of substance

C_0 = Initial content at time point $t = 0$ (at time of batch release)
k = Degradation rate of zero-order reaction
t = Time

As the content of the drug in the medicinal product (assay value) and the amount of degradation products are known at time of batch release (C_0), and the degradation rate (k) specific for each product has been calculated based on the results of stability studies performed at two or three different storage conditions, the assay values and the amount of degradation products at any time point (t) can be estimated, assuming a linear decomposition process.

The shelf-life of any product can then be predicted based on short-term data. The time, when the specified acceptance criteria for assay or degradation products have been reached in the calculation, defines the predicted shelf-life.

The following steps should be completed to predict a retest period or shelf-life:

1. Perform stability studies at two, better three different temperatures, e.g., at 25, 30, and 40 °C.

2. Calculate the resulting linear regression line for each temperature separately.

3. Calculate the different slopes of the linear regression lines as described in **Note 1**.

4. Create an Arrhenius plot using the different slopes as described in **Note 2**.

5. Calculate the slope of the Arrhenius plot, i.e., the degradation rate.

6. Calculate the activation energy E_a and the Arrhenius Factor A as described in **Note 2**.

7. Calculate assay or the amount of degradation products at any time beyond long-term data available as described in **Note 3**.

When linear regression lines are calculated in order to predict shelf-lives, the confidence intervals should always be considered, and a proper statistical analysis should be performed.

4.6 Prediction of Degradation During Shipment and Storage

In case of a slow, linear degradation process, a zero-order reaction kinetic can be applied as described in Eq. 18. This assumption is justified for stable products, where the chemical reaction rate is intentionally reduced by the formulation optimized during pharmaceutical development, including the chemical interaction between the drug and the excipients.

In the following, Eq. 18 is used to calculate the amount of degradation products at the end of defined periods of time, starting from production to the expiry date. This approach supports the decision by the Qualified Person in the EU or by any expert in charge, whether the product has been damaged by temperature excursions recorded during shipment [13, 14].

4.6.1 Phase I: Storage at the Manufacturer's Warehouse

A medicinal product contains a known amount of the degradation product A (C_0) at the time of batch release ($t = 0$). The product is stored at the manufacturer's warehouse until it is picked up by a shipment service provider. The upper limit of the temperature in the warehouse should be taken, when the amount of degradation product A (C_{stor}) at the end of the storage period (t_{stor}) is calculated using Eq. 19:

$$C_{stor} = C_0 + k_{stor} \cdot t_{stor} \qquad (19)$$

C_{stor} = Content of degradation product (%) at the end of storage

C_0 = Initial content (%) at time point $t = 0$ (at time of batch release)

k_{stor} = Degradation rate at the upper temperature limit during storage (%/month)

t_{stor} = Storage time (months)

In countries belonging to climatic zone I or II [15], medicinal products are normally stored at ambient conditions, i.e., 15–30 °C. The MKT in these zones never increases above 25 °C, and, therefore, the degradation rate at 25 °C can be used. For products stored in countries belonging to climatic zone III or IV, the degradation rate at 30 °C should be used [16]. If a less stable product is stored at lower temperatures, the upper limit of that condition should be taken, e.g., for a product stored at 2–8 °C, the degradation rate at 8 °C should be used.

4.6.2 Phase II: Shipment

The next time period would be the time during which the product is shipped from the manufacturer's warehouse to a wholesaler's warehouse in the target country. The amount of degradation product A contained in the product is increasing starting from the value found at the end of the storage at the manufacturer's warehouse (C_{stor}), and can be calculated taking into account the time of shipment (t_{ship}) and the MKT during shipment using Eq. 20:

$$C_{ship} = C_{stor} + k_{ship} \cdot t_{ship} \qquad (20)$$

C_{ship} = Content of degradation product (%) at the end of shipment

C_{stor} = Content of degradation product (%) at the end of storage

k_{ship} = Degradation rate at MKT during shipment (%/month)

t_{ship} = Time of shipment (months)

4.6.3 Phase III: Storage After Shipment

The final phase is the storage of the medicinal product at the wholesaler's warehouse, the pharmacy, and the patient. The temperature during this period is unknown, and, therefore, the upper limit of the recommended (labeled) storage condition should be taken for calculation of the amount of the degradation product A at the labeled expiry date using Eq. 21:

$$C_{exp} = C_{ship} + k_{label} \cdot t_{exp} \tag{21}$$

C_{exp} = Content of degradation product (%) at expiry date

C_{ship} = Content of degradation product (%) at the end of shipment

k_{label} = Degradation rate at the maximum recommended temperature (%/month)

t_{exp} = Time period from end of shipment until expiry date (months)

In the EU Member States, stable products do not show a storage condition on the label [17]. In this case, a temperature of 25 °C should be assumed for the above calculation. This approach is justified as in countries belonging to climatic zone I and II, the MKT never increases above 25 °C.

If the amount of degradation product A at the labeled expiry date is lower than the specified acceptance criterion, the product can continue to be marketed. It can then be assumed that the temperature excursion during shipment did not affect the quality of the product nor did it reduce its shelf-life. The same approach can be applied taking the decrease of the drug during storage and shipment instead of the increase of the degradation products. Examples are provided in **Note 3**.

5 Impact of Humidity

The impact of humidity on active substances and pharmaceutical products can be neglected in this context as humidity requires much more time than temperature to change the quality parameters. The humidity factor can be incorporated to evaluate the impact on products during long-term storage. The time during shipment, however, is too short to have an impact.

6 Notes

Note 1: Calculation of the Slope and Intercept of a Linear Regression Line

The general equation for a line is provided in Eq. 13. The slope of a line can be calculated by using Eq. 22:

$$b = \frac{n \sum xy - (\sum x)(\sum y)}{n \sum x^2 - (\sum x)^2} \tag{22}$$

b = Slope of the line = degradation rate

n = number of time points

y = Assay or amount of degradation product found (%)

x = Storage time (months)

The slope of a line is always positive in case of increasing y-values, e.g., amount of degradation products (y) over the time (x), and negative if the y-values are decreasing, e.g., assay of the drug (y) over the time (x).

The intercept of a line can be calculated by using Eq. 23:

$$a = \frac{\sum y - b \sum x}{n} \tag{23}$$

a = y-Intercept at $x = 0$

y = Assay or amount of degradation product found (%)

x = Storage time (months)

b = Slope of the line = degradation rate

n = Number of time points

Table 6
Amount (y) of degradation product A found at $n = 8$ time points (x) after storage of a medicinal product at 25 °C/60% RH for 36 months

x	y	x^2	xy
0	0.25	0	0.00
3	0.28	9	0.84
6	0.27	36	1.62
9	0.32	81	2.88
12	0.31	144	3.72
18	0.34	324	6.12
24	0.41	576	9.84
36	0.44	1296	15.84
108	2.62	2466	40.86

Example 25° C

The result of analytical tests of a medicinal product stored at 25 °C/ 60% RH for 36 months is presented in Table 6.

Next is the calculation of the sum of all x-values, and the sum of all y-values, followed by the calculation of the values for x^2 at each time point, and the sum of all x^2 values, and finally the calculation of the values for $(x \cdot y)$ at each time point, and the sum of all $(x \cdot y)$-values.

Now the slope (b) of the regression line can be calculated using Eq. 24. The result is:

$$b = \frac{(8 \times 40.86) - (108 \times 2.62)}{(8 \times 2466) - 108^2} = \frac{326.88 - 282.96}{19728 - 11664}$$

$$= \frac{43.92}{8064} = 0.005446 \tag{24}$$

The y-intercept (a) of the linear regression line at $x = 0$ can be calculated using Eq. 25. The result is:

$$a = \frac{2.62 - (0.005446 \times 108)}{8} = \frac{2.62 - 0.58817}{8}$$

$$= \frac{2.0318}{8} = 0.25398 \tag{25}$$

Statistical computer programs facilitate the calculation of stability data (e.g., MATLAB from The MathWorks, Inc.).

Regression analysis of a single batch:

```
clear, clc
close all
% Months on x
months = (0;3;6;9;12;18;24;36);
% Content of Degradation Product A over the time on y
decompA = (0.25,0.28,0.27,0.32,0.31,0.34,0.41,0.44);
n=8
t=tinv(0.95, n-2)
df_num=1
df_den=n-2
F_cri=finv(0.95,df_num,df_den)
```

```
%Linear regression line and ANOVA Table
mdl = LinearModel.fit(months,decompA)
tbl = anova(mdl)
%Plot
plot (mdl)
xlabel('Time [months]')
ylabel('Degradation Product A [%]')
title ('Storage at 25°C/60% RH')
```

Result:

```
Linear regression model:
    y ~ 1 + x1

Estimated Coefficients:
                 Estimate        SE          tStat        pValue


    (Intercept)   0.25397      0.0091679     27.702     1.4632e-07
    x1            0.0054464    0.00052218    10.43      4.553e-05


Number of observations: 8, Error degrees of freedom: 6
Root Mean Squared Error: 0.0166
R-squared: 0.948,  Adjusted R-Squared 0.939
F-statistic vs. constant model: 109, p-value = 4.55e-05

tbl =

                SumSq        DF      MeanSq        F         pValue


    x1         0.029901      1      0.029901    108.79     4.553e-05
    Error      0.0016491     6      0.00027485
```

$$F_{\text{calculated}} = 108.79 > F_{1,n-2}(1\text{-}\alpha) = 5.9874$$

Conclusion: The x- and y-values are linearly related.

Example 30 °C
The result of analytical tests of a medicinal product stored at 30 °C/75% RH for 36 months is presented in Table 7.

In this case, the slope (b) of the regression line using Eq. 22 is $b = 0.0106$, and the y-intercept (a) using Eq. 23 is $a = 0.2670$.

Table 7
Amount (y) of degradation product A found at $n = 8$ time points (x) after storage of a medicinal product at 30 °C/75% RH

x	y	x^2	xy
0	0.25	0	0
3	0.31	9	0.93
6	0.33	36	1.98
9	0.37	81	3.33
12	0.38	144	4.56
18	0.48	324	8.64
24	0.52	576	12.48
36	0.64	1296	23.04
108	3.28	2466	54.96

```
Linear regression model:
   y ~ 1 + x1

Estimated Coefficients:
                  Estimate        SE         tStat       pValue

                  _____      _____     _____    _____

   (Intercept)     0.26696      0.007959     33.543     4.6737e-08
   x1              0.010595     0.00045332    23.373     4.0236e-07


Number of observations: 8, Error degrees of freedom: 6
Root Mean Squared Error: 0.0144
R-squared: 0.989,  Adjusted R-Squared 0.987
F-statistic vs. constant model: 546, p-value = 4.02e-07

tbl =

                 SumSq       DF     MeanSq         F         pValue

                _____     __    _____     _____     _____

   x1           0.11316      1     0.11316      546.28     4.0236e-07
   Error        0.0012429    6     0.00020714
```

$$F_{\text{calculated}} = 546.28 > F_{1,n-2}\,(1\text{-}\alpha) = 5.9874$$

Conclusion: The x- and y-values are linearly related.

Table 8
Amount (y) of degradation product A found at $n = 3$ time points (x) after storage of a medicinal product at 40 °C/75% RH

x	y	x^2	xy
0	0.25	0	0
3	0.36	9	1.08
6	0.46	36	2.76
9	1.07	45	3.84

Example 40 °C
The result of analytical tests of a medicinal product stored at 40 °C/ 75% RH for 6 months is presented in Table 8.

In this case, the slope (b) of the regression line using Eq. 22 is $b = 0.0350$, and the y-intercept (a) using Eq. 23 is $a = 0.2517$.

```
Linear regression model:
    y ~ 1 + x1

Estimated Coefficients:
                    Estimate        SE          tStat       pValue


    (Intercept)     0.25167     0.0037268     67.529      0.0094266
    x1              0.035       0.00096225    36.373      0.017498


Number of observations: 3, Error degrees of freedom: 1
Root Mean Squared Error: 0.00408
R-squared: 0.999,  Adjusted R-Squared 0.998
F-statistic vs. constant model: 1.32e+03, p-value = 0.0175

tbl =

                SumSq       DF      MeanSq        F        pValue


    x1          0.02205     1       0.02205      1323      0.017498
    Error       1.6667e-05  1       1.6667e-05
```

$$F_{\text{calculated}} = 1323 > F_{1,n-2}(1\text{-}\alpha) = 161.45$$

Conclusion: The x- and y-values are linearly related.

Note 2: Calculation of the Arrhenius Plot
The three different slopes of the linear regression line calculated in **Note 1** are to be expressed as natural logarithm $\ln(k)$ at the three different storage temperatures expressed as $1/T$ (°K^{-1})

Table 9
Example: calculation of the Arrhenius plot using the three degradation rates found expressed as ln(k) at three different storage temperatures expressed as 1/T ($^{\circ}K^{-1}$)

	k	ln(k)	T	1/T
25 °C	0.0054	−5.2129	298.16	0.00335
30 °C	0.0106	−4.5469	303.16	0.00330
40 °C	0.0350	−3.3524	313.16	0.00319

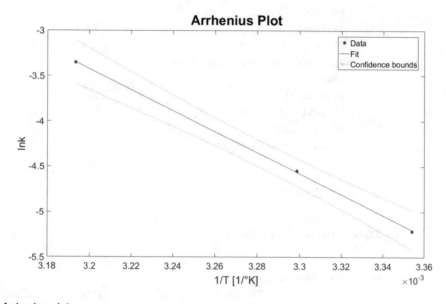

Fig. 13 Arrhenius plot

(*see* Table 9) in order to prepare the Arrhenius plot presented in Fig. 13.

The MATLAB lines look like this:

```
clear, clc
close all
% Regression Analysis for Arrhenius Plot
% Calculation of 1/T at 25C
kelv=273.16;
temp25=25+kelv;
x1=1/temp25
% Calculation of 1/T at 30C
temp30=30+kelv;
x2=1/temp30
% Calculation of 1/T at 40C
temp40=40+kelv;
```

```
x3=1/temp40
% 1/T on x
Temp = (x1;x2;x3)
% k values to lnk values
k = (0.0054464;0.010595;0.035)
% lnk on y
lnk = log(k)

% Linear regression line and ANOVA Table
mdl = LinearModel.fit(Temp,lnk)
tbl = anova(mdl)
n=3
t=tinv(0.95,n-2)
df_num=1
df_den=n-2
F_cri=finv(0.95,df_num,df_den)
%Plot
plot (mdl)
xlabel('1/T (1/°K)')
ylabel('lnk')
title('Arrhenius Plot')
```

Result:

```
Linear regression model:
    y ~ 1 + x1

Estimated Coefficients:
                Estimate        SE         tStat        pValue

    (Intercept)   33.533      0.56776      59.063      0.010778
    x1           -11549       172.96      -66.775      0.0095331


Number of observations: 3, Error degrees of freedom: 1
Root Mean Squared Error: 0.02
R-squared: 1,  Adjusted R-Squared 1
F-statistic vs. constant model: 4.46e+03, p-value = 0.00953

tbl =

                SumSq        DF      MeanSq        F         pValue

    x1          1.7769        1       1.7769     4458.9     0.0095331
    Error       0.0003985     1       0.0003985
```

$F_{\text{calculated}} = 4458.9 > F_{1,n-2}\,(1\text{-}\alpha) = 161.45$

Conclusion: The x- and y-values are linearly related.

As a result, the slope of the Arrhenius plot (b) is found to be $-11{,}549$ using Eq. 14, and the regression line intersects the y-axis at 33.533. Now the activation energy E_a can be calculated (Eq. 26):

$$E_a = -b \cdot R = 11{,}549 \cdot 8.3144 \cdot 10^{-3}\,(\text{kJ/mol})$$
$$= 96.023\ (\text{kJ/mol}) \tag{26}$$

Based on these results, it is possible to calculate the degradation rate (k_{25}) at 25 °C as follows (Eq. 27):

$$\ln(k_{25}) = -11{,}549 \cdot 0.00335 + 33.533 = -5.2012 \tag{27}$$

The result is $k_{25} = 0.0055$ (%/month).

Note 3: The Impact of Temperature Excursions During Shipment

The product given as example above is stable for 24 months when stored at the long term condition of 25 °C/60% RH, it is also stable for more than 12 months when stored at the intermediate condition 30 °C/65% RH, but shows significant change after 6 months on storage at the accelerated condition of 40 °C/75% RH. As a consequence, in the EU the product would be assigned a shelf-life of 24 months with a labeling statement "Store below 30 °C" according to the current CHMP Guideline on Declaration of Storage Conditions [16].

Assuming storage of this product at the manufacturing site in the UK, followed by a shipment to a wholesaler in Spain, the temperature data logger showed two excursions during shipment, and the Qualified Person at the manufacturing site is asked to assess the impact of these excursions on the quality and in particular on the shelf-life of this product.

Phase I: Storage at the Manufacturer's Warehouse

The medicinal product contains a known amount of the degradation product A (C_0) at time of batch release ($t = 0$), i.e., 0.25%. The product is stored at the manufacturer's warehouse at 15–30 °C for 6 months. The degradation rate (k_{25}) at 25 °C calculated (*see* Eq. 28) is now taken to calculate the amount of degradation product A (C_{stor}) at the end of the storage period (t_{stor}) (Eq. 28):

$$C_{\text{stor}} = C_0 + k_{\text{stor}} \cdot t_{\text{stor}}$$
$$= 0.25\ (\%) + 0.0055\ (\%/\text{month}) \cdot 6(\text{months})$$
$$= 0.2831\ (\%) \tag{28}$$

$C_{\text{stor}} = $ Content of degradation product (%) at the end of storage

C_0 = Initial content (%) at time point $t = 0$ (at time of batch release)

k_{stor} = Degradation rate at the upper temperature limit during storage (%/month)

t_{stor} = Storage time (months)

The MATLAB program looks like this:

```
clear, clc
close all

% Calculation of Degradation rate k at 25C
kelv=273.16;
temp25=25+kelv;
x1=1/temp25
ln_k=(-11549*x1)+ 33.533
k=exp(ln_k)
% Estimation of C after 6 months storage at max 25°C
C_0=0.25 % Degradation product A at t=0
t=6 % time (months)
C = C_0 + (k*t)
```

Phase II: Shipment

Next is the first part of the shipment from the manufacturer's warehouse in the UK to a depot in France during summer time. The data logger showed an excursion above 30 °C for less than 60 min, and the MKT provided by the data logger program is 29.3 °C for the shipment period of 47.8 h.

The degradation rate (k_{MKT1}) at the MKT for the first part of the shipment is calculated as follows (Eq. 29):

$$\ln(k_{MKT1}) = -11,549 \cdot 0.0033 + 33.533 = -4.6506 \qquad (29)$$

$$k_{MKT1} = 0.0096 \ (\%/\text{month})$$

The amount of degradation product A at the end of this first part of the shipment can be calculated using (Eq. 30):

$$C_{ship1} = C_{stor} + k_{ship} \cdot t_{ship} = 0.2831 + 0.0096 \cdot 0.0664$$
$$= 0.2837\% \qquad (30)$$

C_{ship1} = Content of degradation product (%) at the end of first shipment

C_{stor} = Content of degradation product (%) at the end of storage

k_{ship} = Degradation rate at MKT during shipment (%/month)

$t_{\text{ship}} = $ Time of shipment (months)

The MATLAB program looks like this:

```
clear, clc
close all

% Calculation of Degradation rate k at MKT during first part of
shipment
kelv=273.16;
tempMKT1=29.3+kelv;

x1=1/tempMKT1
ln_k=(-11549*x1)+ 33.533
k=exp(ln_k)

% Estimation of C after 47.8 h storage at MKT 1
C_0=0.2831 % Degradation product A at the start of shipment 1
t=(47.8/24)/30 % time (months)

C = C_0 + (k*t)
```

During the second part of the shipment from the depot in France to the wholesaler's warehouse in Spain, the data logger showed an excursion above 30 °C for more than 2 h, and the MKT is 32.1 °C for the shipment period of 62.7 h.

The degradation rate (k_{MKT2}) at the MKT for this second part of the shipment is calculated as follows (Eq. 31):

$$\ln(k_{\text{MKT2}}) = -11,549 \cdot 0.0033 + 33.533 = -4.3003 \qquad (31)$$

$$k_{\text{MKT2}} = 0.0136 \ (\%/\text{month})$$

The amount of degradation product A at the end of this second part of the shipment can be calculated using (Eq. 32):

$$\begin{aligned} C_{\text{ship2}} = C_{\text{stor}} + k_{\text{ship}} \cdot t_{\text{ship}} &= 0.2837 + 0.0136 \cdot 0.0871 \\ &= 0.2849\% \end{aligned} \qquad (32)$$

$C_{\text{ship2}} = $ Content of degradation product (%) at the end of second shipment

$C_{\text{stor}} = $ Content of degradation product (%) at the end of storage
$k_{\text{ship}} = $ Degradation rate at MKT during shipment (%/month)
$t_{\text{ship}} = $ Time of shipment (months)

The MATLAB program looks like this:

```
clear, clc
close all

% Calculation of Degradation rate k at MKT during second part
of shipment
kelv=273.16;
tempMKT2=32.1+kelv;
x1=1/tempMKT2

ln_k=(-11549*x1)+ 33.533
k=exp(ln_k)

% Estimation of C after 62.7 h storage at MKT 2
C_0=0.2837 % Degradation product A at the start of shipment 2
t=(62.7/24)/30 % time (months)

C = C_0 + (k*t)
```

Phase III: Storage After Shipment

Finally, the product is stored at the wholesaler's warehouse in Spain at a MKT below 25 °C until it is distributed to a pharmacy and used by the patient. The degradation rate to be used is the same as the one calculated for the storage at the manufacturer's warehouse in the UK, i.e., $k_{25} = 0.0055$ (%/month). The amount of degradation product A at the end of the labeled shelf-life can be calculated using Eq. 33:

$$C_{exp} = C_{ship} + k_{label} \cdot t_{exp}$$
$$= 0.2849 + 0.0055 \cdot 17.8465 = 0.3832\% \qquad (33)$$

C_{exp} = Content of degradation product (%) at expiry date

C_{ship} = Content of degradation product (%) at the end of shipment

k_{label} = Degradation rate at the maximum recommended temperature (%/month)

t_{exp} = Time period from end of shipment until expiry date (months)

The MATLAB program looks like this:

```
clear, clc
close all

% Calculation of Degradation rate k at 25C
kelv=273.16;
temp=25+kelv;
x1=1/temp
```

```
ln_k=(-11549*x1)+ 33.533
k=exp(ln_k)


% Estimation of C at the expiry date
C_0=0.2849 % Degradation product A after 2nd shipment
t=24-(6+((47.8/24)/30)+((62.7/24)/30)) % time (months)


C = C_0 + (k*t)
```

As a result, the product would not be OOS at the end of the expiry date of 24 months after its production, as the amount of the degradation product A would not be above the specified acceptance criterion of not more than 0.45%. The short-term excursions of the temperature above 30 °C during shipment did not affect the quality of the product on the market, and would not shorten its shelf-life.

References

1. EU Directive 2001/83/EC, Article 79 and 80 (2001). https://ec.europa.eu/health/sites/health/files/files/eudralex/vol-1/dir_2001_83_consol_2012/dir_2001_83_cons_2012_en.pdf

2. European Commission Guidelines on Good Distribution Practice of Medicinal Products for Human Use (2013/C 343/01 – corr) (2013). http://eur-lex.europa.eu/LexUriServ/LexUriServ.do?uri=OJ:C:2013:343:0001:0014:EN:PDF

3. Irish HPRA Guide to Control and Monitoring of Storage and Transportation Temperature Conditions for Medicinal Products and Active Substances (IA-G0011-2) (2017). https://www.hpra.ie/docs/default-source/publications-forms/guidance-documents/ia-g0011-guide-to-control-and-monitoring-of-storage-and-transportation-conditions-v1.pdf?sfvrsn=16

4. US Regulations 21 CFR 211.142 (b), 203.32, 205.50

5. USP 40 - General Chapter <1079> "Good Storage and Distribution Practices for Drug Products"

6. Health Canada Guidelines for Temperature Control of Drug Products during Storage and Transportation GUI-0069 (2011). http://www.hc-sc.gc.ca/dhp-mps/alt_formats/pdf/compli-conform/gmp-bpf/docs/GUI-0069-eng.pdf

7. WHO Technical Report Series 957 (2010) Annex 5 WHO Good Distribution Practices for Pharmaceutical Products (revised). http://apps.who.int/medicinedocs/documents/s17059e/s17059e.pdf

8. WHO Technical Report Series 961 (2011) Annex 9 Model guidance for the storage and transport of time- and temperature-sensitive pharmaceutical products. http://apps.who.int/medicinedocs/documents/s18652en/s18652en.pdf

9. Muth JE (2006) Basic statistics and pharmaceutical statistical applications. Chapman & Hall/CRC, Boca Raton, London, New York

10. ICH Guideline Q1E - Evaluation for Stability Data - developed by the appropriate ICH Expert Working Group in 2003 http://www.ich.org/fileadmin/Public_Web_Site/ICH_Products/Guidelines/Quality/Q1E/Step4/Q1E_Guideline.pdf

11. ICH Guideline Q1A(R2) - Stability Testing of New Drug Substances and Products, developed by the appropriate ICH Expert Working Group in 2003.http://www.ich.org/fileadmin/Public_Web_Site/ICH_Products/Guidelines/Quality/Q1A_R2/Step4/Q1A_R2__Guideline.pdf

12. Grimm W (1993) Storage Conditions for Stability Testing in the EC, Japan and USA Drug Dev Ind Pharm 19(20):2795–2830

13. Zahn M (2006) Temperature control and product quality of medicines in transit. Regul Aff J 17(11):731–736

14. Zahn M (2011) Temperature excursions during shipment and storage. In: Baertschi SW

(ed) Pharmaceutical stress testing: predicting drug degradation, 2nd edn. Informa Healthcare, London

15. Zahn M (2008) Global stability practice. In: Huynh-Ba K (ed) Handbook of stability testing in pharmaceutical development. Springer, New York

16. Zahn M et al (2006) A risk-based approach to establish stability testing conditions for tropical countries. J Pharm Sci 95:946–965. Erratum 96:2177 (2007)

17. CHMP Guideline on declaration of storage conditions (CPMP/QWP/609/96/Rev2) (2007). http://www.ema.europa.eu/docs/en_GB/document_library/Scientific_guide line/2009/09/WC500003468.pdf. All websites accessed 03 Mar 2018

Chapter 13

Stability Testing Parameters and Issues for Nanotechnology-Based Drug Products

Kamla Pathak and Satyanarayan Pattnaik

Abstract

Stability is one of the critical aspects in ensuring safety and efficacy of drug products, and hence its assessment has gained a paramount importance in the pharmaceutical industry. However, the stability problems and assessment of stability of drug-loaded nanoformulations remain a very challenging aspect in the pharmaceutical field. The stability issues of drug nanoparticles could arise during manufacturing, storage, and shipping. Though, recent advancement in analytical technology has offered ample tools for stability assessment of nanopharmaceuticals, they have their own limitations in terms of efficiency. In this chapter, we summarize various stability testing parameters, techniques used in their evaluation and the issues related to stability testing of nanotechnology based drug products.

Key words Nanoparticle, Nano-formulation, Nanotechnology, Stability testing, Nano-pharmaceuticals

1 Introduction

With significant attention focused on nanoscience and nanotechnology in recent years, nanomaterials based drug delivery has been propelled to the forefront by researchers from both academia and industry [1–3]. Various nanostructured materials have been produced and applied to drug delivery, such as nanoparticles [4], nanocapsules [5], nanotubes [6], micelles [7], microemulsions [8], and liposomes [9]. In general, the term "nanoparticles" refers to particles with size less than 100 nm. However, submicron particles are also commonly referred as nanoparticles in the field of pharmaceutics and medicine [10–14]. Nanoparticles are categorized as nanocrystals [2, 10], polymeric [15], liposomal [9], and solid lipid nanoparticles (SLN) [16], depending on their composition, function, and morphology. Stability is one of the critical aspects in ensuring safety and efficacy of drug products. The stability issues of drug nanoparticles could arise during manufacturing, storage, and shipping. For example, in intravenously administered

Sanjay Bajaj and Saranjit Singh (eds.), *Methods for Stability Testing of Pharmaceuticals*, Methods in Pharmacology and Toxicology, https://doi.org/10.1007/978-1-4939-7686-7_13, © Springer Science+Business Media, LLC, part of Springer Nature 2018

nanosuspensions, formation of larger particles (>5 µm) could lead to capillary blockade and embolism [17], and thus drug particle size and size distribution need to be closely monitored and controlled during storage. High temperature produced during manufacturing can modify crystallinity of the drug particles [12]. The stability studies for new drug products are usually performed following the guidelines of International Conference on Harmonisation (ICH) of Technical Requirements for Pharmaceuticals for Human Use. The procedure of performing the stability studies for new drug products, new dosage forms, and biotechnology based products are outlined in the ICH guidelines Q1A(R2), Q1C, and Q5C. Although a large number of studies on stability testing of nanoformulations have appeared in the primary pharmaceutical literature, there have not been many comprehensive reviews on the topic of the techniques employed for their stability evaluation. The objective of this chapter is to bring together and analyze reported studies involving stability testing of nanoproducts, with focus on the techniques used for evaluation of their stability parameters.

2   General Stability Testing Parameters for Drug Nanoformulations

The nanoparticle drug formulations are obviously different from other pharmaceutical products due to their size factor. In their case, nanometric size is a defining characteristic, therefore, accurately quantifying the size is important. Commonly used techniques for size determination often fail in the submicrometer range. For instance, submicron particles are too small for direct imaging using optical microscopy. Reversibly, most light scattering sizing tools used for nanoparticles are not suitable for objects larger than micrometer range. Because of their unique properties, nanoparticles are employed in applications uncommon for suspensions. Conventional suspensions unlike nanosuspensions, have larger suspended particles, hence are not delivered via intravenous route. Small particle size of nanoformulations allows them to be delivered via intravenous administration as a solid material. This renders characterization of the upper end of size distribution of nanopharmaceuticals important from the view point of safety, i.e., the potential for embolism. However, in certain cases, the characterization of a nanoparticle system is similar to doing the same with a macroscopic analyte. Determining the state of solid within the particle using thermal or X-ray methods is not much different so long as the possibility of size-induced artifacts is evaluated.

2.1 Particle Size, Size Distribution, and Morphology

The particle size is defined not only by the size of the average, but also by the way in which "average" is defined. Mean, median, and mode are equally valid descriptors. In addition, the population itself can be defined by the number or volume of particles present, and these are only two of the various weighting schemes that can be employed. Another important issue is the width or shape of the distribution. It may be polydisperse or narrow and may be skewed or symmetric. The information content expressed in a complete size distribution usually exceeds greatly than that can be extracted from the available experimental signal. Subtle differences in the experiment can translate to large variations in the result obtained, thus complicating the problem of determining the size distribution. The shape of the particle itself is also important as its nature affects the experimental observation directly. For instance, a spherical particle will scatter light differently from one that is rectangular, but it also influences the abscissa of the size distribution (e.g., projected area, Feret's diameter) [18]. Lastly, the results for average size distribution can depend on how they were acquired. This is the trivial case of instrumental design, in which data handling and extraction routines vary among instruments of the same type, the ones from different manufacturers. A more significant situation arises when variation results from the differences in physical principles underlying the measurements. For example, a multi-angle light scattering experiment relies on the interaction of the photons with the electric field of the particle, whereas dynamic light scattering is based on the time-dependent interference pattern generated by particles in motion. Both are light scattering experiments, so the principles of measurement can vary significantly even among methods that might seem similar to the casual user of analytical information.

A variety of techniques, including photon correlation spectroscopy (PCS), also known as dynamic light scattering (DLS); and laser diffraction (LD), also known as low-angle laser light scattering (LALLS); coulter counter etc., are commonly used to measure the particle size and size distribution. The analytical tools to measure the particle size of nano-drug products and their limitations are summarized in Table 1. The PCS/DLS is widely used to determine the size and size distribution of small particles suspended in a liquid medium. The mean particle size and polydispersity index (PDI) are the two measured parameters of this technique. A PDI value of 0.1–0.25 indicates a narrow size distribution, while a PDI greater than 0.5 refers to a broad distribution [17]. However, this technique fails to measure size of dry powders and its measurement range is too narrow (3 nm to 3 μm) to detect the interference from the microparticles (>3 μm) within the nano-formulation. Photon cross-correlation spectroscopy (PCCS) is an extension of the well-established PCS. The key principle of PCCS is 3D cross-correlation technique. In a special scattering geometry, the cross-correlation of the scattered light allows for the precise separation of the single and multiple scattered fractions. With PCCS, the multiple scattering is completely suppressed, and hence this enables PCCS to extend the evaluation method of PCS to opaque suspensions and emulsion. Laser diffraction has a much wider detection range (20 nm to

Table 1
Common tools to analyze particle size of nano-drug formulations and their limitations

Tools/techniques	Assessed parameter	Limitations
Photon correlation spectroscopy/dynamic light scattering	Size, size distribution	Narrow measurement range A small quantity of small sized particles can easily be "hidden" in a much larger quantity of large size particles Not applicable to dry powders/concentrated suspensions
Laser diffraction	Size, size distribution	Particles >5 μm not detectable Accuracy of measurements for nonspherical particles is doubtful Results vary significantly with optical parameters
Photon cross-correlation spectroscopy	Size, size distribution	Narrow measurement range Not applicable to dry powders
Coulter counter	Size	Measurements below 1–2 μm are difficult Test particles should be electrical insulators
Acoustic spectroscopy	Size, surface charge	Unsuitable for analyzing dilute suspensions (<1% w/v) Air bubbles can interfere with measurements
Turbidimetry	Size, size distribution	Failure of Beer's law due to multiple and dependent scattering Require a lot of mathematical modeling Applies only to spherical shaped particles
Nuclear magnetic resonance spectroscopy	Size	Not useful for particles <0.5 μm
Scanning electron microscope/transmission electron microscope	Size, morphology	Analysis time can be very long Sample preparation is time consuming, expensive, and requires considerable technical expertise
Atomic force microscope	Size, morphology	Produces single scan image size Scanning speed is slower than SEM

2000 μm) and it can be used to evaluate both suspension and dry powder samples. The typical LD characterization parameters are LD50, LD90, and LD99, indicating that 50%, 90%, or 99% of the particles are below the given size, respectively. LD is especially suitable for characterizing parenteral and pulmonary suspensions due to its wide measurement range. LD can detect the presence of microparticles (>5 μm), which are detrimental to parenteral nano-suspensions. However, LD provides only relative size distribution. The coulter counter, on the other hand, measures the absolute number of particles per volume unit for the different size classes, and is more precise than the LD. Although PCS, LD, and coulter counter techniques provide rapid measurement of particle size and size distribution, they do not have the capability in evaluating particle morphology.

Acoustic spectroscopy is another approach, which measures the attenuation of sound waves as a means of determining size through the fitting of physically relevant equations [6]. Moreover, the oscillating electric field generated by the movement of charged particles under the influence of acoustic energy provides information on the surface charge [19]. Turbidimetry is an ensemble method applied in determination of size of the nanoparticles [20]. Significantly for non-absorbing particles, turbidity is complement to light scattering because it represents the amount of incident radiation not reaching the detector. This approach requires tiny amounts of sample and can be easily executed using a spectrophotometer. However, the lack of commercial implementation requires the researchers to carry out appropriate calculations on their own.

Nuclear magnetic resonance (NMR) spectroscopy can be used to determine both the size and the qualitative nature of nanoparticles. The selectivity afforded by chemical shift complements the sensitivity to molecular mobility to provide information on the physicochemical status of components within the nanoparticle [21]. Pulsed field gradient methods allow diffusivity of the entire particle to be quantified and compared to produce 2-D, diffusion ordered plots in which the colloidal behavior and chemical speciation are leveraged simultaneously. The diffusion coefficient has also been used as a surrogate for size of the nanoparticle [22].

Direct visualization techniques like scanning electron microscopy (SEM), transmission electron microscopy (TEM), and atomic force microscopy (AFM) are widely used for assessment of the particle shape or morphology. TEM has a smaller size limit of detection, is a good validation for other methods, and affords structural information via electron diffraction, but staining is usually required, and one must be cognizant of the statistically small sample size and the effect that vacuum can have on the particles. Very detailed image can result from freeze-fracture approaches in which a cast is made of the original sample [23]. However, it is very challenging and time-consuming to measure a significant number of particles to achieve statistical size distribution using these techniques. Moreover, they usually require additional sample preparation such as coating that could be invasive to the particles, potentially causing some changes in particle properties.

2.2 Sedimentation/ Creaming

Visual observation of settling of suspended particles over a period of time has been the traditional method to evaluate sedimentation or creaming. Sedimentation or flocculation volume can be obtained as a quantitative evaluation of suspension stability by measuring the volume of the settled or creamed particle layer relative to the total suspension volume within a specific time. A higher flocculation volume indicates a more stable suspension. The relatively modern approaches to evaluate sedimentation/creaming include laser back scattering [24] and near-infrared transmission [25].

2.3 Particle Surface Charge

Laser doppler electrophoresis is commonly used to measure zeta potential (ZP). This technique evaluates electrophoretic mobility of suspended particles in the medium. Absolute value of ZP above 60 mV yields excellent stability, while 30 mV, 20 mV, and less than 5 mV generally results in good stability, acceptable short-term stability, and fast particle aggregation, respectively. This rule is only valid for pure electrostatic stabilization or in combination with low-molecular weight surfactants, and is not valid when high molecular weight stabilizers/polymers are present [26].

2.4 Crystalline State

Powder X-ray diffraction (PXRD) and differential scanning calorimetry (DSC) have been routinely used to assess the crystallinity of the drug nanoparticles [2, 27]. XRD differentiates amorphous and crystalline nanoparticles as well as different polymorphic phases of the particles, while DSC is often used as a supplementary tool to XRD. Crystalline particles usually have a sharp melting peak which is absent in amorphous materials [28]. The melting point can also be utilized to differentiate different polymorphs. Transitions in relative crystallinity due to instability are assessed with these analytical tools. X-ray scattering is another technique that finds application in lipid lattice structure examination of the particles. The X-ray beam passed through the sample is obtained by a synchrotron. A main advantage is the possibility to perform the experiment on colloidal suspensions in their native state. Both small-angle X-ray scattering (SAXS) and wide-angle X-ray scattering (WAXS) find application in the physical stability characterization of nanoformulations.

2.5 Chemical Stability and Drug Content

High performance liquid chromatography (HPLC) is the most common characterization technique used to evaluate chemical stability that provides precise quantitative analysis on the degradation and impurities. Mass spectrometry (MS) is often coupled with HPLC to identify the molecular structure of impurities. Some other techniques such as FTIR and NMR can also be used for chemical stability assessment. However, they are not as precise and sensitive as HPLC, and thus not widely used for stability assessment. Drug content estimation over a period of time under stability conditions again is a very useful parameter to assess the stability of nanoformulations. Standard quantitative assay techniques may be followed like UV visible spectrophotometry, spectrofluorometry, and HPLC.

2.6 Drug Release and Leakage

To assess stability of most drug products, including nanoparticles based drug delivery systems, drug release is an important consideration. In general, drug release rate depends on various factors like solubility of drug, desorption of the surface-bound/adsorbed drug, drug diffusion through the nanoparticle matrix or system, nanoparticle matrix or system erosion/degradation and combination of erosion/diffusion processes. Thus, solubility, diffusion, and biodegradation of the matrix materials govern the release process. In the case of nanospheres, where the drug is uniformly distributed, the release occurs by diffusion or erosion of the matrix under sink conditions. If the diffusion of the drug is faster than matrix erosion, the mechanism of release is largely controlled by a diffusion process. The rapid initial release or "burst" is mainly due to drug particles over the surfaces, which diffuse out of the drug polymer matrices. Often, the drug release and its kinetics are affected by the type of in vitro dissolution technique adopted in the study. Care should be taken while selecting the dissolution technique, the components of the dissolution media, and formulation specific conditions, e.g., one of the most preferred methods is with a dialysis bag. However, the bag, can sometimes retard the diffusion and interact with drug molecules. In select nanoformulations (e.g., liposomes, nano-capsules), drug leakage studies have to be performed additionally. For quantitative analysis of the drug leakage, clinically used single photon emission computed tomography imaging agents (e.g., Tc-99m mebrofenin) or fluorescent markers (e.g., 6-carboxyl fluorescein) are encapsulated in the nanoformulations as an indicator. Fluorescence quenching measurements have been used to detect leakage of hydrophilic fluorescent molecules from liposomes.

2.7 Kinetics of Drug Release from Nanoparticles

The knowledge of the mechanism and kinetics of drug release from the nanoparticle systems indicates their performance. Drug release involves mass transfer phenomenon involving diffusion of the drug from higher to low concentration regions in the surrounding biological fluid. Though drug release data are applied basically for quality control; understanding of physicochemical aspects of drug delivery systems and their release mechanisms, and predicting behavior of systems in vivo, are very useful tools to assess the stability of nanoformulations. However, there are difficulties in modeling drug release data, as there is a great diversity in the physical form of nanoparticles with respect to size, shape, arrangement of the core and the coat. Other properties of core include solubility, diffusivity, partition coefficient, and properties of coat are porosity, tortuosity, thickness, crystallinity, and inertness.

2.8 Ex Vivo and In Vivo Stability

It is also very important and challenging to assess the stability of nanotechnology based products under conditions that resemble in vivo environment. It is essential to understand whether and how the different body environments influence stability of nanoformulations, so as to design optimal products, and to identify their fate after administration. One of the important parameters is stability, and the level of aggregation of nanoparticles in physiological conditions (e.g., plasma) or different media, important for biotechnological and biological applications (e.g., culture media). Few studies [29, 30] have revealed stability issues of nanoparticles in different culture media, depending on ionic and protein composition, consequently affecting their characteristic and functionality in vitro and in vivo. It was shown that stable nanoparticles in water or low-ionic buffer form large aggregates in physiological or similar conditions [29, 30]. Nanoparticle stability in serum and tissue homogenates mimics a typical persistence in the body. Homogenates represent the best possibility to get an idea of the effect of the organs or body fluids on the particles. If nanoparticles aggregate in serum homogenate for instance, this would mean that they could aggregate also upon injection in blood. Apart from clogging of bold vessels, the drug delivery properties of nanoparticles would be affected due to aggregation. Drug release from single particle is different than the drug release from particle agglomerate, as the drug has to diffuse through different "layers" of particles. Moreover, if the particle size is larger than a certain threshold, the formulation residence time in the body would be affected due to uptake by white cells. Stability in given media is a complex combination of surface properties of nanoparticles, media composition, and nanoparticle concentration; therefore, characterization of nanoparticles in physiologically relevant media is crucial for understanding their interaction with biological systems [31].

The absolute rates of aggregation can be experimentally determined by turbidity or size measurements, or are numerically calculated using stability ratio approach. The confirming experiments must be performed in such a way that the data correspond to the early stage of aggregation, because these methods take into account only the early time of aggregation where single particles collide and form doublets. Under such conditions, the selection of particle size and concentration, and electrolyte type and concentration becomes challenging, especially when using nanoparticles, because of their size and relatively small light scattering properties.

To perform different ex vivo studies in which the samples are quite diluted, DLS may not be suitable because of the samples' opacity (biological samples are usually opaque) and the presence of various other particulate substances, similar in size to the nanoparticles. Spectrophotofluorimetry is commonly employed to evaluate the nanoparticle biodistribution. A correlation between particle fluorescence and colloidal stability may be a useful tool to assess nanoformulation stability [32]. However, polymer degradation and dye release can significantly bias the spectrophotofluorimetry analysis, while this is not an issue with DLS.

During the delivery process for tumor targeting, after extravasation into tumor tissue, nano-formulation (per se liposomes) remain within tumor stroma as a drug-loaded depot and eventually are subject to enzymatic degradation and/or phagocytic attack, leading to release of drug for subsequent diffusion to tumor cells. Therefore, the temporal profiles of biodistribution and stability of nanoformulated contrast agents/drug carriers in vivo are critical in determining the imaging/therapeutic efficacy and the necessity for advanced design of activatable controlled release.

Non-invasive molecular imaging techniques are excellent tools to investigate in vivo stability or fate of nanoparticles [33]. Multi-modal hybrid technologies such as positron emission tomography (PET)/computed tomography (CT) or PET/magnetic resonance imaging (MRI) were recently developed giving the chance to examine the pharmacological profiles of nanoparticles [33]. By verifying the physical residence of nanoparticles in tissues that are co-localized with the imaging contrast, it can be assured that an appropriate interpretation of nanoparticle biodistribution is done using the aforementioned noninvasive imaging modalities. Polymer-drug conjugates for possible drug delivery can be radiolabeled to investigate their biodistribution via PET imaging [34]. PET, with its possibility to detect and quantify picomolar amounts of a radiotracer, has emerged as one of the most powerful imaging techniques for assessing in vivo stability of the nanoformulations.

Microdialysis systems have been proposed as a platform for dynamic monitoring of the nanoparticle stability in vivo [35]. Since the microdialysis probe contains a membrane with a specific molecular weight cutoff, it possesses a selective permeability for molecules with different sizes at locus of tissue, in the close vicinity of the probe. If the contrast agent or drug tagged nanoparticles on site can maintain their morphological stability, their size will be too large to be selectively collected through the microdialysis membrane (see Fig. 1). On the contrary, the contrast agents or drug molecules leaching from the disintegrated nanoparticles, due to their small size, can easily diffuse through the probe membrane and be collected in microdialysates for further analysis (see Fig. 2).

Site-specific labeling with spin probes and fluorophores combined with electron paramagnetic resonance (EPR) spectroscopy and fluorescence resonance energy transfer (FRET) measurements also provide insights into the molecular architecture and dynamics within nanoparticles. These analytical methods have proved to be very useful for determining nanoparticle stability in blood and have allowed quantitative analysis of the dynamic changes in assembly structure, local stability, and cargo diffusion of micellar nanoparticles [36].

2.9 Microbial Stability

Microbial stability assessment is specifically important for parenterally administered nanoformulations. The US FDA recommends two types of pyrogen tests: (i) limulus amebocyte lysate (LAL) based assay, sensitive to even pictogram quantities of endotoxin, and (ii) rabbit pyrogen test (an in vivo test, which has the capability

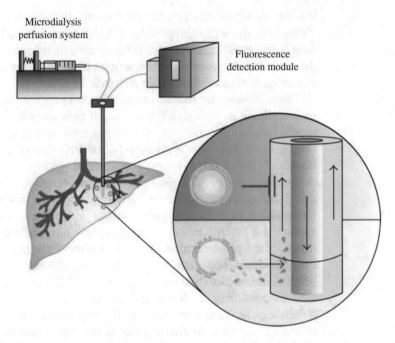

Fig. 1 The microdialysis probe with total diameter of 360 μm and molecular size cutoff at 100 KDa was in situ implanted for simultaneous measurements of fluorescence intensity of extracellular fluid. If the liposomes are ruptured, the encapsulated carboxyfluorescein (CF) molecules will be leaching out and collected by microdialysis probe. Thus, the stability of liposomes on site in liver can be dynamically assessed by the change of fluorescence intensity in microdialysates. (Adapted from Ref. 35)

to identify various pyrogenic substances). Catalytic nanoparticles, such as dendrimers, might cause false-positive pyrogenicity determinations with the LAL test, if they activate the LAL proteolytic cascade and generate a colorimetric product. Other nanoparticles might quench absorbance at the assay wavelength or adsorb endotoxin on their surfaces, leading to a false negative pyrogenicity determination. Most nanoparticles have the potential to interfere with the LAL assay and only a few particle types do not interfere with this standard test.

Though autoclaving is feasible for few nanoformulations, it causes melting of the particles and favors possible aggregation for lipid based formulations; and alters HLB values of polyethoxylated surfactants leading to their physical instability [37, 38]. Gamma-sterilization is not recommended in lipid based nanoformulations due to possibilities of formation of free radicals leading to chemical instability [39]. Though physical removal of microorganisms by filtration is a soft and feasible technique for a selected group of nanoformulations [40], it is not applicable for nanoparticles having larger size (where drug is adsorbed over the particle surface) and formulations with high viscosity. However, high hydrostatic pressure, which has documented evidence of microbial stabilization of

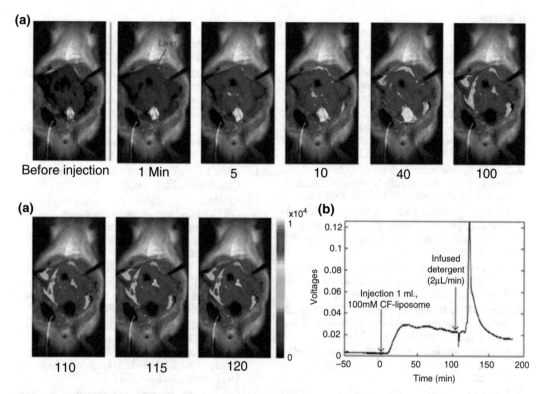

Fig. 2 (**a**) The time-lapse optical imaging of liposome containing higher CF concentration at 100 mM illustrated no augmentation of fluorescence intensity in liver throughout the imaging course; the consistent self-quenching of fluorescence implicated the liposomes on site in liver remained their intact liposomal integrity. (**b**) At later phase of imaging course, the lysis buffer of Triton X-100 was locally infused at 2 μL/min via microdialysis probe. It caused the rupture of liposomal lipid integrity, resulting in an immediate increase of CF fluorescence intensity measured in the microdialysate (Adapted from Ref. 35)

food products (e.g., fruit juices, sea foods) may be another alternate for sterilization of nanosuspensions/nanoemulsions [41].

3   Conclusions

The stability problems and assessment of stability related to drug-loaded nanoformulations remain a very challenging issue in the pharmaceutical field. The recent advancement in analytical technology has proved to be a boon for stability assessment of pharmaceutical products, including very special group of nanotechnology based formulations. Diverse characterization tools are now available but with their inherent limitations in terms of efficiency. Though physicochemical characterization techniques have gained a lot of attention by the researchers, there is a surge need for more work to be done for stability assessment in vivo.

References

1. Pathak K, Akhtar N (2016) Nose to brain delivery of nanoformulations for neurotherapeutics in Parkinson's disease: defining the preclinical, clinical and toxicity issues. Curr Drug Deliv. 13(8):1205–1221 (Epub ahead of print)

2. Pattnaik S, Swain K, Rao JV, Varun T, Subudhi SK (2015) Aceclofenac nanocrystals for improved dissolution: influence of polymeric stabilizers. RSC Adv 5(112):91960–91965

3. Pathak K, Raghuvanshi S (2015) Oral bioavailability: issues and solutions via nanoformulations. Clin Pharmacokinet 54(4):325–357

4. Panyam J, Labhasetwar V (2003) Biodegradable nanoparticles for drug and gene delivery to cells and tissue. Adv Drug Deliv Rev 55 (3):329–347

5. Couvreur P, Fattal E, Legrand P et al (2002) Nanocapsule technology: a review. Crit Rev Ther Drug Carrier Syst 19(2):99–134

6. Bianco A, Kostarelos K, Prato M (2005) Applications of carbon nanotubes in drug delivery. Curr Opin Chem Biol 9(6):674–679

7. Kwon GS, Okano T (1996) Polymeric micelles as new drug carriers. Adv Drug Deliv Rev 21 (2):107–116

8. Lawrence MJ, Rees GD (2000) Microemulsion-based media as novel drug delivery systems. Adv Drug Deliv Rev 45 (1):89–121

9. Allen TM, Moase EH (1996) Therapeutic opportunities for targeted liposomal drug delivery. Adv Drug Deliv Rev 21(2):117–133

10. Pattnaik S, Swain K, Manaswini P et al (2015) Fabrication of aceclofenac nanocrystals for improved dissolution: process optimization and physicochemical characterization. J Drug Deliv Sci Tech 29:199–209

11. Yang W, Peters JI, Williams RO III (2008) Inhaled nanoparticles—a current review. Int J Pharm 356:239–247

12. Keck CM, Müller RH (2006) Drug nanocrystals of poorly soluble drugs produced by high pressure homogenisation. Eur J Pharm Biopharm 62:3–16

13. Gao L, Zhang D, Chen M (2008) Drug nanocrystals for the formulation of poorly soluble drugs and its application as a potential drug delivery system. J Nanopart Res 10:845–862

14. Sung JC, Pulliam BL, Edwards DA (2007) Nanoparticles for drug delivery to the lungs. Trends Biotechnol 25(12):563–570

15. Soppimath KS, Aminabhavi TM, Kulkarni AR, Rudzinski WE (2001) Biodegradable polymeric nanoparticles as drug delivery devices. J Control Release 70(1–2):1–20

16. Muller RH, Mäder K, Gohla S (2000) Solid lipid nanoparticles (SLN) for controlled drug delivery—a review of the state of the art. Eur J Pharm Biopharm 50(1):161–177

17. Patravale VB, Date AA, Kulkarni RM (2004) Nanosuspensions a promising drug delivery strategy. J Pharm Pharmacol 56:827–840

18. Allen T (1997) Particle measurement, 5th edn. Chapman & Hall, London

19. Amziane A, Belliard L, Decremps F et al (2011) Ultrafast acoustic resonance spectroscopy of gold nanostructures: towards a generation of tunable transverse waves. Phys Rev B 83:014102

20. Kourti T (2006) Turbidimetry in particle size analysis. Encyclopedia of Analytical Chemistry. Published online: 15 Sep 2006, doi: https://doi.org/10.1002/9780470027318.a1517

21. Matyus SP, Braun PJ, Wolak-Dinsmore J et al (2015) HDL particle number measured on the Vantera®, the first clinical NMR analyzer. Clin Biochem 48(3):148–155. https://doi.org/10.1016/j.clinbiochem.2014.11.017

22. Valentini M, Vaccaro A, Rehor A et al (2004) Diffusion NMR spectroscopy for the characterization of the size and interactions of colloidal matter: the case of vesicles and nanoparticles. J Am Chem Soc 126:2142–2147

23. Leo E, Brina B, Forni F et al (2004) In vitro evaluation of PLA nanoparticles containing a lipophilic drug in water-soluble or insoluble form. Int J Pharm 278:133–141

24. Johnson KA (2007) Interfacial phenomena and phase behaviour in metered dose inhaler formulations. In: Hickey AJ (ed) Inhalation aerosols: physical and biological basis for therapy, 2nd edn. Informa Healthcare, New York, pp 347–372

25. Kuentz M, Röthlisberger D (2003) Rapid assessment of sedimentation stability in dispersions using near infrared transmission measurements during centrifugation and oscillatory rheology. Eur J Pharm Biopharm 56 (3):355–361

26. Mishra PR, Shaal LA, Müller RH et al (2009) Production and characterization of hesperetin nanosuspensions for dermal delivery. Int J Pharm 371:182–189

27. Pattnaik S, Swain K, Mallick S et al (2011) Effect of casting solvent on crystallinity of ondansetron in transdermal films. Int J Pharm 406:106–110

28. Pattnaik P, Swain K, Rao V et al (2015) Polymer co-processing of ibuprofen through compaction for improved oral absorption. RSC Adv 5(91):74720–74725

29. Maiorano G, Sabella S, Sorce B et al (2010) Effects of cell culture media on the dynamic formation of protein-nanoparticle complexes and influence on the cellular response. ACS Nano 4(12):7481–7491. https://doi.org/10.1021/nn101557e

30. AC S, Grubbs J, Qian S et al (2012) Probing nanoparticle interactions in cell culture media. Colloids Surf B Biointerfaces 95:96–102. https://doi.org/10.1016/j.colsurfb.2012.02.022

31. Shaikh MV, Kala M, Nivsarkar M (2016) Development and optimization of an ex vivo colloidal stability model for nanoformulations. AAPS PharmSciTech 18(4):1288–1292

32. Lazzari S, Moscatelli D, Codari F et al (2012) Colloidal stability of polymeric nanoparticles in biological fluids. J Nanopart Res 14(6):920

33. Stockhofe K, Postema JM, Schieferstein H et al (2014) Radiolabeling of nanoparticles and polymers for PET imaging. Pharmaceuticals (Basel) 7(4):392–418

34. Herth MM, Barz M, Moderegger D et al (2009) Radioactive labeling of defined HPMA-based polymeric structures using (18F) FETos for in vivo imaging by positron emission tomography. Biomacromolecules 10:1697–1703

35. Jeng C-C, Cheng S-H, Ho JA, et al (2011) Dynamic probing of nanoparticle stability in vivo: a liposomal model assessed using in situ microdialysis and optical imaging. J Nanomat 2011: Article ID 932719, 8 pages

36. Li Y, Budamagunta MS, Luo J et al (2012) Probing of the assembly structure and dynamics within nanoparticles during interaction with blood proteins. ACS Nano 6(11):9485–9495

37. Choi KO, Aditya NP, Ko S (2014) Effect of aqueous pH and electrolyte concentration on structure, stability and flow behaviour of non-ionic surfactant based solid lipid nanoparticles. Food Chem 147:239–244

38. Schwarz C, Mehnert W, Lucks JS et al (1994) Solid lipid nanoparticles (SLN) for controlled drug delivery. I. Production, characterization and sterilization. J Control Release 30(1):83–96

39. Basaran E, Demirel M, Sirmagül B et al (2010) Cyclosporine-a incorporated cationic solid lipid nanoparticles for ocular delivery. J Microencapsul 27(1):37–47

40. Konan YN, Gurny R, Allémann E (2002) Preparation and characterization of sterile and freeze-dried sub-200 nm nanoparticles. Int J Pharm 233(1–2):239–252

41. Brigger I, Armand-Lefevre L, Chaminade P et al (2003) The stenlying effect of high hydrostatic pressure on thermally and hydrolytically labile nanosized carriers. Pharm Res 20(4):674–683

Chapter 14

Stability Testing Issues and Test Parameters for Herbal Medicinal Products

Gulshan Bansal, Jasmeen Kaur, Nancy Suthar, Sarabjeet Kaur, and Rahul Singh Negi

Abstract

With increase in demand for herbal medicinal products, the supply of such drugs and products has increased tremendously in the market, particularly in the developing world. To keep a check on the quality, safety, and efficacy of these products, drugs regulators across the globe have issued international as well as national level guidelines specific for such products. Shelf-life assignment of these products is one of the critical parameters for ensuring their quality, safety and efficacy. These guidelines across the globe recommend assigning of the shelf-life to these products on the basis of stability testing. But performing such testing on herbal products is not as convenient as with synthetic drug products. The major issues pertaining to reliable and effective conduct of stability testing on herbal medicinal products are significant variations of quality of herbal raw material responsible for batch-to-batch variation; lack of identification and availability of therapeutic markers; changing chromatographic fingerprints due to inter- and intra-molecular interactions among the phytoconstituents, and stability of the latter. In addition to these, selection of test parameters exerts a considerable influence on reliability of data generated for assessment of the shelf-life. Because therapeutic activity of a herbal medicinal product is not ascribed solely to particular marker(s), monitoring of both chemical parameters and intended biological activity(ies) is suggested to be a part of stability testing program of herbal medicinal products.

Key words Herbal medicinal products, Markers, Stability parameters, Shelf-life, Phytoconstituents, Storage

1 Introduction

About 70–95% of the population in developing countries depends upon herbs and herbal medicinal products to meet their primary healthcare needs. These products are increasingly being used in developed countries as well [1]. This growth in herbal medicinal product usage is witnessed internationally and has grown in past 15 years tremendously. Many proprietary herbal medicinal products, majority of these polyherbal, are available for the treatment of almost any kind of disease. Production of herbal substances, preparations and products in large volumes has raised questions

Sanjay Bajaj and Saranjit Singh (eds.), *Methods for Stability Testing of Pharmaceuticals*, Methods in Pharmacology and Toxicology, https://doi.org/10.1007/978-1-4939-7686-7_14, © Springer Science+Business Media, LLC, part of Springer Nature 2018

on their quality, safety, and efficacy (QSE). Drug regulatory authorities across the globe have laid down guidelines for manufacture of herbal substances, preparations and products to assure their QSE. The United States Food and Drug Administration (USFDA) has laid down very stringent criterion for approval of any herbal medicinal product that is claimed to have specific biological or therapeutic effects [2]. European countries allow use of herbal substances, their preparations and products as medicinal products, provided these are duly standardized [3–11]. Many other countries such as Australia, Canada, China, India, Japan, and Saudi Arabia also approve herbal products as medicinal agents, provided these meet the three attributes of QSE. Nevertheless, assuring QSE of a herbal medicinal product at release does not ensure consistent therapeutic effects and/or safety of the product during its shelf-life because the chemical and/or therapeutic attributes of herbal substance, preparation and the product itself may be altered due to exposure to different chemical or environmental conditions during their storage/shelf-life. Therefore, it is expected by all agencies that systematic stability studies are carried on all types of herbal materials and products to confirm their QSE through storage till the shelf-life.

2 Stability Testing of Herbal Materials and Medicinal Products

The stability testing of herbal medicinal products is as important as that of synthetic drug products. But it is much more difficult and challenging for the former. In a synthetic drug product, the active pharmaceutical ingredient is well defined qualitatively as well as quantitatively, and its content is directly related to the therapeutic effectiveness of the product. Therefore, the actives serve as direct markers for stability testing of the product, to establish its shelf-life. In contrast to it, a herbal drug substance, preparation or medicinal product is a very complex heterogeneous mixture of chemicals belonging to different categories (such as alkaloids, terpenoids, flavonoids, organic acids, carbohydrates and glycosides, saponins, amino acids, and others). All these chemicals are also liable to degrade, similar to synthetic drugs, under the influence of varied environmental factors such as temperature, light, air, moisture, pH, and others. It implies that the contents of these phytochemicals are most likely to change during the shelf-life of the product causing possible negative effects on the QSE. Many studies are reported on stability of different herbal substances, preparations and products under a variety of environmental factors (see Table 1), which support this argument that herbal materials are also chemically unstable. Furthermore, therapeutic actions of a herbal medicinal product are usually a function of additive or synergistic actions of chemically diverse phytoconstituents. So, any change in content of a specific

Table 1
Some reports on stability testing of herbal substances/preparations/products

Herbal substance/preparation/product	Condition(s)	Change(s) observed	Reference
Zingiber officinale, 6-Gingerol	>25 °C Alkaline pH	Unstable Good for stability	[12]
Aleurites moluccana leaves extract formulation	Heat and moisture	Degradation of swertisin and 2-*O*''-rhamnosyl swertisin is dependent on concentration of extract in formulation	[13]
Andrographis paniculata whole plant extract	Air oxidation	Andrographolide degrades	[14]
Azadirachta indica emulsifiable concentrate	High temperature	Azadirachtin A decreases by 90–98%	[15]
Bacopaside I and bacoside A₃	>60 °C	Both are degraded	[16]
Calendula officinalis flowers tincture	25 °C/60% RH, 24 months 40 °C/75% RH; 80 °C/100 °C	Flavonoid content remains constant Flavonoid content decreases	[17]
Caesalpinia pulcherrima flowers extract	75 ± 25% RH	Antioxidant activity decreases	[18]
Cassia alata leaves extract	Sun drying Varied pH	Kaempferol-3-gentiobioside is completely lost Anticryptococcal activity decreases with increasing pH	[19] [20]
Cinnamomum camphora leaves extract	Visible light pH 3 pH 3-11	Significant decrease in activity Activity is maximum Activity decreases by 10%	[21]
Clerodendrum infortunatum 2.5% and 5% leaves extract gel	25 °C ± 2 °C/60% RH ± 5% RH; 30 °C ± 2 °C/65% RH ± 5% RH; 40 °C ± 2 °C/75% RH ± 5% RH	2.5% extract gel is more stable (pH, viscosity, appearance, and spreadability) than the gel with 5% extract	[22]
Curcuma longa dried rhizome	Light	Lipid soluble fraction photosensitive in terms of *ar*-turmerone, turmerone, and curlone	[23]
Echinacea purpurea flowers extract	High temperature	Alkamide content decreases	[24]
Ginkgo biloba, *Hypericum perforatum*, *Piper methysticum* formulations	High humidity Sunlight	Degradation of markers is accelerated Unstable	[25]

(continued)

Table 1
(continued)

Herbal substance/preparation/product	Condition(s)	Change(s) observed	Reference
Hippophae rhamnoides juices and berries	≥25 °C	Total ascorbic acid content is significantly decreased (≥20%)	[26]
Hypericum perforatum extract and beverages	Acidic pH	Hypericin, pseudohypericin, hyperforin, and adhyperforin degrade	[27]
Ocimum sanctum leaves extract	Varied pH	Activity is significantly higher at pH 7 than at acidic pH	[28]
Olea europaea oil	20 °C; light	Extensive degradation of pheophytin	[29]
Orthosiphon stamineus leaves extract	≥60 °C	Sinensetin and rosemarinic acid content decreases	[30]
Ginsenosides Rb1, Rb2, Rg1	pH < 7	Ginsenosides degrade readily in aqueous solution	[31]
Parthenolide	75% pH 5–7 pH 1 or 9	Complete degradation Slow degradation (40–60% after 80 days) Rapid degradation (90% within 5 h)	[32, 33]
Piper nigrum fruits oil	Air oxidation	Terpenoids in essential oil are oxygenated	[34]
Plantago lanceolata dried leaves	75% RH 0 and 45% RH	Aucubin, catalpol, and acteoside content decrease by 95.7, 97, and 70.5% No significant change in contents	[35]
Rosemary extract	Air	Carsonic acid gets oxidized	[36]
Stevia rebaudiana carbonated beverages and leaves extract	60 °C Sunlight	Rebaudioside and stevioside are lost Rebaudiside is photo-sensitive and stevioside is photostable	[37] [38]

marker or a set of specific markers during stability testing of a herbal drug substance, preparation or medicinal product may not transcend to similar change in its therapeutic effectiveness. It entails that quantitative monitoring of specific marker(s) during stability studies of herbal materials/products may not form a firm basis of establishing their shelf-life, during which they are expected to elicit consistent therapeutic effectiveness.

3 Global Regulations

Drugs regulatory agencies across the globe such as World Health Organization (WHO), European Medicines Agency (EMEA), and International Conference on Harmonisation (ICH) recommend the submission of stability data of any medicinal product prior to its approval. WHO and EMEA have issued specific guidelines, i.e., "Stability testing of active pharmaceutical ingredients and finished pharmaceutical products" [8], and "Stability testing of herbal medicinal products and traditional herbal medicinal products" [39], respectively, for this purpose. WHO's "Supplementary guideline for the manufacture of herbal medicines" explicitly require that any specifically proposed shelf-life of a herbal material or herbal preparation should be supported by stability data generated under the specified storage conditions [40]. In addition to these, EMEA has issued other guidelines too, for assessment of quality of herbal medicinal products, which include "Quality of herbal medicinal products/traditional herbal medicinal products" [5], "Test procedures and acceptance criteria for herbal substances, herbal preparations and herbal medicinal products/traditional herbal medicinal products" [6], "Markers used for quantitative and qualitative analysis of herbal medicinal products and traditional herbal medicinal products" [41], and "Quality of combination herbal medicinal products/traditional herbal medicinal products" [42]. USFDA also states in its guideline entitled "Stability Testing Guidelines for Dietary Supplements" that an expiration date, if any on a product, should be supported by appropriately generated stability data [43]. Many other countries individually or regional groups have issued their own set of guidelines on stability testing (see Table 2) to ensure that patients get herbal medicinal products that are safe and efficacious [44].

The approaches in different guidelines to achieve QSE include assay of markers (active or analytical), biological assays, and/or chromatographic chemoprofiling or fingerprinting of control and stability samples of a product stored under the defined stability test conditions (see Table 3). Nevertheless, according to both EMEA and WHO, a herbal medicinal substance or herbal preparation is regarded as an active substance. Therefore, mere assay of marker compound(s) may not reflect the true stability

Table 2
Regulatory guidelines on stability testing of herbal products across the globe, other than from USFDA, EMEA and WHO

Country/ group of countries	Regulatory authority	Guidelines/administrative laws	Year of implementation/ amendment/ revision
ASEAN countries	ASEAN Traditional Medicine and Health Supplement (TMHS) Product Working Group	ASEAN Guidelines on Stability and Shelf-life of Traditional medicines and Health Supplements [45]	2013
Australia	Therapeutic Goods Administration	Australian Regulatory Guidelines for Complementary Medicines [46]	2011
Austria	Austrian Medicines and Medical Devices Agency	Austrian Medicines Act [10]	2002
Brazil	Brazilian Health Surveillance Agency (ANVISA)	Guideline to Herbal Medicine Registration RDC 14/10 [47, 48]	2004
Canada	Natural Health Products Directorate	Quality of Natural Products Guide [49]	2012
China	State Food and Drug Administration	Regulations for the Protection of TCM Products	1992
		Drug Administration Law of P.R. China	2001
		Regulations for Implementation of the Drug Administration Law of P.R. China	2002
		Provisions for Drug Registration [44, 50]	2007
Ghana	Food and Drugs Authority	Guideline for Registration of Herbal Medicinal Products in Ghana [51]	2013
Ireland	Irish Medicinal Board (IMB)	Traditional Herbal Medicinal Products Registration Scheme [52]	2007
India	Department of AYUSH	Drug and Cosmetic (Amendment) Act [53]	2005
Indonesia	Ministry of Health Republic of Indonesia	National Policy on Traditional Medicine (KOTRANAS) [54]	2007
Japan	Pharmaceutical and Medical Devices Agency	Guideline on Data Requirements for Ethical Kampo Formulation [55]	2013
Kenya	Pharmacy and Poisons Board of Kenya	Registration of Herbal and Complementary products: Guidelines to Submission of Applications. [56]	2010

(continued)

Table 2
(continued)

Country/ group of countries	Regulatory authority	Guidelines/administrative laws	Year of implementation/ amendment/ revision
Kuwait	Pharmaceutical and Herbal Medicines Registration and Control Administration	Documents and Materials Required for Registration of Herbal Products [57]	1997
Malaysia	Drug Control Authority	National Policy on Traditional and Complementary Medicine [58]	2001
New Zealand	The New Zealand Medicines and Medical Devices Safety Authority(Medsafe)	New Zealand Regulatory Guidelines for Medicines [59]	2011
Philippines	Food and Drugs Administration (formerly, Bureau of Food and Drugs), Department of Health	Guidelines on the Registration of Traditionally used Herbal Products Guidelines on the Registration of Herbal Medicines [60]	2004
Rwanda	Ministry of Health	MOH Guidelines on Submission of Documentation for Registration of Human Pharmaceutical Products [61]	2014
Saudi Arabia	Saudi Food and Drug Authority	Data Requirements for Herbal and Health Products Submission: Content of the Dossier [62]	2012
SADC countries	Southern African Development Community (SADC)	SADC Guidelines for Stability Testing [63]	2004
Singapore	Health Sciences Authority	Health Supplement Guidelines [64]	2012
Switzerland	Swissmedic	Requirements of Quality Documentation for Asian Medicinal Products [11]	2007
Tanzania	Tanzania Food and Drugs Authority	Guidelines for Application for Registration of Traditional Medicinal Products. [65]	2014
Uganda	National Drug Authority	Guidelines for Regulation of Traditional/Herbal Medicines (local) [66]	2009
United Arab Emirates	Ministry of Health, Dept. of Pharmacy and Drug Control	Summary of Requirements for Registration of Herbal Products [67]	2007
United Kingdom	Medicines and Healthcare products Regulatory Agency	Traditional Herbal Medicines Registration Scheme [9]	2011
Zambia	Pharmaceutical Regulatory Authority	Guidelines on Application for Registration of Herbal Medicines [68]	2004

Table 3
Recommended conditions for stability testing according to WHO and other guidelines

Study	Storage condition	Minimum period covered by data at submission	Testing frequency
Long-term	25 °C ± 2 °C/60% RH ± 5% RH or 30 °C ± 2 °C/65% RH ± 5% RH or 30 °C ± 2 °C/75% RH ± 5% RH	12 months	0, 3, 6, 9, 12, 18, 24 months and then annually
Intermediate	30 °C ± 2 °C/65% RH ± 5% RH	6 months	0, 6, 9 and 12 months
Accelerated	40 °C ± 2 °C/75% RH ± 5% RH	6 months	0, 3 and 6 months

characteristics of the product. It is for this reason, regulatory guidelines recommend that stability of herbal medicinal product should be assessed in terms of stability of not only the known therapeutic marker(s), but also other constituents (as maximum as possible) by appropriate techniques, such as chromatographic fingerprint analysis in addition to the other tests like the study of physical, chemical, and microbiological parameters. The content of known therapeutic constituent(s) during the proposed shelf-life should not vary by ±5% of the declared assay value, unless justified. However, the content of marker in a herbal medicinal product having unknown therapeutic constituent(s) should not vary by >±10% of the initial assay value during the proposed shelf-life.

4   Issues in Stability Testing of Herbal Materials and Medicinal Products

Despite the specific regulatory recommendations and scientific expertise available across the globe for conducting stability studies, stability assesments in dossier submissions of herbal medicinal products are usually not based on sound and systematic stability studies. Various issues that may be considered responsible for this noncompliance in stability testing are related to quality of herbal raw materials, marker selection for analytical studies, possible inter-constituent interactions, and selection of monitoring parameters during stability testing.

4.1 Quality of Herbal Raw Material

In synthetic drug products, the raw materials are of definite chemical composition and purity, and variation in quality or purity of these raw materials in different batches of any synthetic drug product is negligible. The stability data generated through systematic studies on select batches act as supporting data for other batches of that product. The shelf-life determined by stability testing of initial batches of a product also applies to subsequent batches of the product, provided there is no change in master formula and formulation process. However, the same cannot be said about a herbal material and product because they are a complex heterogeneous mixture of varied phytoconstituents. Due to such chemical complexity, the composition of a herbal medicinal product is not fully characterized. Moreover, the phytoconstituents in a drug substance, preparation or product often work synergistically in delivering therapeutic effects. These facts entail that all constituents in a herbal medicinal product responsible for its particular therapeutic activity are not identified and/or quantified for the want of reference standards. Further, batch-to-batch consistency in a herbal medicinal product is dependent upon the quality of raw material. A herb or herbal substance from different cultivators of different geographical location or harvested at different times during a year cannot have same concentrations of phytoconstituents in it. It implies that different batches of a herbal raw material are most likely to have variable quality attributes, and shelf-life of a product determined through stability testing of one set of batches cannot necessarily extrapolate to other batches. Various determinants, directly or indirectly, govern the content and nature of phytoconstituents in a herbal raw material, as discussed below.

4.1.1 Polyonymous Drugs

In traditional literature, a herb is known by many names in different or, for that matter, even in the same languages. Sometimes, the use of one name for two different herbs as per local tradition may lead to use of two botanically different herbs for same herbal preparation. As a case, both *Centella asiatica* and *Bacopa monnieri* are used as brahmi in many places in India. Similarly, two different plants, namely *Boerhaavia diffusa* and *Trianthema portulacastrum* are known as Punarnava [69]. The use of two different herbs under one common name may result in altogether different quality attributes and pharmacological effects of the herbal medicinal product.

4.1.2 Processing Methods

A herb is a heterogeneous mixture of resins, sterols, lignins, tannins, alkaloids, carbohydrates, glycosides, terpenoids, and others. Knowledge of the desired phytoconstituent(s), which is exerting the desired action(s), is important for selecting the right processing method. For example, red ginseng is steam dried whereas white ginseng is air-dried. Both are different in terms of phytoconstituent content, and therapeutic effect. Red ginseng exhibits more potent anticancer properties than white ginseng because of rare ginsenosides, such as ginsenosides Rh2 and Rg3. Contents of these anticancer specific ginsenosides are governed by the processing method of ginseng. Drying of red ginseng at higher steaming temperature yields nonpolar ginsenosides, which are potent in anticancer activity, whereas the drying at lower temperature yields polar ginsenosides, which are weak anticancer agents [70, 71]. Therefore, the knowledge of various drying techniques, extraction methodologies, and storage conditions for a particular herb are important considerations that may affect the efficacy of the product. So, it becomes imperative on the part of manufacturer or supplier to know about the phytochemical composition of the herb or herbal substance to select the right processing method for formulation of the material so that desired quality attributes are retained [72].

4.1.3 Contamination of Raw Material

A herbal substance may be contaminated with other plant parts, fungal infestation, microbial toxins, pesticides, heavy metal, etc. Such contaminations have potential to result in intoxication of final medicinal product. Improper storage and handling of herbal substance by unskilled manpower (which is true in most cases) may also result in contamination of herbal preparations or the medicinal products. Microbial contamination may lead to degradation of certain constituents due to catalytic activity of microbial enzymes. Therefore, monitoring of microbial load in a herbal substance/preparation/herbal medicinal product should be an integral part of stability testing protocol. Pesticide residues and heavy metal contaminants are other unwanted components present in a herbal material and product, which apart from toxic manifestations, can also react with markers causing a possible alteration in chemical composition of the product [69, 73].

4.1.4 Adulteration and Substitution

The supply of genuine herbal raw materials is usually low in comparison to their demand by herbal drug industry. To cope up with the increased demand, malpractices like adulteration and substitution are prevalent. Herbs are adulterated with inferior substitutes for profit-making. *Actaea racemosa,* which is used to relieve the symptom of menopause, is adulterated with cheap variants of Actaea species [74]. *Panax ginseng* is usually adulterated with other varieties of ginseng (*Panax quinquefolium, Panax pseudoginseng, Eleutherococcus senticosus*). The safety profiles of such species have not been studied so far, and their usage may result in adverse reactions [75, 76]. Star anise (*Illicium anisatum*) is substituted by bastard anise (*Illicium verum*), which is poisonous in nature [77]. *Bacopa monnieri* is mentioned as brahmi in traditional literature, but it is substituted with *C. asiatica,* which is known as mandookparni [78]. Both the herbs have been reported to have memory-enhancing activities, but their phytochemical properties are different. Shankhpushpi is known as any of the four herbs, i.e., *Convolvulus pluricaulis, Canscora decussata, Evolvulus alsinoides* and *Clitorea ternatea* in Compendium of Indian Medicinal Plants [79]. However, all these four herbs are found to be phytochemically different, and hence are expected to have different biological profiles. Therefore, use of any of the four herbs as shankhpushpi by various manufacturers adds to the complications in quality determination of the product. Such substitution practices and/or use of variety or species of a herb, other than those specified in traditional system of medicine, can severely affect therapeutic efficacy as well as safety of the product. Hence, authenticity of the raw material is one of the major determinants of safety and efficacy of botanical medicines.

4.1.5 Improper Agricultural Practices

Efficacy of a herbal drug product depends upon the content of desired phytoconstituent(s) in the raw material. It requires skill and knowledge to decide on the germplasm, part of the plant and age of the plant to be harvested to get maximum yield along with the season of harvesting and post-harvesting processing methods. Active constituent of any herbal material is significantly affected by manipulation in any of these variables. Geographical locations, type of soil, rainfall and storage conditions too have a significant effect on the phytoconstituent yield [73]. With rise in demand of medicinal herbs, these are grown haphazardly, giving lesser consideration to the conditions appropriate for good yield of desired phytoconstituents. For instance, content of aloe-emodin, rhein, and emodin vary significantly with the difference in altitude of collection [80]. An instance is even known where organic farming resulted in higher yield of carotenoids and minerals in comparison to conventional farming [81].

4.2 Selection of Marker(s)

The selection of markers for assessment of shelf-life of a herbal material/product is the most challenging task during rational stability testing. A critical study of the available physicochemical stability reports on herbal materials and products reveals that different research groups have used different markers for stability testing of a herbal substance, preparation or the medicinal product. For stability studies on *Actaea racemosa*, Budukh et al. used cimiracemoside-A, actein, and 27-deoxyactein (triterpenes) as markers [82], whereas Jiang et al. used cimiracemoside-F, 3-epi-26-deoxyactein, actein (triterpenes), and polyphenols as markers [83]. Comparative analysis of these two studies reveals that polyphenols are unstable compared to triterpenes at higher temperatures. Therefore, shelf-life of *A. racemosa* with respect to polyphenolic content is shorter than that with respect to triterpene content. Similarly, stability studies on *Echinacea purpurea* were conducted using alkamide and cichoric acid [84] as well as using alkamides [24]. Cichoric acid is very unstable compared to alkamides, which again implies two different shelf-lives for the same herb. Another case is of stability studies on *Calendula officinalis*, wherein one research group used total carotenoid content as marker [85], whereas others used the flavonoid content [17, 86]. Both the markers are chemically diverse, which may reflect different shelf-lives of *C. officinalis*. These literature reports suggest that there is wide variability in (i) susceptibility of different classes of makers to chemical change during shelf-life, and (ii) selection of markers for monitoring of stability of herbal materials/products. Therefore, the major question, which needs to be answered in the very first place, in assessment of shelf-life of a herbal drug substance, preparation or medicinal product, is that "which phytoconstituent is to be selected for monitoring during stability testing, so that a reliable shelf-life of the herbal material/product can be established"?

The sole purpose of consuming any herbal medicinal product is to get specific therapeutic and/or nutritional benefits, and these benefits are functions of individual, additive, or synergistic actions of its different phytoconstituents. Therefore, an ideal stability studies protocol for such a product should involve quantitative analysis of marker(s), whose levels can be extrapolated to its intended purpose(s). For instance, withanolides in *Withania somnifera* are related to immunomodulatory activity [87]; rebaudiside and stevioside are related to sweetness of *Stevia rebaudiana* [88]; curcumin is responsible for anti-inflammatory activity of *Curcuma longa* [89]; and hyperforin is chiefly responsible for antidepressant activity of *H. perforatum* [90]. Nonetheless, knowing the biologically active constituent in a herbal material may not be sufficient, because most herbal medicinal products are composed of a cocktail of herbal substances or preparations. In such cases, it is usually not possible to ascribe a particular biological activity to a set of active markers. In this regard, the WHO's Supplementary guidelines on good manufacturing practices for the manufacture of herbal medicines states that "...it is often not feasible to determine the stability of each active ingredient. Moreover, because the herbal material, in its entirety, is regarded as the active ingredient, a mere determination of the stability of the constituents with known therapeutic activity will not usually be sufficient. Chromatography allows tracing of changes, which may occur during storage of a complex mixture of biologically active substances contained in herbal materials. It should be shown, as far as possible, e.g. by comparisons of appropriate characteristic/fingerprint chromatograms, that the identified active ingredient (if any) and other substances present in the herbal material or finished herbal product are likewise stable and that their content as a proportion of the whole remains within the defined limits" [40].

The US FDA has also included biological assay as one of the quality control parameters [2]. In light of these regulatory recommendations, it becomes imperative to assess shelf-life of a herbal material and product in terms of chemical stability as well as biological activity. But out of the huge pool of reports on stability studies on herbal substances, preparations and products, only a few studies are conducted with respect to both marker compound and biological activity. For instance, immunomodulatory activity of *W. somnifera* is found to vary proportionally to the concentration of withanolide [87]; decrease in free radical scavenging activity of *Bacopa monnieri* corresponds well with decrease in concentration of bacopaside I [91]; free radical scavenging activity of *Orthosiphon stamineus* extract is proportional to the content of polyphenols [30]; and antiangiogenic activity of *Matricaria chamomilla* extract is directly related to flavonoids and apigenin-7-O-glucoside content [92]. However, contrary to these correlating reports, some studies have defied a correlation between stability of a selected marker and a particular biological activity tested during the stability studies. Exposure of *Olea europaea* to high temperature causes decrease in pheophytin (marker), but the antioxidant activity is increased [29]. Change in azadirachtin A content in *Azadirachta indica* formulations does not conform to similar changes in antibacterial and anti-diabetic activities [15]. Determination of biological half-life (in terms of antibacterial activity) and chemical half-life (in terms of allicin) of garlic extracts indicates that allicin alone is not responsible for antibacterial activity of the extract [93]. Therefore, shelf-life assignment to a herbal medicinal product to ensure consistent therapeutic efficacy and safety should be based on systematic stability testing that include evaluation of physical and chemical stabilities as well as the intended biological activity of the stability samples by appropriate in vitro and/or in vivo methods.

4.3   Drug–Drug Interactions

As discussed above repeatedly, a herbal drug substance, preparation or medicinal product contains numerous phytoconstituents of different chemical classes. These constituents may undergo various inter- as well as intra-molecular reactions under the influence of varied environmental conditions, such as heat, humidity, air and/or light during processing, formulation and storage of the material. These possible interactions between different groups of constituents (*see* Fig. 1) may result in a product with altered therapeutic and toxicity profile. Tannins cause precipitation of alkaloids [94]. Proteins and polysaccharides form reversible complexes with polyphenols via H-bonding and hydrophobic interactions causing a decrease in the activity due to free polyphenols [95]. Water-soluble glycosides increase the water solubility of tannins via non-covalent interactions, as observed in paeniflorin and glycyrrhizin [96]. Heavy metal ions form mono-dentate and bi-dentate complexes with polysaccharides, tannins, and lignins [97]. Complex formation too has an effect on overall efficacy of the product. Monoherbal products of *Convolvulus pluricaulis* can be monitored for their anxiolytic activity using scopoletin as a marker, but the presence of *Centella asiatica* interferes with this activity of scopoletin. It has been suggested that phytoconstituents of *Centella asiatica* may be involved in complex formation with scopoletin [98].

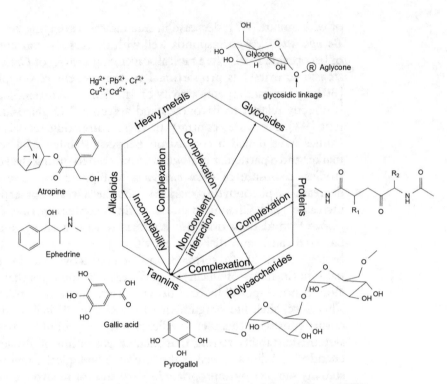

Fig. 1 Possible inter-molecular interactions among different phytoconstituents [99]

4.4 Stability of Phytoconstituents

Herbal medicinal products are also exposed to varied stress conditions before and during production process as well as during storage. Phytoconstituents can degrade under the influence of these stress conditions (*see* Fig. 2), which may, in turn, alter the therapeutic efficacy of the products. Curcumin undergoes extensive degradation under alkaline conditions to give furilic acid and vanillin [100]. Phenolic compound like gallic acid are sensitive to alkaline and acidic environment. Thus, the products containing gallic acid should be maintained at neutral pH [101, 102]. Flavonol glycosides (quercetin, kaempferol, and isorhamnetin) in *Ginkgo biloba* are highly unstable to basic, oxidative, and thermal stressors, but stable under acidic conditions [103–105]. Camphene, Δ^3-carene, limonene and α-terpinene undergo dehydrogenation, epoxidation, double bond cleavage, allylic oxidations and rearrangements, when heated in the presence of air [106]. These chemical changes are not perceptible from any possible alteration in physical attributes of the product, and can be monitored by studying the changes in chemical fingerprints using sophisticated analytical techniques.

4.5 Selection of Analytical and Statistical Techniques

Chemical analysis can be performed for reliable prediction of shelf-life by only careful selection of analytical techniques and sample preparation. The contents of markers in a herbal substance/preparation/product vary from extremely low to appreciable amounts.

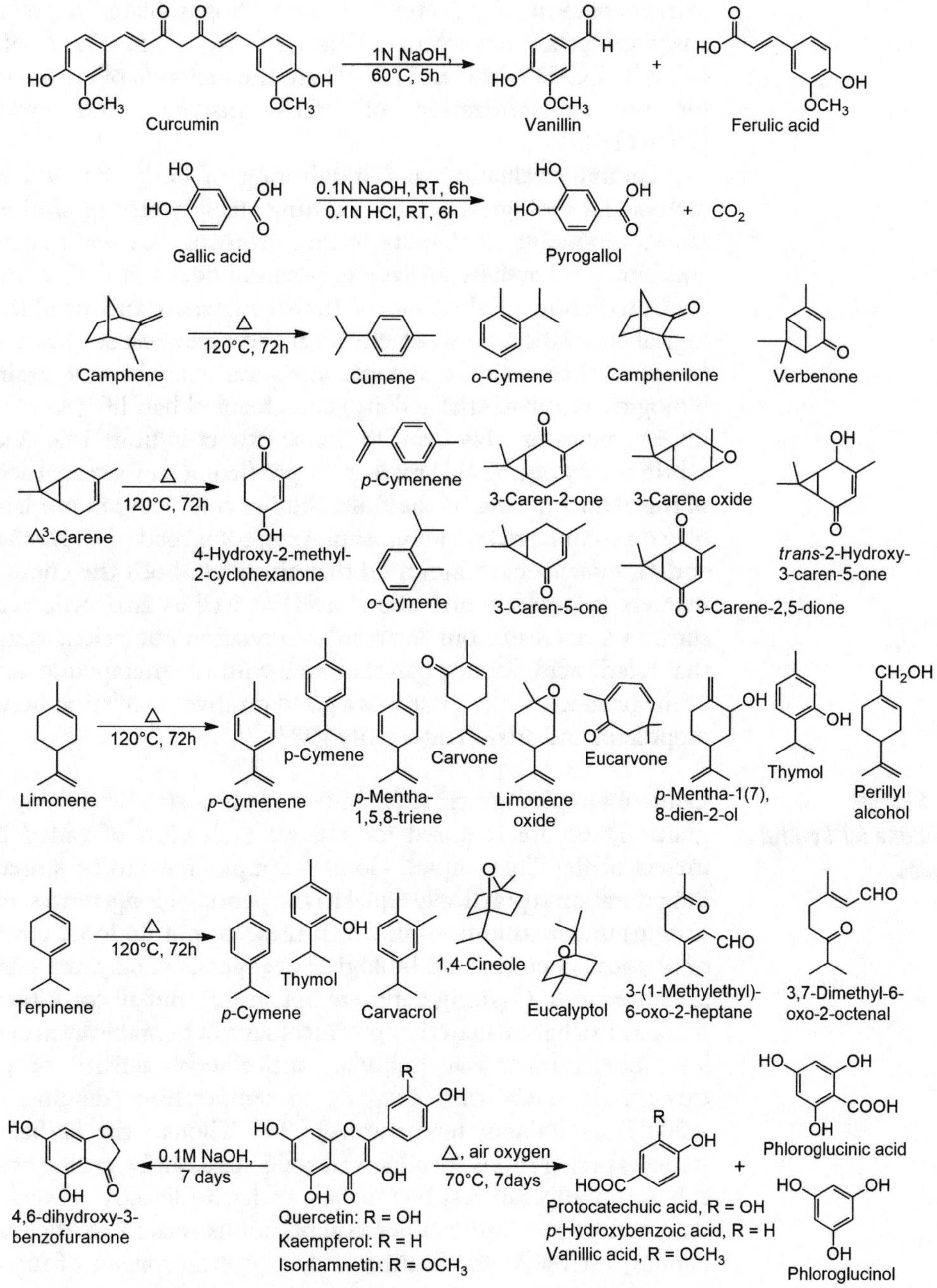

Fig. 2 Stress degradation products of various phytoconstituents

Also, the chemical diversity of these markers range from being non-chromophoric (such as sugars, steroids, and fatty acids) to strongly UV absorbing (such as flavonoids and phenolics). Therefore, the analytical technique selected for comprehensive chemical analysis or chemical profiling should be able to detect maximum possible number of markers as well as the biologically important markers present in even trace amounts. Sophisticated hyphenated analytical techniques such as LC-MS, LC-IR, LC-DAD, LC-NMR, GC-MS, LC-UV-MS, and LC-RI are the methods of choice so far for the standardization of herbal materials and products [107–113].

Though evaluation and monitoring of both chemical parameters and biological activities during stability testing are important components of stability testing protocol, but mere chemical and biological activity analysis in isolation does not suffice for the true prediction of shelf-life of herbal materials and products. A logical correlation between chemical and biological studies should be established using a suitable statistical analysis. For example, biological (antibacterial activity) and chemical half-life (Azadirachtin A) studies on *Azadirachta indica* extract indicate that Azadirachtin A may not be sole marker for predicting antibacterial activity of the extract during its shelf-life. Studies conducted in our laboratory on commercial shankhpushpi syrup composed of *C. pluricaulis* and *C. asiatica* have indicated that although, both the content of markers (scopoletin and asiatic acid) as well as anxiolytic activity showed a decrease, but Pearson's correlation coefficient suggests that asiatic acid did not correlate well with the therapeutic activity of the product, while there was a good positive correlation between scopoletin and anxiolytic activity [98].

4.6 Storage Conditions for Control Samples

Control samples are critically important in a stability testing program. These are required for relative evaluation of varied parameters of stability samples. Control samples have to be stored for long durations (practically equal to the period of long-term stability testing) under conditions in which these do not undergo any kind of physical, chemical and biological change. Generally, the samples are stored at 4 °C (refrigeration temperature). But all constituents/markers in a herbal material/product may not be stable even at such low temperature. For example, antibacterial activity of garlic extracts decreases with decrease in temperature (ranging from −20 °C to ambient temperature) [93]. Though the herbal substances/preparations/products in solid state can be stored at even sub-zero temperatures, but storage of herbal liquids at such low temperature can cause other complications related to thermodynamics, such as crystallization and/or polymorphism of markers. Therefore, selection of appropriate storage temperature for control samples can also be equally challenging.

5   Test Parameters

Herbal raw materials usually do not come with a certificate of analysis. Therefore, it becomes imperative on the part of the product manufacturer to conduct various tests on the raw material to assure its identity and quality prior to the production of herbal medicinal products. Those tests become a guiding force for selecting appropriate tests for monitoring of stability of the product. Broadly, these tests can be classified into physical, chemical, biological, and microbiological. The physical test parameters include, but not limited to, color, odor, moisture content, various pharmacopoeial tests such as tablet hardness, friability, disintegration time, dissolution time, and viscosity for different formulations. The chemical parameters are aimed to evaluate varied constituents/ markers qualitatively and/or quantitatively through chemical tests and/or chromatographic techniques. The purpose of biological tests is to ascertain the consistent therapeutic activities as well as efficacy of the product during its shelf-life. Herbal materials and products, due to their carbohydrate and moisture contents, can be an excellent medium for assisting growth of microbes. Contamination of herbals with hazardous microbes at any stage from harvesting to final product development can lead to serious consequence. Therefore, microbiological tests are also an important component of the herbal medicinal products stability program to evaluate the their microbial purity [114]. Evaluation of all these four test parameters constitutes an ideal stability testing protocol for herbal products to establish their shelf-life. Regulatory guidelines recommend that any herbal product should be subjected to accelerated stability testing (at 40 °C/75% RH) for 6 months, intermediate stability testing (at 30 °C/65% RH) for 6–12 months, and long-term stability testing (at 25–30 °C/60–75% RH) for a period equal to the proposed shelf-life of the product as mentioned in Table 3. However, intermediate stability testing is not required when the conditions for long-term testing are same as those for intermediate ones [7]. Meta-analysis of literature reports of stability studies on different types of herbal materials/products reveals that there is a wide variation in conditions employed (temperature of −80 to 100 °C, relative humidity of 0 to 100%, and duration of a few hours to 3 years). Same is the situation with parameters for assessment of shelf-life. Out of these, only 23% studies comply with storage conditions and sampling schedule recommended for accelerated stability studies, and only a negligible proportion (<1%) of the studies comply with conditions recommended for long-term and accelerated stability studies (*see* Table 4). Also, only 8% of the studies comply with all the parameters required for shelf-life assessment, regardless of the stability conditions employed. Figures 3 and 4 show the status of analysis of these studies. Some studies are conducted by analyzing physical parameters only, and hence provide only minimal information about stability of the products. Most of the laboratories have analyzed only chemical aspect of the stability of the product using active/analytical markers or by fingerprint analysis, without providing any correlation with the therapeutic efficacy. Therefore, there is almost total noncompliance with the

Table 4
Studies conducted in partial or complete compliance with WHO guidelines

Herb/ phytoconstituent/ herbal product	Stability condition, duration in months (Mo)	Findings	Ref.
Actaear acemosa formulations	40 °C/75% RH, 6 Mo; 25 °C/60% RH, 6 Mo; 50 °C, 1 Mo	Triterpene glycoside content falls under accelerated condition	[83]
Centella asiatica whole plant extract	40 °C/75% RH, 6 Mo	Physically stable; total phenolic content, content of kaempferol and asiatic acid, and antioxidant and AChE inhibitory activities decrease	[115]
Hypericum perforatum	40 °C/75% RH, 6 Mo; 25 °C/65% RH, 6 Mo	Chemically unstable at higher humidity and temperature	[116]
K-Gin capsules (contains *Panax ginseng*)	25 °C/75% RH; 35 °C/75% RH; 40 °C/75% RH, 24 Mo	Chemically and physically stable	[117]
Peppermint oil and caraway oil	40 °C/75% RH, 1 Mo	Physically stable	[118]
Piper longum	40 °C/75% RH, 6 Mo; 30 °C/65% RH, 6 Mo; Real time study, 6 Mo	TPC and antioxidant activity decreases; Better activity and higher TPC in long-term stability samples	[119]
Senna leaves	25 °C/60% RH; 30 °C/60% RH; 40 °C/75% RH	Content of sennosides decreases at higher temperature and humidity	[120]
Shankhpushpi syrups	40 °C/75% RH, 6 Mo; 30 °C/65% RH, 12 Mo	Physically stable; TPC, scopoletin and asiatic acid content decreases significantly; antioxidant, AChE inhibitory and anxiolytic activity decreases	[121, 122]
Withania somnifera root extract	40 °C/75% RH, 6 Mo; 30 °C/65% RH, 6 Mo	Physically unstable; Withaferin A and withanolide A content decreases	[87]
Topical gel of *Sesbania grandiflora* leaf extract	25 °C/60% RH, 3 Mo; 30 °C/65% RH, 3 Mo; 40 °C/75% RH, 3 Mo	No change in physicochemical parameters	[123]

recommended conditions and test parameters in generation of stability data of different herbal materials/products. In order to get complete picture about the therapeutic stability of a herbal medicinal product over its claimed shelf-life, physicochemical as well as biological activity(ies) of the product must be evaluated during its stability testing. Such a comprehensive accelerated stability testing has been reported on different extracts (fresh as well as commercially available) of *Centella asiatica* [115], which is an

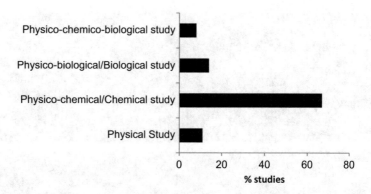

Fig. 3 Studies following physical, chemical, and/or biological test parameters

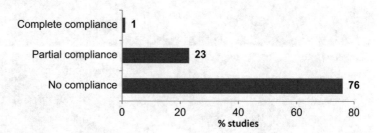

Fig. 4 Extent of compliance of stability studies on herbal materials/products to WHO guidelines

important herbal preparation in any herbal medicinal product aimed to treat central nervous system disorders such as anxiety and memory loss, and is used as a substitute of *B. monnieri* in Ayurveda. Its primary active constituents are asiaticosides, asiatic acid, madecassoside, madecassic acid, kaempferol, and β-sitosterol. Amongst these, asiaticoside derivatives are reported to be responsible for prevention of Alzheimer's disease [124], and β-sitosterol is also reported to be associated with multiple activities. Ethanol extract preparations of its root, petioles, and leaves act as potent antioxidants [125]. The LC-UV and HPTLC monitoring of stability samples reveals that content of asiatic acid and kaempferol decreases gradually over 6 months [115]. In addition to these markers, HPTLC fingerprint of the extracts are also generated. Though the markers contents are found to decrease, but there are significant visible changes in the fingerprints in stability samples withdrawn over 6 months (Fig. 5). The antioxidant and acetylcholine esterase (AChE) inhibitory activities also decrease gradually over 6 months with respect to the respective control. The decrease is more prominent in commercial extract than in fresh extract, and the preservative is found to slow the progression of this decrease. Furthermore, Pearson's correlation analysis of data of chemical tests and biological activities has revealed a linear positive

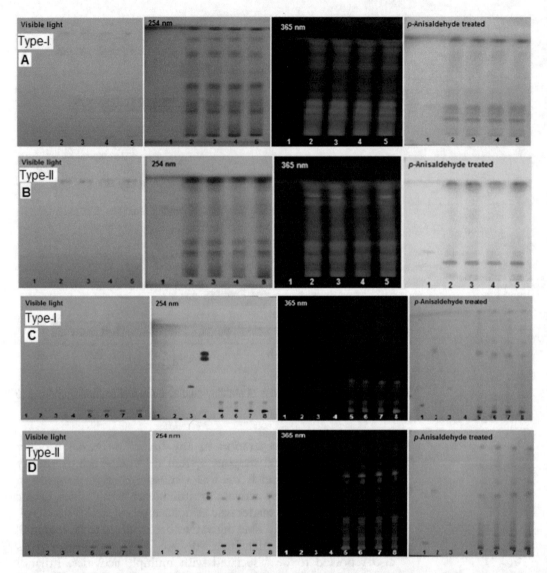

Fig. 5 HPTLC fingerprints of control and stability samples commercial extract (Type-I) and fresh extract (Type-II) of *C. asiatica*. Figures **a** and **b** show the profiles of standard solutions of asiaticoside (1), control sample (2) and stability samples of extracts after 1 month (3), 3 months (4), and 6 months (5) under accelerated conditions. The mobile phase was Chloroform:Glacial acetic acid:Methanol:Water (5.5:3:0.5:0.4). The Figures **c** and **d** show the profiles of standard solutions of asiatic acid (1), β-sitosterol (2), kaempferol (3), methyl paraben and propyl paraben mixture (4), of control samples (5) and stability samples of the extracts after 1 month (6), 3 months (7), and 6 months (8) under accelerated conditions. The mobile phase was chloroform:toluene:ethyl acetate:formic acid (5.5:2:1:0.2). The plates were visualized in visible light, UV light (254 and 365 nm), and in visible light after treatment with *p*-anisaldehyde

correlation between the different chemical and biological parameters, on the basis of which the total phenolic content, asiatic acid, and kaempferol in *C. asiatica* are suggested as chemical markers to assess chemical as well as therapeutic shelf-lives of herbal products containing *C. asiatica*. Microbial load in the product is also necessary to be monitored during its shelf-life to ensure safety from microbial contaminations.

6   Conclusions and Perspectives

Shelf-life assessment of herbal medicinal products is as important as that of synthetic drug products. Though this class of products has been contributing significantly in healthcare system globally, particularly in developing countries, and the drug regulators across the globe have issued specific guidelines for establishing their shelf-life on the basis of systematically generated stability data, yet their stability testing have been hitting many roadblocks. The lack of knowledge of therapeutic markers; non-availability of known therapeutic markers at the commercial scale; problems related to batch-to-batch variation in herbal raw materials due to mistaken identities of many herbs; varied agriculture practices, contamination of raw material due to heavy metals, microbes, pesticides, fertilizers; and practices of adulteration and substitution have been identified as major hurdles in effective implementation of the guidelines. The other issue in this regard is selection of appropriate test parameters for testing of stability samples, even if the above-mentioned hurdles are removed. Selection of test parameters is broadly governed by the nature of the active constituents and the formulation category. The therapeutic marker(s) in a herbal medicinal product may be known, but its monitoring by sensitive analytical method(s) may not necessarily be extrapolated to the monitoring of its therapeutic efficacy. It is because of the fact that in addition to the therapeutic marker(s), a herbal material/medicinal product contains numerous other types of constituents that may interact with each other and/or with the marker(s) resulting in formation of newer compounds in the product during shelf-life. These new compounds may affect the therapeutic potential of the product positively, negatively or differently or even may not have any effect. These compounds may also appear in the chromatographic fingerprint of the stability sample, thus posing severe analytical challenges. Therefore, testing of physical and all chemical parameters during stability studies on a herbal medicinal product cannot give an unequivocal opinion about its therapeutic shelf-life. It necessitates the inclusion of biological assays in the stability testing program of herbal medicinal products, as also suggested by WHO guidelines. But the major challenge in achieving this target is lack of ready availability of reliable in vitro models for fast evaluation of biological activities during the testing. Another requirement of the in vitro model is that the data provided by it should be extrapolatable to the in vivo model for the tested activity. Though use of cell lines seems to be an answer to this problem, but extensive resources and super-skilled manpower limits their use in routine stability testing programs.

Here, biotechnology, or appropriately nanobiotechnology, can play an important role by inventing novel enzyme based or other in vitro models that can create an environment similar to the in vivo one.

References

1. Robinson MM, Zhang X (2011) The world medicines situation. Traditional medicines: global situation, issues and challenges. World Health Organization, Geneva

2. USFDA (2004) Guidance for industry: botanical drug products. Department of Health and Human Services, United States Food and Drug Administration, Rockville MD. https://www.fda.gov/downloads/drugs/guidancecomplianceregulatoryinformation/guidances/ucm458484.pdf

3. CPMP (2003) Stability testing of new drug substances and products. CPMP/ICH/2736/99, Committee for Proprietary Medicinal Products, European Medicines Agency, London, UK

4. CPMP (2003) Guideline on stability testing: stability testing of existing active substances and related finished products. CPMP/QWP/122/02 Rev1 corr, Committee for Proprietary Medicinal Products, European Medicines Agency, London, UK

5. CPMP (2011) Quality of herbal medicinal products/ traditional herbal medicinal products. CPMP/QWP/2819/00 Rev2, Committee for Medicinal Products for Human Use, European Medicines Agency, London, UK

6. CPMP (2011) Guideline on specifications: test procedures and acceptance criteria for herbal substances, herbal preparations and herbal medicinal products/traditional herbal medicinal products. CPMP/QWP/2820/00 Rev2, Committee for Medicinal Products for Human Use, European Medicines Agency, London, UK

7. ICH (2003) Stability testing of new drug substances and products. International Conference on Harmonization, Q1A(R2), IFPMA, Geneva

8. WHO (2009) Stability testing of active pharmaceutical ingredients and finished pharmaceutical products. WHO technical report series, No. 953. World Health Organization, Geneva

9. UK (2014) Medicines, medical devices and blood regulation and safety-guidance. Medicines and Healthcare Product Regulatory Agency, London, UK

10. Austria (2009) Austrian medicines and medical devices agency. http://www.basg.gv.at/en/about-us/basg-and-ages-mea/quality-management/. Accessed Apr 2016

11. Switzerland (2012) Registration and harmonisation in the area of medical products in Switzerland. Swiss Agency for Therapeutic Products, Swissmedic, Bern, Switzerland

12. Phadke M, Sane RT, Menon SN, Hijli PS, Shah M, Patel PH (1998) Accelerated stability study on gingerol from *Zingiber officinale* using high performance thin layer chromatographic method. Toxicol Lett 95:152

13. Cesca TG, Faqueti LG, Rocha LW, Meira NA, Meyre-Silva C, deSouza MM, Quintao NLM, Silva RML, Cechinel Filho V, Bresolin TMB (2012) Antinociceptive, anti-inflammatory and wound healing features in animal models treated with a semisolid herbal medicine based on *Aleurites moluccana* L. Willd. Euforbiaceae standardized leaf extract. Semisolid Herbal J Ethnopharmacol 143(1):355–362

14. Garg C, Sharma P, Satija S, Garg M (2016) Stability indicating studies of *Andrographis paniculata* extract by validate HPTLC protocol. J Pharmacog Phytochem 5(6):337–344

15. Kumar L, Parmar BS (2000) Effect of emulsion size and shelf-life of Azadirachtin A on the bioefficacy of neem (*Azadirachta indica* A. Juss) emulsifiable concentrates. J Agric Food Chem 48(8):3666–3672

16. Phrompittayarat W, Wittaya-areekul S, Jetiyanon K, Putalun W, Tanaka H, Ingkaninan K (2008) Stability studies of saponins in *Bacopa monnieri* dried ethanolic extract. Planta Med 74(14):1756–1763

17. Bilia AR, Bergonzi MC, Gallori S, Mazzi G, Vincieri FF (2002) Stability of the constituents of calendula, milk-thistle and passion flower tinctures by LC-DAD and LC-MS. J Pharm Biomed Anal 30(3):613–624

18. Soisuwan S, Mapaisansin W, Samee W, Brantner AH, Kamkaen N (2010) Development of peacock flower extract as anti-wrinkle formulation. J Health Res 24(1):29–34

19. Moriyama H, Iizuka T, Nagai M, Miyataka H, Satoh T (2003) Anti inflammatory activity of heat-treated *Cassia alata* leaf extract and its flavonoid glycoside. Yakugaku Zasshi J Pharm Soc Japan 123(7):607–611

20. Ranganathan S, Balajee SAM (2000) Anti-cryptococcus activity of combination of

extracts of *Cassia alata* and *Ocimum sanctum*. Mycoses 43(7-8):299–301

21. Chen Y, Dai G (2012) Antifungal activity of plant extracts against *Colletotrichum lagenarium*, the causal agent of anthracnose in cucumber. J Sci Food Agr 92(9):1937–1943

22. Das S, Haldar PK, Pramanik G (2011) Formulation and evaluation of herbal gel containing *Clerodendronin fortunatum* leaves extract. Int J Pharm Tech Res 3(1):140–143

23. Jain V, Prasad V, Pal R, Singh S (2007) Standardization and stability studies of neuroprotective lipid soluble fraction obtained from *Curcuma longa*. J Pharm Biomed Anal 44 (5):1079–1086

24. Al-Jabari M, Al-Bawab A, Abdoh AA (2008) Stability study of the natural extract of *Echinacea purpurea* in aqueous solutions. Dirasat: Pure Sci 35(1):27–37

25. Marais A (2001) Increased-rate stability studies for St. John's Wort (*Hypericum perforatum*), *Ginkgo biloba* and Kava Kava (*Piper methysticum*) under unfavourable environmental conditions, University of Pretoria, 302. https://repository.up.ac.za/bitstream/handle/2263/23083/00front.pdf?sequence=1&isAllowed=y. Accessed 22 Aug 2016

26. Gutzeit D, Baleanu G, Winterhalter P, Jerz G (2008) Vitamin C content in sea buckthorn berries (*Hippophaë rhamnoides* L. ssp. *rhamnoides*) and related products: a kinetic study on storage stability and the determination of processing effects. J Food Sci 73(9): C615–C620

27. Ang CY, Hu L, Heinze TM, Cui Y, Freeman JP, Kozak K, Luo W, Liu FF, Mattia A, DiNovi M (2004) Instability of St. John's wort (*Hypericum perforatum* L.) and degradation of hyperforin in aqueous solutions and functional beverage. J Agric Food Chem 52 (20):6156–6164

28. Juntachote T, Berghofer E (2005) Antioxidative properties and stability of ethanolic extracts of holy basil and galangal. Food Chem 92(2):193–202

29. Psomiadou E, Tsimidou M (2002) Stability of virgin olive oil, photo-oxidation studies. J Agric Food Chem 50(4):722–727

30. Akowuah GA, Zhari I (2010) Effect of extraction temperature on stability of major polyphenols and antioxidant activity of *Orthosiphon stamineus* leaf. J Herbs Spices Med Plants 16(3-4):160–166

31. Miyamoto E, Odashima S, Kitagawa IS, Tsuji A (1984) Stability kinetics of ginsenosides in aqueous solution. J Pharm Sci 73(3):409–410

32. Jin P, Madieh S, Augsburger LL (2007) The solution and solid state stability and excipient compatibility of parthenolide in feverfew. AAPS Pharm Sci Tech 8(4):200–205

33. Jin P, Madieh S, Augsburger LL (2008) Selected physical and chemical properties of feverfew (*Tanacetum parthenium*) extracts important for formulated product quality and performance. AAPS PharmSci Tech 9 (1):22–30

34. Orav A, Stulova I, Kailas T, Muurisepp M (2004) Effect of storage on the essential oil composition of *Piper nigrum* L. fruits of different ripening states. J Agric Food Chem 52 (9):2582–2586

35. Gonda S, Tóth L, Gyémánt G, Braun M, Emri T, Vasas G (2012) Effect of high relative humidity on dried *Plantago lanceolata* L. leaves during long-term storage: effects on chemical composition, colour and microbiological quality. Phytochem Anal 23(1):88–93

36. Schwarz K, Ternes W, Schmauderer E (1992) Antioxidative constituents of *Rosmarinus officinalis* and *Salvia officinalis*. Part III. Stability of phenolic diterpenes of rosemary extracts under thermal stress as required for technological processes. Eur Food Res Technol (*formerly* Z Lebensm Unters Forsch) 195 (2):104–107

37. Chang SS, Cook JM (1983) Stability studies of stevioside and rebaudioside A in carbonated beverages. J Agric Food Chem 31 (2):409–412

38. Gardana C, Scaglianti M, Simonetti P (2010) Evaluation of steviol and its glycosides in *Stevia rebaudiana* leaves and commercial sweetener by ultra-high-performance liquid chromatography-mass spectrometry. J Chromatogr A 1217(9):1463–1470

39. EMEA (2010) Reflection paper on stability testing of herbal medicinal products and traditional herbal medicinal products. EMEA/HMPC/3626/09, Committee on Herbal Medicinal Products, European Medicines Agency, London, UK

40. WHO (2006) Supplementary guidelines on good manufacturing practices for the manufacture of herbal medicines. WHO Technical Report Series, No. 937. World Health Organization, Geneva.

41. EMEA (2008) Reflection paper on markers used for quantitative and qualitative analysis of herbal medicinal products and traditional herbal medicinal products. EMEA/HMPC/253629/07, Committee on Herbal Medicinal Products, European Medicines Agency, London, UK

42. EMEA (2008) Quality of combination herbal medicinal products/traditional herbal medicinal products. EMEA/HPMC/CHMP/CVMP/214869/2006, Committee on Herbal Medicinal Products, European Medicines Agency, London, UK

43. USFDA (2003) Current good manufacturing practice in manufacturing, packing, or holding dietary ingredients and dietary supplements. Proposed rule, United States Food and Drug Administration, Rockville, MD

44. Bansal G, Kaur I, Kaur J (2017) Herbal health products quality through stability studies: a global regulatory concern. Appl Clin Res Clin Trials Reg Affairs 4(1):26–35

45. ASEAN (2005) ASEAN guidelines on stability and shelf-life of traditional medicines and health supplements. Adopted at 20th ASEAN traditional medicines and health supplements scientific committee meeting (ATSC) 26–29 August 2013, Bangkok and endorsed at 20th ACCSQ traditional medicines and health supplements product working group (TMHSPWG) meeting 15–16 November 2013, Yogyakarta, Indonesia

46. Australia (2011) Australian regulatory guidelines for complementary medicines—Part IV: general guidance. Therapeutic Goods Administration, Australia

47. Brazil (2005) Guidelines for registration/listing of herbal medicines and related products directorate of registration and regulatory affairs. Brazil NAFDAC/RR/006/00, Brazil

48. Carvalho ACB, Perfeito JPS, Leandro VCS, Ramalho LS, Marques RFO, Silveira D (2011) Regulation of herbal medicines in Brazil: advances and perspectives. Braz J Pharm Sci 47(3):467–473

49. Canada (2015) Quality of natural products guide. Natural and non-prescription health products directorate. Health Canada, Ottawa, Canada

50. Schroeder T (2002) Chinese regulation of traditional Chinese medicine in the modern world: can the Chinese effectively profit from one of their most valuable cultural resources? Pacific Rim Law Policy J 11(3):687–716

51. Ghana (2013) Guideline for registration of herbal medicinal products in Ghana. Food and Drugs Authority, Accra, Ghana

52. Ireland (2012) Guide to traditional herbal medicinal products registration scheme. Irish Medicinal Board, Dublin, Ireland

53. Drug and Cosmetic Act (1940) Ministry of Health and Family Welfare, New Delhi, India.

54. Indonesia (2007) National policy on traditional medicine. Ministry of Health, Jakarta, Indonesia

55. Maegawa H, Nakamura T, Saito K (2014) Regulation of traditional herbal medicinal products in Japan. J Ethnopharmacol 158 (Part B):511–515

56. Kenya (2010) Registration of herbal and complementary products: guidelines to submission of applications. Pharmacy and Poisons Board, Nairobi, Republic of Kenya

57. Kuwait (1997) Pharmaceutical & herbal medicines registration & control administration: documents and materials required for registration of herbal products. Drug and Food Control, Ministry of Health, Safat, Kuwait

58. Jayaraj P (2010) Regulation of traditional and complementary medicinal products in Malaysia. Int J Green Pharm 4(1):10–14

59. New Zealand (2011) New Zealand medicines and medical devices safety authority. New Zealand Regulatory Guidelines for Medicines. Medsafe, Wellington, New Zealand

60. Phillipines (2004) Guidelines on the registration of traditionally-used herbal products. Administrative Order No. 184, Phillipines.

61. Rwanda (2014) MOH Guidelines on submission of documentation for registration of human pharmaceutical products. Ministry of Health, Kigali, Republic of Rwanda

62. Saudi Arabia (2012) Data requirements for herbal & health products submission: content of the Dossier. Saudi Food and Drug Authority, Riyadh, Saudi Arabia.

63. South Africa (2004) Guideline for stability testing. Southern African Development Community, Botswana, Southern Africa

64. Singapore (2015) Regulatory guidance: health supplements guidelines. Health Sciences Authority, Singapore

65. Tanzania (2014) Guidelines for application for registration of traditional medicinal products. Tanzania Food and Drugs Authority, Dar es Salaam, Tanzania.

66. Uganda (2009) Guidelines for regulation of traditional/herbal medicines (local) in Uganda. National Drug Authority, Kampala, Uganda.

67. UAE (2007) Summary of requirements for registration of herbal products. Drug Control Department, Ministry of Health, Abu Dhabi, United Arab Emirates.

68. Zambia (2004) Guidelines on application for registration of Herbal Medicines. Pharmaceutical Regulatory Authority, Lusaka, Zambia

69. Dubey NK, Kumar R, Tripathi P (2004) Global promotion of herbal medicine: India's opportunity. Curr Sci 86(1):37–41

70. In G, Ahn N-G, Bae B-S, Lee M-W, Park H-W, Jang KH, Cho D-G, Han CK, Park CK, Kwak Y-S (2017) *In situ* analysis of chemical components of induced by steaming between fresh ginseng, steamed ginseng, red ginseng. J Ginseng Res 41(3):361–369

71. Lee SM, Bae B-S, Park H-W, Ahn N-G, Cho D-G, Cho Y-L, Kwak Y-S (2015) Characterization of Korean red ginseng (*Panax ginseng* Meyer): history, preparation method, chemical composition. J Ginseng Res 39 (4):354–391

72. Mosihuzzaman M, Choudhary MI (2008) Protocols on safety, efficacy, standardization, documentation of herbal medicine (IUPAC Technical Report). Pure Appl Chem 80 (10):2195–2230

73. Mukherjee PK, Rai S, Kumar V, Mukherjee K, Hylands PJ, Hider RC (2007) Plants of Indian origin in drug discovery. Exp Op Drug Disc 2(5):633–657

74. Verbitski SM, Gourdin GT, Ikenouye LM, McChesney JD, Hildreth J (2014) Detection of Actaea racemosa adulteration by thin-layer chromatography and combined thin layer chromatography bioluminescence. J AOAC Int 91(2):268–275

75. Chan TY, Critchley JA (1996) Usage and adverse effects of Chinese herbal medicines. Hum Exp Toxicol 15(1):5–12

76. Inamdar N, Edalat S, Kotwal VB, Pawar S (2008) Herbal drugs in milieu of modern drugs. Int J Green Pharm 2(1):2–8

77. Razic S, Dogo S, Slavkovic L (2006) Investigation on bioavailability of essential and toxic elements in plants and soils. J Nat Med 62:340–344

78. Sudha S, Kumaresan S, Amit A, David J, Venkataraman BV (2002) Anti-convulsant activity of different extracts of *Centella asiatica* and *Bacopa monnieri* in animals. J Nat Rem 2 (1):33–41

79. Rastogi and Mehrotra (1990) Compendium of Indian medicinal plants, vol I. PID, New Delhi, pp 8, 49, 53, 75, 96, 114, 222, 286, 434

80. Tabin S, Kamili AN, Ganie SA, Zargar O, Sharma V, Gupta RC (2016) Genetic diversity and population structure of Rheum species in Kashmir Himalaya based on ISSR markers. Flora 223:121–128

81. Pérez-López AJ, López-Nicolas JM, Núñez-Delicado E, Amor FMD, Carbonell-Barrachina AA (2007) Effects of agricultural practices on color, carotenoids composition, and minerals contents of sweet peppers, cv. Almuden. J Agric Food Chem 55 (20):8158–8164

82. Budukh PP, Avery BA, Wyandt CM (2003) Short term stability testing of selected commercial black Cohosh formulations. www.aapsj.org/abstracts/Am_2003/AAPS2003-000344.PDF

83. Jiang B, Kronenberg F, Balick MJ, Kennelly EJ (2013) Stability of black cohosh triterpene glycosides and polyphenols: potential clinical relevance. Phytomedicine 20(6):564–569

84. Livesey J, Awang DVC, Arnason JT, Letchamo W, Barrett M, Pennyroyal G (1999) Effect of temperature on stability of marker constituents in *Echinacea purpurea* root formulations. Phytomedicine 6(5):347–349

85. Bernatoniene J, Masteikova R, Davalgiene J, Peciura R, Gauryliene R, Bernatoniene R, Majiene D, Lazauskas R, Civinskiene G, Velziene S, Muselik J, Chalupova Z (2011) Topical application of *Calendula officinalis* (L.): formulation and evaluation of hydrophilic cream with antioxidant activity. J Med Plant Res 5(6):868–877

86. Akhtar N, Khan BA, Mahmood T, Parveen R, Qayum M, Anwar M, Shahiq-uz-zaman FM (2010) Formulation and evaluation of antisebum secretion effects of sea buckthorn w/o emulsion. J Pharm Bioallied Sci 2(1):13–17

87. Patil D, Gautam M, Jadhav U, Mishra S, Karupothula S, Gairola S, Jadhav S, Patwardhan B (2010) Physicochemical stability and biological activity of *Withania somnifera* extract under real-time and accelerated storage conditions. Planta Med 76(5):481–488

88. Tanaka O (1982) Steviol-glycosides: new natural sweeteners. TrAC Trends Anal Chem 1 (11):246–248

89. Akram M, Uddin S, Ahmed A, Usmanghani K, Hannan A, Mohiuddin E, Asif M (2010) Curcuma longa and Curcumin: a review article. Rom J Biol-Plant Biol 55(2):65–70

90. Barnes J, Anderson LA, Phillipson JD (2001) St John's wort (*Hypericum perforatum* L.): a review of its chemistry, pharmacology and clinical properties. J Pharm Pharmacol 53 (5):583–600

91. Srivastava P, Raut HN, Puntambekar HM, Upadhye AS, Desai AC (2010) Stability studies of crude plant material of *Bacopa monnieri* and its effect on free radical scavenging activity. J Phytology 2(8):103–109

92. Srivastava JK, Gupta S (2009) Extraction, characterization, stability and biological

activity of flavonoids isolated from chamomile flowers. Mol Cell Pharmacol 1(3):138–147

93. Fujisawa H, Suma K, Origuchi K, Kumagai H, Seki T, Ariga T (2008) Biological and chemical stability of garlic-derived allicin. J Agric Food Chem 56(11):4229–4235

94. Fear CM (1929) The alkaloid test of tannins. Analyst 54(639):316–318

95. McManus JP, Davis KG, Beart JE, Gaffney SH, Lilley TH, Haslam E (1985) Polyphenol interactions. Part 1. Introduction; some observations on the reversible complexation of polyphenols with proteins and polysaccharides. J Chem Soc Perkin Trans 11 (9):1429–1438

96. Tanaka T (1999) Structure, property, and function of plant polyphenol. Foods Food Ingredients J Japan:64–70

97. Martin-Dupont F, Gloaquen V, Guilloton M (2006) Study of chemical interaction between barks and heavy metal cation in the sorption process. J Environ Sci Health 41(2):149–160

98. Nancy, Bansal G (2017) Stability testing of some commercially available CNS active herbal products. Unpublished results.

99. Bansal G, Suthar N, Kaur J, Jain A (2016) Stability testing of herbal drugs: challenges, regulatory compliance and perspectives. Phytother Res 30(7):1046–1058

100. Wang L, Lu N, Zhao L, Qi C, Zhang W, Dong J, Hou X (2016) Characterization of stress degradation products of curcumin and its two derivatives by UPLC-DAD-MS/MS. Arabian J Chem. https://doi.org/10.1016/j.arabjc.2016.02.003

101. Damle M, Dalavi N (2015) Development and validation of stability indicating HPLC method for determination of ellagic and gallic acid in Jambul seeds (Syzygium cumini). Int J Appl Sci Biotechnol 3(3):434–438

102. Hemingway RW, Hillis WE (1971) Behavior of ellagitannins, gallic acid, and ellagic acid under alkaline conditions. TAPPI J 54 (6):933–936

103. Jin Y, Zhang W, Meng Q, Li D, Garg S, Teng L, Wen J (2013) Forced degradation of flavonol glycosides extracted from Ginkgo biloba. Chem Res Chin Univ 29(4):667–670

104. Ravber M, Pecar D, Gorsek A, Iskra J, Knez Z, Skerget M (2016) Hydrothermal degradation of rutin: identification of degradation products and kinetics study. J Agric Food Chem 64(48):9196–9202

105. Zenkevich IG, Eshchenko AY, Makarova SV, Vitenberg AG, Dobryakov YG, Utsal VA (2007) Identification of the products of oxidation of Quercetin by air oxygen at ambient temperature. Molecules 12(3):654–672

106. McGraw GW, Hemingway RW, Ingram LL, Canady CS, McGraw WB (1999) Thermal degradation of terpenes: camphene, Δ^3-carene, limonene, α-terpinene. Environ Sci Technol 33(22):4029–4033

107. Anjamma M, Bhavani L (2017) GC-MS analysis of Momordica charantia and Momordica dioica fruit and root methanolic extracts. Int J Pharmacog Phytochem Res 9(6):808–813

108. Ashraf K, Mujeeb M, Ahmad A, Ahmad N, Amir M (2015) Determination of curcuminoids in Curcuma longa Linn. by UPLC/Q-TOF–MS: an application in turmeric cultivation. J Chromatogr Sci 53(8):1346–1352

109. Saracini E, Tattini M, Traversi ML, Vincieri FF, Pinelli P (2005) Simultaneous LC-DAD and LC-MS determination of ellagitannins, flavonoid glycosides, acyl-glycosyl flavonoids in Cistus salvifolius L. leaves. Chromatographia 62(5-6):245–249

110. Tatsis EC, Boeren S, Exarchou V, Troganis AN, Vervoort J, Gerothanassis IP (2007) Identification of the major constituents of Hypericum perforatum by LC/SPE/NMR and/or LC/MS. Phytochemistry 68 (3):383–393

111. Trivedi MK, Branton A, Trivedi D, Nayak G, Lee AC, Hancharuk A, Sand CM (2017) LC-MS, GC-MS, NMR spectroscopic analysis of Withania somnifera (Ashwagandha) root extract after treatment with the energy of consciousness (The Trivedi Effect®). Eur J Biophys 5(2):27–37

112. Tuenter E, Ahmad R, Foubert K, Amin A, Orfanoudaki M, Cos P, Maes L, Apers S, Pieters L, Exarchou V (2016) Isolation and structure elucidation by LC-DAD-MS and LC-DAD-SPE-NMR of cyclopeptide alkaloids from the roots of Ziziphus oxyphylla and evaluation of their antiplasmodial activity. J Nat Prod 79(11):2865–2872

113. Wang PH, Zhang YB, Yang XW, Zhao DQ, Wang YP (2016) Rapid characterization of ginsenosides in the roots and rhizomes of Panax ginseng by UPLC-DAD-QTOF-MS/MS and simultaneous determination of 19 ginsenosides by HPLC-ESI-MS. J Ginseng Res 40(4):382–394

114. WHO (2007) WHO guidelines for assessing quality of herbal medicines with reference to contaminants and residues. World Health Organization, Geneva

115. Kaur I, Suthar N, Kaur J, Bansal Y, Bansal G (2016) Accelerated stability studies on dried extracts of Centella asiatica through chemical, HPLC, HPTLC, biological activity analyses. J Evid Based Complementary Altern Med 21(4):NP127–NP137

116. Koyu H, Haznedaroglu MZ (2011) Investigation of impact of storage conditions on *Hypericum perforatum* L. dried total extract. J Food Drug Anal 23(3):545–551

117. Babiker LB, Gadkariem EA, Alashban RM, Aljohar HI (2014) Investigation of stability of Korean ginseng in herbal drug product. Am J Appl Sci 11(1):160–170

118. Sachan AK, Sachan NK, Kumar S, Sachan A, Gangwar SS (2010) Evaluation and standardization of essential oils for development of alternative dosage forms. Eur J Sci Res 46 (2):194–203

119. Srivastava P, Raut HN, Puntambekar HM, Desai AC (2011) Effect of storage conditions on free radical scavenging activities of crude plant material of *Piper longum*. J Phytology 3 (6):23–27

120. Goppel M, Franz G (2004) Stability control of senna leaves and senna extracts. Planta Med 70(5):432–436

121. Jain A, Kaur J, Nancy BY, Saini B, Bansal G (2017) WHO guided real time stability testing on Shankhpushpi syrup. J Pharm Technol Res Management 5(1):1–19

122. Nancy BY, Bansal G (2015) HPLC-UV/FD methods for scopoletin and asiatic acid: development, validation and application in WHO recommended stability testing of herbal drug products. Biochem Anal Biochem 4(4):1–8

123. Dwivedi S, Gupta S (2012) Formulation and evaluation of herbal gel containing *Sesbania grandiflora* (L.) Poir. leaf extract. Acta Chim Pharm Indica 2(1):54–59

124. Mook-Jung I, Shin JE, Yun SH, Huh K, Koh JY, Park HK, Jew SS, Jung MW (1999) Protective effects of asiaticoside derivatives against beta-amyloid neurotoxicity. J Neurosci Res 58(3):417–425

125. Hamid AA, Md. Shah Z, Muse R, Mohamed S (2002) Characterisation of antioxidative activities of various extracts of *Centella asiatica* (L) Urban. Food Chem 77(4):465–469

Chapter 15

Stability Testing Considerations for Biologicals and Biotechnology Products

Christine P. Chan

Abstract

This chapter discusses common issues and general approaches to studying the stability of biologicals for product development, covering key required studies for product registration and post-approval process changes. Several commonly used stability-indicating test methods for proteins are discussed with procedural details. Design considerations of accelerated stability and forced degradation (stress testing) studies for support of manufacturing operations and comparability demonstrations are outlined.

Key words Protein stability, Protein structure, Monoclonal antibodies, Forced degradation studies, Stress testing, Stability-indicating assays

1 Introduction

Stability testing programs are an integral part of pharmaceutical product development. In the case of biologicals, due to complexity of the molecular structure as well as the manufacturing process, the design and execution of these studies require thorough planning and coordination through the various stages of development to product registration as well as post-approval life cycle management. There are over 1000 biotechnology products (i.e., medicines and vaccines produced using biological processes) in various stages of preclinical and clinical development for many currently unmet medical needs [1]. These biotherapeutics encompass a broad range of molecular types, including monoclonal antibodies (e.g., full-length, conjugated to small molecule drugs, and variations of domain scaffolds), vaccines, recombinant proteins, cell therapies, gene therapies, antisense oligonucleotides, and short-interfering RNA molecules. The structural features of these biopharmaceuticals are diverse and highly complex. For example, most protein drugs are large molecules consisting of multiple domains that contribute to different biological functions for drug efficacy. Maintaining drug stability throughout the manufacturing process,

Sanjay Bajaj and Saranjit Singh (eds.), *Methods for Stability Testing of Pharmaceuticals*, Methods in Pharmacology and Toxicology, https://doi.org/10.1007/978-1-4939-7686-7_15, © Springer Science+Business Media, LLC, part of Springer Nature 2018

transport, storage, and delivery to patients remains very challenging. Most biopharmaceutical product types have common structural features and may allow some level of platform development approaches. However, there are often unique issues for each product candidate that is addressed in a case-by-case manner over the course of formulation and stability program development. In this chapter, study design and considerations for biologics stability programs are discussed using examples from protein-based products which are the most common biopharmaceuticals.

2   Protein Instability Issues

Protein instability can result from chemical and/or physical perturbations on the structure. Chemical degradation includes peptide backbone fragmentation, oxidation, N-terminal cyclization, deamidation and isomerization, racemization, glycation, and disulfide rearrangement [2]. Physical instability may arise from conformational, colloidal, and interfacial mechanisms that affect the higher order structure (HOS) of the individual molecules as well as the population interactions. These changes can lead to unfolding and denaturation, surface adsorption, aggregation, and precipitation of the biotherapeutics, which in turn may cause loss of activity and efficacy as well as potentially increase the risk of unwanted immunogenicity. It is well recognized that proteins are only marginally stable with relatively small free energy differences between the folded and partially unfolded states [3]. During commercial manufacturing, the protein is subjected to different environmental stresses that may result in different modes of instability [4]. Chemical modifications and physical instability are often linked. Oxidation of a protein may lead to HOS perturbation [5], and conversely HOS changes may lead to more rapid modifications of amino acids previously buried within a folded protein. It is often not possible to clearly discern the individual kinetics and relationships between chemical and physical instabilities. Careful studies are thus needed to characterize the degradation profiles for each protein of interest.

A key challenge in protein-based therapeutics development is the inherent product heterogeneity resulting from posttranslational modifications (PTM) during cell culture as well as the chemical and physical changes in structure during manufacturing and storage. In addition, process residuals such as host cell proteins (e.g., proteases [6], lipases [7]) and low-level impurities [8] (e.g., peroxides, metal ions, and nonmetallic leachables) can vary between process lots affecting the product quality attributes and stability to different degrees. Extensive process development efforts are thus required to establish an integrated control strategy to consistently manufacture a well-defined and well-controlled spectrum of molecular species for a given biopharmaceutical. A diverse array of assays are applied to derive structure and function information to establish product knowledge space, particularly with regard to criticality of product attributes impacting stability, safety, and efficacy. The selection of the final formulation in many cases involves a balancing act. Multiple product critical quality attributes (CQAs) need to be maintained within their respective acceptable ranges for defined safety and efficacy by a robust final formulation. Well-designed long-term stability and forced degradation studies (FDS) are important to support the establishment of drug product shelf-life as well as the limits of manufacturing variations and acceptable excursions [9].

3   Stability Studies: Protocols and Test Methods

General requirements for a stability data package in the registration application for biologicals follows the same key ICH Q1A (R2) [10] guideline as for small molecules, with additional considerations outlined in the annex ICH Q5C [11]. Long-term, real-time, real-condition stability studies are required for establishment of product shelf-life. Accelerated stability studies are conducted at a temperature higher than the intended formulation/storage condition and expected to provide useful support data for establishing the expiration date, provide product stability information, as well as help elucidate the degradation profile of the drug substance or drug product. FDS (stress testing) are conducted using different modes of stress (e.g., pH shift, heat, chemical oxidation, light exposure, mechanical stress, and cycles of freeze-thaw) under extreme conditions. The intent is to identify the likely degradation products, which further helps in determination of the intrinsic stability of the molecule and gain understanding of the primary degradation mechanisms. Table 1 summarizes the standard stability study conditions based on ICH Q1A(R2) recommendation. As indicated in ICH Q5C [11], it should be noted "that those conditions may not be appropriate for biotechnological/biological products. Conditions should be carefully selected on a case-by-case basis".

Table 1
Typical stability study conditions based on ICH Q1A(R2)

Long-term storage condition	Accelerated storage condition
5 °C ± 3 °C	25 °C ± 2 °C/60% RH ± 5% RH
25 °C ± 2 °C/60% RH ± 5% RH	40 °C ± 2 °C/75% RH ± 5% RH
−20 °C ± 3 °C and below	Case-by-case; 5 °C ± 3 °C or 25 °C ± 2 °C to cover potential excursions

Given the high cost of drug development, most protein product candidates are subjected to early evaluation of manufacturability at the transition from discovery to development phase. For monoclonal antibodies, this set of experiments typically includes short-term stability studies at 2–8, 25, and 40 °C, freeze-thaw studies, limited FDS (e.g., exposure to low and high pH, light, and oxidative reagents), and determination of the viscosity of high concentration samples [12]. These results provide basic understanding of the colloidal properties and prevalent degradation mechanisms of a molecule, with focus on detecting gross changes in the protein that may compromise stability and potency.

Accelerated stability studies are broadly used during development to make formulation choices, assess suitability of proposed stability-indicating methods, and support expiry dating of clinical trial materials. Due to complexity of degradation mechanisms (e.g., aggregation), protein stability at long-term low temperature storage is not always predictable based on studies at higher temperature [13, 14]. While the overall degradation profile observed would follow the combined kinetics of the individual molecular instabilities, the relative contribution of the different degradation mechanisms may change at different temperatures. Overall, non-Arrhenius kinetics is observed in most cases [15, 16]. Despite the lack of direct correlation of accelerated stability and long-term stability (*see* Table 1) for most proteins, accelerated study results remain relevant in demonstrating product integrity upon excursion/accidental exposure in commercial manufacturing and transport. Overall, it is important to derive some understanding and mechanistic linkage of degradation products observed in the accelerated and FDS to those observed in the long-term studies. Extended characterization tools are needed in addition to the routine release and stability-monitoring tests [16, 17].

3.1 Example Drug Substance Stability Protocol

It is now common to store bulk protein drug substance (DS) in the frozen state since freezing slows degradation rates, reduces risk of microbial contamination, and simplifies transportation. Colder temperatures (ca. −80 °C) afford improved long-term stability because of reduced molecular mobility, but for practical reasons, most DS are stored in warmer freezers (ca. −20 °C). Table 2 summarizes an example stability protocol where the bulk DS is stored at −20 °C for up to 2 years, then thawed and refrigerated before filling into glass vials at the drug product manufacturing site. The long-term stability study samples stored at −20 °C would be in a reduced-size container but of the same material as the bulk freezer bags. Samples are withdrawn at designated time points, and subjected to full testing (the "a" samples). The 5 °C condition is serving as the accelerated condition here. However, this does not adequately represent the worst-case scenario for potential excursion of the DS. In this example, a second arm is added to the stability study as summarized in the bottom of Table 2 [18]. A subset of DS

Table 2
Time/temperature schedule for drug substance stability program

Storage condition	Time in months							
	0	1	3	6	9	12	18	24
−20 °C	ab	a	a	ab	a	ab	a	ab
5 °C		a	a	a	a	a		

Storage condition for "b" samples after thaw	Time in months					
	0	1	2	3	6	9
5 °C		a	a	a	a	a	a
25 °C		a	a	a	a	a	

Note: *Top* DS storage at two temperatures; *bottom* storage temperatures after thaw of −20 °C DS vials, pulled at time points designated as "b"
a - full testing at designated time points; b - remove portion of DS vials, thaw and test at designated time points

samples are removed from frozen storage at designated time points (the "b" samples), thawed according to the thawing instructions specific to the DS and container size, stored at two holding temperatures, and then subjected to full testing out to the designated maximum hold time. The 5 °C data demonstrate stability throughout the DP manufacturing hold time and the 25 °C data support potential temperature excursions. In addition, this protocol allows assessment of the potential cumulative effects of frozen bulk storage plus short-term heat stress on degradation.

Small-scale freeze-thaw cycling experiments conducted in early development are useful for rapid formulation definitions, but do not reflect the impact of the rates of freezing and thawing at large-scale. In addition, these experiments do not capture the long-term consequences of storage in the frozen state. It is generally recognized that proteins are most susceptible to freeze-thaw damages during the transition period between solution and solid [19]. Frozen state aggregation behavior is most affected by phase separation, crystallization of cryoprotectants, and mobility. Accelerated stability study at a different temperature is thus not relevant. Scale-appropriate studies for frozen DS are typically conducted as part of the formulation and process development [20].

3.2 Example Drug Product Stability Protocol

Biopharmaceutical drug products are provided as lyophilized powder which requires reconstitution before administration or in liquid form for ease-of-use by patients. If the drug product is further diluted in the clinic for infusion, in-use stability studies need to be conducted to support the administration protocol. Table 3

Table 3
Time/temperature schedule for drug product stability program

	Time in months								
Storage condition	0	1	2	3	6	9	12	18	24
2–8 °C		a	a		a	a	a	a	a	a
25 °C		a	a	a	a	a				

Note: a - full testing at designated time points

Table 4
Typical assay set used for stability studies of protein-based biopharmaceuticals

Appearance and color
pH
Total protein content
Purity by SEC
Purity by CE-SDS, reduced and non-reduced
Charge variant analysis by CE-IEF
Potency by bioassay

summarizes an example stability protocol where the drug product vial is stored at 2–8 °C for up to 2 years. The 25 °C condition serves as the accelerated condition.

3.3 Stability Testing Methods

Testing at each time point of the stability studies should include monitoring of product attributes that are susceptible to change during storage and are likely to influence quality, safety, and efficacy. Table 4 shows a typical testing set for protein biotherapeutics. In general, tests for appearance and color, pH and protein content are expected in the protocol for all time points. Tests for bioburden, endotoxin, sterility (or container closure integrity testing), particulates and other formulation-specific tests may also be included at selected time points (e.g., T0 and end of study).

The stability-indicating methods for a given protein product are developed through the course of development based on product knowledge accumulated over time from early real-time, accelerated and FDS performed on the various process development lots as the program progressed. Test method validations should be completed before applying them to generate formal real-time stability data on multiple representative drug product lots for shelf-life definition. It is important to recognize that individual analytical methods often have inherent limitations due to principles of detection and sample preparation requirements (e.g., concentration and buffer changes, chemical derivatization, and interaction with separation matrix) and may provide only partial or perturbed profile of protein degradation. A comprehensive approach using orthogonal and complementary analytical tools is thus important. The four methods highlighted below represent the most commonly used tests applied for stability monitoring of proteins.

3.3.1 Size-Exclusion High Performance Liquid Chromatography (SEC)

SEC is the industry standard method for monitoring relative amounts of monomer, aggregates, and fragments of protein products. The strength of the method lies in the high precision and robustness, ease of use and compatibility with quality control environment.

Method: The classical column for monoclonal antibody analysis is the Tosoh TSK Gel G3000SWXL 7.8 × 3000 mm column. Isocratic separations are carried out in 150 mM potassium phosphate buffer, pH 7 at a flow rate of 0.5 mL/min with column temperature at 25 °C. Samples are diluted with the mobile phase to 0.25 mg/mL, centrifuged for 2 min at $5100 \times g$ to remove particles, and 10–50 μL injected for each analysis. UV detection can be performed at 280 nm and/or 220 nm [21]. The area percentages of total high molecular weight species (HMWS, peaks eluting before the monomer main peak), monomer (main peak) and low molecular weight species (LMWS, peaks eluting after the monomer main peak) are calculated and reported as area % of total area (*see* **Note 1**).

There may be issues of perturbation of the sample during SEC analysis and concerns include sample dilution, change of solvent conditions, interaction with resins and column frit as well as shear-induced disruption or denaturation which may dissociate but also possibly create aggregates [22]. The use of an orthogonal technique such as analytical ultracentrifugation in sedimentation velocity mode (AUC-SV) to qualify the routine SEC assay for size distribution information is thus very important. The commercialization of shorter and narrower columns packed with reduced particle sizes has allowed improvement in the resolution and throughput. Additional characterization of protein aggregation can be achieved by coupling SEC with various detectors, including refractive index (RI), ultraviolet (UV), multi-angle laser light scattering (MALLS), and viscometer (IV). There are also newer applications of hyphenating SEC with mass spectrometry (MS) detectors [23].

3.3.2 Capillary Electrophoresis-Sodium Dodecyl Sulfate (CE-SDS)

Capillary electrophoresis (CE) carried out using automated instrumentation is routinely used for assessment of product purity based on size and charge attributes. In CE-SDS, bare fused silica capillaries are used in conjunction with polymeric sieving matrix to separate samples pre-treated with SDS. The SDS coats proteins to yield an even distribution of charge per unit mass, allowing size-based separation of the proteins in a sample. In a typical purity assessment for monoclonal antibodies (mAb), samples are analyzed under non-reducing as well as reducing conditions.

Method: Non-reduced samples are prepared by mixing 150 µL of the purified mAb sample and 50 µL of a 4% (w/w) SDS solution containing 160 mM iodoacetamide. For reduced samples, 150 µL of the purified mAb sample is mixed with 50 µL of 4% (w/w) SDS solution and 10 µL of 0.1 M dithiothreitol. Final target mAb concentration is 1 mg/mL. Samples are heated in a water bath at 65 °C for 10 min and 100 µL of the non-reduced or reduced samples are aliquoted into a sample tube for electrophoretic separation in the PA800 instrument (SCIEX). Separations are performed using a short bare fused silica capillary (50 µm ID with a 30.2 cm total length and 20.2 cm effective length from the sample introduction inlet to the detector window), with detection at 220 nm. Prior to each CE run, the capillary is rinsed at 70 psi with 0.1 M NaOH (3 min), 0.1 M HCl (1 min), and deionized water (1 min). The CE-SDS polymer solution (or CE-SDS running buffer) is then loaded into the capillary at 50 psi for 15 min from the outlet side. Samples are injected electrokinetically at 10 kV for 10 s. The CE analysis is conducted at −15 kV for 30 min. Typically the current obtained is ~32.5 µA when the capillary temperature is maintained at 40 °C [24]. Relative peak area percentages are calculated for reporting.

This is a replacement method for the classical SDS-PAGE (SDS-polyacrylamide gel electrophoresis), offering enhanced reproducibility and easier quantitation. Sensitivity by on-line UV detection is equivalent to Coomassie Blue staining while pre-derivatization by fluorescent dye coupled with LIF (laser-induced fluorescence) detection is equivalent to silver staining [24]. Available commercial kits covering a size range of 10–200 kDa are mostly optimized for analysis of monoclonal antibodies, their subunit chains as well as related fragments and non-dissociable aggregates [25]. Due to differences in protein stability, it is important to optimize or verify the sample preparation parameters for individual proteins to ensure there are no artifacts introduced by the protocol [26].

3.3.3 Capillary Electrophoresis-Isoelectric Focusing (CE-IEF)

In isoelectric focusing electrophoresis (IEF), proteins are separated based on migration to a position of zero net charge (corresponding to its pI) within a pH gradient formed by ampholyte solutions. Instrumentation employing imaging technology to acquire IEF data within capillaries allows fast run time and robust reproducibility [27]. IEF offers high separation efficiencies and is routinely used for profiling charge isoforms.

Method: Samples are diluted with an ampholyte mixture containing methylcellulose, broad range ampholytes (pH 3–10), and pI markers. Final target mAb concentration is 0.5 mg/mL. The sample mix is centrifuged at 2000 × g for 5 min to remove bubbles and a 150 μL aliquot is then transferred to a glass autosampler vial for analysis. The IEF separation can be conducted on an iCE3 instrument (Protein Simple) using a silica capillary coated with fluorocarbon in a cartridge. The catholyte consists of 0.1 M NaOH in 0.1% methylcellulose and the anolyte consists of 0.08 M phosphoric acid in 0.1% methylcellulose. Samples are injected into the capillary using pressure (1000 mbar) and a pre-focus voltage of 1500 V is applied for 1 min to remove salts. A focus voltage of 3000 V is applied for 8 min to create the pH gradient, with spectral image collected approximately every 34 s [28]. Since it is often not possible to fully resolve product charged variants, peak entities are monitored as peak groups, e.g., acidic, main, and basic.

This method is now the standard charge variant profiling method for product release, replacing the gel-based IEF method and often preferred over the ion-exchange HPLC method due to robustness. During IEF, proteins lose surface charge while being focused into very concentrated sample zones. Adding a solubilizing agent (e.g., urea) can eliminate aggregates and improve separation and reproducibility. Adding narrow pH-range ampholytes can further improve resolution of isoforms with similar pIs [29]. Fluorescence detection mode allows improved sensitivity and lower baseline noise.

Electrophoretic mobility on CE often does not correlate with chromatographic retention on HPLC due to their different separation mechanisms. Given the many different possible combinations of PTMs on a protein, complete resolution of variant peaks in a single analysis is difficult to achieve. Thus, it is common to use both CE and HPLC methods in conjunction. Characterization of variant peaks of a product is usually accomplished through fractionation using the HPLC method, with subsequent individual peak analysis via the CE-IEF method. In parallel, detailed structural analysis by LC-MS can be performed to determine the common posttranslational modifications. The IEF method has been used to monitor C-terminal lysine processing, N-terminal cyclization, deamidation, glycosylation variants, and disulfide variants [2].

3.3.4 Potency by Binding ELISA (Enzyme-Linked Immunosorbant Assay)

Most quality control lab assays utilize the plate-based ELISA format to monitor binding of biopharmaceuticals such as monoclonal antibodies (immunoglobulin G, IgG) to their intended target receptors.

Method: For direct binding ELISA, the 96-well plates are coated with the appropriate target solution overnight at 4 °C. Plates are washed with phosphate-buffered saline containing 0.05%

polysorbate 20 and blocked with a blocking buffer for 1 h at 30 °C. For the primary incubations, various concentrations of sample IgG are added to the pre-coated plates. The amount of bound sample IgG is measured by commercially available anti-human IgG labeled with horseradish peroxidase (HRP). The enzymatic reaction can be developed using colorimetric or chemiluminescence substrates depending on required sensitivity. A qualified standard IgG material is included to generate a calibration curve and quantitative analysis is completed using nonlinear regression analysis [12] (*see* **Note 2**).

3.4 Specification Setting

For product attributes that are known to change over time (e.g., potency, degradation products), shelf-life limits need to be established in addition to the release limits. The difference between the release and shelf-life limits should account for the degradation during shipping, the degradation during long-term storage and a margin to account for the uncertainty in the estimated degradation, the analytical uncertainty and if feasible also batch-to-batch variation. These terms should be estimated from long-term stability data using statistical methods. Accelerated stability data might be helpful depending on the protein degradation pathways. Further discussions on approaches can be found in ICH guidances Q6B [30] for specification setting and Q1E [31] for stability data evaluation as well as published reviews [32, 33].

4 Stability Studies for Comparability Demonstration

Comparability exercises are commonly required at certain milestones during drug development as well as after product registration when changes are implemented into the manufacturing process. The goal is to evaluate and demonstrate that there is no change in product quality and stability profiles that might impact safety and efficacy [34, 35]. Long-term and accelerated stability data of process validation lots are often required except for low risk minor changes. Partial results of an ongoing long-term study are often acceptable in submissions, with commitment to report completed studies later.

FDS are commonly included in comparability evaluations. The expectation is that small differences between materials may be amplified and detectable under high stress conditions over a short period of time (several weeks). The regulatory guidelines are currently very general. There are few guidelines (e.g., ICH Q1B) which define standard conditions for studying photostability [36] to no procedural instructions on the practical approach to FDS. The design of the study in terms of selection of stress conditions, duration of stress studies, and extent of degradation varies depending on instability of the protein and intended applications [37, 38].

Pre- and post-change materials can be assessed through profile comparisons to illustrate similar modes of degradation, and rate comparisons for a subset of key attributes where appropriate. In the latter case, an equivalence test is used, with the establishment of a meaningful equivalence margin ($\pm\Delta$slope) based on the effect size derived from product historical data [39].

5   Conclusion

Biopharmaceuticals have complicated structures and complex manufacturing processes. Design of the stability programs is more challenging than for the development of small molecule products. Thorough considerations of the accumulated understanding of product stability profile, typical process variations, and assay variabilities are key to establishing shelf-life limits for specific product attributes and progressive evaluation of comparability throughout the product life cycle.

6   Notes

1. The SEC method for each product is often established through fractionation and isolation techniques to explore and confirm the nature of the main monomer peak, major HMWS and LMWS. These fractions are analyzed using orthogonal methods such as charge variant analysis, electrophoretic methods as well as further structural characterization by LC-MS.

2. For biopharmaceuticals requiring binding function for efficacy, a potency assay using the ELISA format is most common. Quality control of protein reagents (i.e., the target molecule preparation from in-house source, the enzyme-conjugated anti-human IgG reagent from commercial sources), the blocking reagent (which may or may not contain proteins) and implementation of automated liquid handling are important for maintaining consistent assay performance in the long-term. Receptor binding kinetics of IgGs are typically characterized during discovery phase using surface plasmon resonance-based systems. While the assay steps are simpler in this method, the high cost of the instrumentation does not allow broad use in the QC labs for routine stability monitoring.

References

1. Pharmaceutical Research and Manufacturers of America Report (2013) Medicines in development biologics. www.phrma.org/sites/default/files/pdf/biologics2013.pdf

2. Liu H, Ponniah G, Zhang HM et al (2014) In vitro and in vivo modifications of recombinant and human IgG antibodies. MAbs 6 (5):1145–1154

3. Dill KA (1990) Dominant forces in protein folding. Biochemistry 29:7133–7155

4. Manning MC, Chou DK, Murphy BM et al (2010) Stability of protein pharmaceuticals: an update. Pharm Res 27:544–575

5. Liu D, Ren D, Huang H et al (2008) Structure and stability of human IgG1 Fc as a consequence of methionine oxidation. Biochemistry 47:5088–5100

6. Gao SX, Zhang Y, Stansberry-Perkins K et al (2011) Fragmentation of a highly purified monoclonal antibody attributed to residual CHO cell protease activity. Biotechnol Prog 108:977–982

7. Dixit N, Salamaat-Miller N, Salinas PA, Taylor KD, Basu SK (2016) Residual host cell protein promotes polysorbate 20 degradation in a sulfatase drug product leading to free fatty acid particles. J Pharm Sci 105:1657–1666

8. Wang W, Ignatius AA, Thakkar SV (2014) Impact of residual impurities and contaminants on protein stability. J Pharm Sci 103:1315–1330

9. Wurth C, Demeule B, Mahler HC, Adler M (2016) Quality by design approaches to formulation robustness—an antibody case study. J Pharm Sci 105:1667–1675

10. ICH Q1A(R2) (2003) Stability testing of new drug substances and products. Fed Regis 68 (225):65717–65718

11. ICH Q5C (1996) Quality of biotechnological products: stability testing of biotechnological/biological products. Fed Regis 61:36466–36474

12. Yang X et al (2013) Developability studies before initiation of process development. Improving manufacturability of monoclonal antibodies. MAbs 5(5):787–794

13. Brader ML et al (2015) Examination of thermal unfolding and aggregation profiles of a series of developable therapeutic monoclonal antibodies. Mol Pharm 12:1005–1017

14. Thiagarajan G, Semple A, James JK, Cheung JK, Shameem M (2016) A comparison of biophysical characterization techniques in predicting monoclonal antibody stability. MAbs 8 (6):71088–71097

15. Wang W, Roberts CJ (2013) Non-Arrhenius protein aggregation. AAPS J 15:840–851

16. Drenski MF, Brader ML, Alston RW, Reed WF (2013) Monitoring protein aggregation kinetics with simultaneous multiple sample light scattering. Anal Biochem 437:185–197

17. Maity H, Lai Y, Srivastava A et al (2012) Principles and applications of selective biophysical methods for characterization and comparability assessment of a monoclonal antibody. Curr Pharm Biotechnol 13:2078–2101

18. Mazzeo A, Carpenter P (2009) Stability studies for biologics. In: Huynh-Ba K (ed) Handbook of stability testing in pharmaceutical development. Springer Science+Business Media, LLC, New York. https://doi.org/10.1007/978-0-387-85627-8. 17

19. Bhatnagar BS, Bogner RH, Pikal MJ (2007) Protein stability during freezing: separation of stresses and mechanisms of protein stabilization. Pharm Dev Technol 12:505–523

20. Singh SK, Kolhe P, Mehta AP, Chico SC, Lary AL, Huang M (2011) Frozen state storage instability of a monoclonal antibody: aggregation as a consequence of trehalose crystallization and protein unfolding. Pharm Res 28:873–885

21. Bond MD et al (2010) Evaluation of a dual-wavelength size exclusion HPLC method with improved sensitivity to detect protein aggregates and its use to better characterize degradation pathways of an IgG1 monoclonal antibody. J Pharm Sci 99:2582–2597

22. Philo JS (2006) Is any measurement method optimal for all aggregate sizes and types? AAPS J 8:E564–E571

23. Fekete S, Beck A, Veuthey JL, Guillarme D (2014) Theory and practice of size exclusion chromatography for the analysis of protein aggregates. J Pharm Biomed Anal 101:161–172

24. Salas-Solano O, Tomlinson B, Du S, Parker M, Strahan A, Ma S (2006) Optimization and validation of a quantitative capillary electrophoresis sodium dodecyl sulfate method for quality control and stability monitoring of monoclonal antibodies. Anal Chem 78:6583–6594

25. Nunnally B et al (2006) A series of collaborations between various pharmaceutical companies and regulatory authorities concerning the analysis of biomolecules using capillary electrophoresis. Chromatographia 64:359–368

26. Zhang J, Burman S, Gunturi S, Foley JP (2010) Method development and validation of capillary sodium dodecyl sulfate gel

electrophoresis for the characterization of a monoclonal antibody. J Pharm Biomed Anal 53:1236–1243

27. Guo A, Camblin G, Han M, Meert C, Park S (2008) Role of CE in biopharmaceutical development and quality control. Separation Sci Tech 9:357–399

28. Rustandi RR, Peklansky B, Anderson CL (2014) Use of imaged capillary isoelectric focusing technique in development of diphtheria toxin mutant CRM197. Electrophoresis 35:1065–1071

29. Salas-Solano O et al (2012) Robustness of iCIEF methodology for the analysis of monoclonal antibodies: an interlaboratory study. J Sep Sci 35:3124–3129

30. ICH Q6B (1999) Specifications: test procedures and acceptance criteria for biotechnological/biological products. Fed Regis 64 (159):44928–44935

31. ICH Q1E (2004) Evaluation for stability data. Fed Regis 69(110):32010–32011

32. Schofield TL (2009) Vaccine stability study design and analysis to support product licensure. Biologicals 37:387–396

33. Capen R et al (2012) On the shelf-life of pharmaceutical products. AAPS Pharm Sci Tech 13:911–918

34. ICH Q5E (2005) Comparability of biotechnological/biological products subject to changes in their manufacturing process. Food Drug Administration 70(125):37861–37862

35. Chan CP (2016 July/August) Analytical strategies for comparability in bioprocess development. BioPharma Asia, p 26–33

36. ICH Q1B (1997) Stability testing: photostability testing of new drug substances and products. Fed Regis 62(95):27115–27122

37. Tamizi E, Jouyban A (2016) Forced degradation studies of biopharmaceuticals: selection of stress conditions. Eur J Pharm Biopharm 98:26–46

38. Chan CP (2016) Forced degradation studies: current trends and future perspectives for protein-based therapeutics. Expert Rev Proteomics 13:651–658

39. Burdick RK, Sidor L (2013) Establishment of an equivalence acceptance criterion for accelerated stability studies. J Biopharm Stat 23:730–743

INDEX

Sanjay Bajaj and Saranjit Singh (eds.), *Methods for Stability Testing of Pharmaceuticals*, Methods in Pharmacology and Toxicology,
https://doi.org/10.1007/978-1-4939-7686-7, © Springer Science+Business Media, LLC, part of Springer Nature 2018

Printed in the United States
By Bookmasters